ORTHOPEDIC SURGERY

Edited by **Zaid Al-Aubaidi** and **Andreas Fette**

Orthopedic Surgery
Edited by Zaid Al-Aubaidi and Andreas Fette

Published by InTech
Janeza Trdine 9, 51000 Rijeka, Croatia

Publishing Process Manager Vedran Greblo

Technical Editor Teodora Smiljanic

Cover Designer InTech Design Team

Additional hard copies can be obtained from orders@intechopen.com

Orthopedic Surgery, Edited by Zaid Al-Aubaidi and Andreas Fette
p. cm.
ISBN 978-953-51-0231-1

For EU product safety concerns:
IN TECH d.o.o., Prolaz Marije Krucifikse Kozulić 3, 51000 Rijeka, Croatia,
info@intechopen.com or visit our website at intechopen.com.

Meet the editors

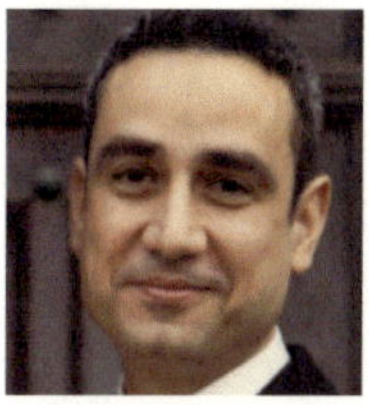

Dr. Zaid Al-Aubaidi was born in Iraq 1969, but is now a Danish citizen. He graduated from Baghdad University in 1993, where he practiced to 1998. Then he traveled to Denmark, and practiced since then. Dr. Al-Aubaidi finished his residency program in 2007 and had one year fellowship in paediatric orthopedics. Since 2009, he has been working at the Odense university hospital as a consultant orthopaedic surgeon and at the same time enjoying an academic position at the University of Southern Denmark. His special interest is; traumatology, deformity correction and paediatric spine. Regarding overseas activities, Dr. Al-Aubaidi have been in Africa 3 times, Switzerland, Germany, China and Canada. During his research career he has 15 published papers.

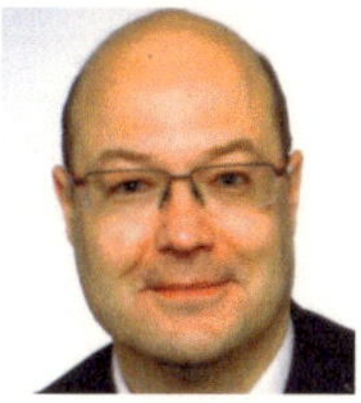

Professor Dr Andreas Fette earned his medical degree at Johannes-Gutenberg-University Mainz, Germany. He is a National and European Board accredited surgeon and pediatric surgeon. During his clinical career Dr Fette has been serving in renowned pediatric surgical centres and in most remote hospitals of the developing world. Pediatric hand surgery has always been one of his favourite subject. During his academic career Dr Fette published 70 peer reviewed papers, 12 book chapters, besides 180 international lectures and 70 workshops and tutorials. He has been awarded post graduate and master degrees from different universities, followed by Medical School professorship, University of Pécs, Hungary, besides being a well recognized international congress chair and visiting professor in the whole field of pediatric surgery.

Contents

Preface

Looking into the fascinating field of orthopedic surgery, pediatric hand surgery is surely one of our most challenging subspecialties. It is often difficult to quickly find the correct diagnosis and treatment in pediatrics, and surely the surgical anatomy of the growing hand is amazingly complex. In addition, some diagnoses are rare and less often mentioned in common surgical textbooks.

I graduated from Baghdad University, school of medicine in 1993. At that time, the standard texts in basic and clinical medical science were available only in the form of hard copies, books. I can remember that these books were heavy, expensive, and not least hard to get. The access to journals was only available in hard copy forms. Registration and being a member was a prerequisite for that. Being a medical student with almost no income made this almost impossible.

Since that time, I thought; this was wrong! I believed, and still do, that knowledge and science although invaluable, should be accessible for everyone. As we are dealing with medical science, the accessibility is even more important. This would mean a better knowledge for doctors and hence better treatment for patients. Through the last years, I had the chance to work in Africa for short periods. I have seen the willingness of the local doctors to give the right and best treatment for their patients. Beside the deficiency of postgraduate education and guidance, missing text books and essential medical journals are obstacles that make it very difficult for these doctors to accomplish their goal.

To share our inspiration we would like to present the following chapters;

Obsolete or chronic traumatic paraplegia is still a difficult medical problem at present time. So what factors then affect the recovery of the nerves functions? Through 17 anatomical studies and operative observations, and can nerve transplantation help in regaining some function? Chapter 1 will be able to answer these questions.

Degenerative spondylolisthesis has long been recognized as a cause of chronic low back pain. The mechanism of pain in degenerative spondylolisthesis has been confirmed by demonstrating the disc lesion pre-operatively by X-rays and MR imaging usually treated with surgical interbody fusion. With advances in minimal access technology using operating microscope, PLIF can now be performed through a minimally invasive. In chapter 2 the authors present a novel surgical technique and clinical outcomes of the unilateral micro-PLIF for degenerative spondylolisthesis. The distal forearm and surrounding soft tissues are commonly affected by acute and chronic disorders. In children, the use of ultrasonography allows the chondral parts of the epiphyseal region to be better evaluated without exposure to radiation than using standard radiographic techniques. The aim of this study in chapter 3 is to demonstrate the normal ultrasonographic findings in the distal forearm region in children.

Epidermolysis bullosa, form an entity of rare congenital diseases with an extraordinary susceptibility of the epithelium and skin to even minimal injury. This epidermal tears lead to blister formation and finally into serious wounds, leaving behind disabling scars and contractions, sometimes even leading to early death. The authors offer the reader of chapter 4 an exciting overview into the treatment of this disease

Compartment Syndrome, is a serious condition of various etiology and clinical presentation. The diagnosis of Compartment Syndrome of the forearm usually needs emergency surgery to prevent disabling sequelae. A comprehensive overview about this pediatric hand surgical challenge will be given by Andreas Fette in chapter 5.

Total hip replacement is the most common practiced and most effective surgical interventions introduced in the last 50 or so years in medicine. Bearing in mind that the use of artificial hips is more rigorous in younger patients and that life expectancy continues to increase, it is time that the question of possible adverse long term effects following implantation needs to be addressed. In chapter 6 the proposed links between hip replacements and carcinogenesis to date would be discussed.

Fractures of the acetabulum are increasing in the same speed of the increasing in motor vehicle accidents. The importance of the acetabulum is clear as being the weight bearing surface of the hip joint. If anatomical reduction and stable internal fixation not done, it can end with painful hip joint due to early osteoarthritis. In chapter 7 the author will present the indications and techniques to perform total hip arthroplasty in this group of patients.

After the discovery of biological effects of bisphosphonates more than 30 years ago, they have now become indispensable in medicine for the treatment of skeletal complications of malignancy, Paget's disease, osteoporosis, multiple myeloma, hypercalcemia and fibrous dysplasia. Chapter number 8 will review history, classification, pharmacokinetics, clinical relevance, the mechanism of action and adverse effects.

Tissue trauma produces a temporary rise in circulating concentrations of various tissue proteins as well as acute phase inflammation related analytes. Measurement of biomarkers in orthopaedic surgeries has been undertaken to evaluate the impact of the surgical trauma. Reading the chapter; Biochemical Measurement of Injury and Inflammation in Musculoskeletal Surgeries in chapter number 9, would illuminate the importance of these markers in orthopaedic surgery.

Musculoskeletal injuries are the most frequent indication for operative management in most centers. Trauma management of the poly-traumatized patient includes, besides resuscitation, early stabilization of long-bones and pelvic fractures. Chapter number 10, will discuss the following; orthopedic trauma anesthesia issues: Pre-operative evaluation, airway management, intra-operative monitoring, anesthetic agents and techniques, intra-operative complications and last but definitely not least post-operative pain management

Since the evolution of internet technology, there has been increasing interest in the concept of online publications. Unfortunately, most of these online publications need registration with fees, in order to be able to use it. I believe that many of the third world and limited income countries' doctors are in need for accessible online medical science.

The concept of InTech online publication, have met all the ambitions and will provide a free online access. I started editing the book during my career in Denmark, Odense University hospital. Choosing studies and chapters and editing them was not an easy job, but I am quite happy with the final result. I tried to select the chapters and studies that can provide new knowledge or enrich the reader's knowledge with an up to date science.

We would like to thank the staff of InTech, especially Mr. Verdan Greblo the publishing process manager, for the care and hard work that made the publication of this book possible.

Yours sincerely

Dr. Zaid Al-Aubaidi
Associate professor, MD. MB.CH.B, Orthopaedic surgery specialist, Subspecialty in paediatric orthopaedic, Odense University Hospital
Denmark

Dr. Andreas Fette
University of Pécs, Medical School
Hungary

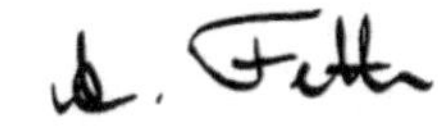

Part 1

Spine

1

Microsurgical Management and Functional Restoration of Patients with Obsolete Spinal Cord Injury

Zhang Shaocheng
Department of Orthopaedics, Changhai Hospital
The 2nd Military Medical University Shanghai
China

1. Introduction

Obsolete or chronic traumatic paraplegia is still a difficult medical problem at present time. Many patients with manifestations of post-injury changes in the spinal cord may have similarly normal images when observed with imaging technology like the MRI. These normal imaging results, however, do not indicate that the spinal cord is intact. Indeed, apart from compression and instability, a great difference in the sensory and motor function recovery is always seen among patients though they may have similar MRI imaging changes. So what factors then affect the recovery of the nerves functions? Through anatomical studies and operative observations, we have found that adhesions in the (**endorhachis**), the traction of the fibrous strip, traumatic scars, (**mollescence**), and cysts are among the main reasons. Elimination of most of these factors has been shown to benefit patients by increasing their potentials for functional recovery. Authur Dr.Zhang Shaocheng who as a survival and a member of medical team , his experiences with the treatments of patients who sustained either incomplete or complete spinal cord injury from the Tangshan (Hebei provence, China) earthquake in 1976; as well as numerous patients with spinal cord injuries from various causes in present time, have also led to the concept that additional functional recovery do occur in patients after using specialized microsurgical techniques like dural sheath slitting, nerve segments implantations among others which form the basis for this publication. The author is privileged to disclose that the Tangshan earthquake, herein mentioned, claimed the lives of 250,000 persons, over 240,000 persons sustained various type of traumatic injuries, and about 6,000 persons manifested either paraplegia or quadriplegia and related complications associated with spinal cord injuries.

Some patients received previous non-specific treatments before attending our services, while others were treated by us first hand. Records of patients thus treated with these specialized microsurgical techniques show early nerve function recovery compared with results from their prior non-specific treatment. Prior MRI studies done on these patients showed that the spinal cords had no severe damages. During the operation, any impediments to functional recovery of the spinal cord such as bone compression or unstable canales spinalis stenosis were eliminated.

Patients with chronic high-level complete spinal cord injury suffer from spastic paralysis as well as bowel and bladder dysfunctions, which cannot be improved by drug treatment or physical therapy. It has been reported from the works of doctors in many countries, based on their decades of clinical experiences, that connecting normal peripheral nerve with root-injured brachial plexus could improve some nerve functions. This mature technology inspired the author to help restore some neurological functions in patients with chronic high-level complete spinal cord injury by connecting normal peripheral nerves, from above the paralysis level, with peripheral nerves around paralyzed parts. As limb muscles are spastic and peripheral nerves, their dominating regeneration capacity, after spinal cord injury occurring later and higher than that of brachial plexus injury, so the prognosis of patients with chronic spinal cord injury is better than that of brachial plexus nerve root injury, given the same operation. Furthermore, after the donor nerve grows to the target muscles, nerve impulses causing target muscle contraction can also stimulate the high-tension coordinating muscle that can be trained to improve limb function.

However, the amount of the neurological function that paraplegic and quadriplegic patients need to regain is much more than what brachial plexus injury patients need, and the number of donor nerve is relatively in shortage. Therefore, only a few nerve functions can be regained. How to connect donor nerve with target nerve fiber accurately is the key. Another important issue to consider is how to maintain and take advantage of appropriate muscle tension and pathological contraction, and prevent target muscles from atrophying after surgery until new nerve fibers grow into the receptor nerve. The response to these concerns can be seen in our surgical approach where we wedge cut the outer membrane of donor nerve fiber and some perineurium of receptor nerve, and cut off some nerve fibers selectively in the muscle to maintain appropriate tension. Finally the donor nerve was embedded into the incision on the receptor nerve, and the outer membranes of the two were sutured together. We term this procedure as nerve **insert** grafting surgery (Fig.1 Fig.2) and the clinical results are quite satisfactory**.**

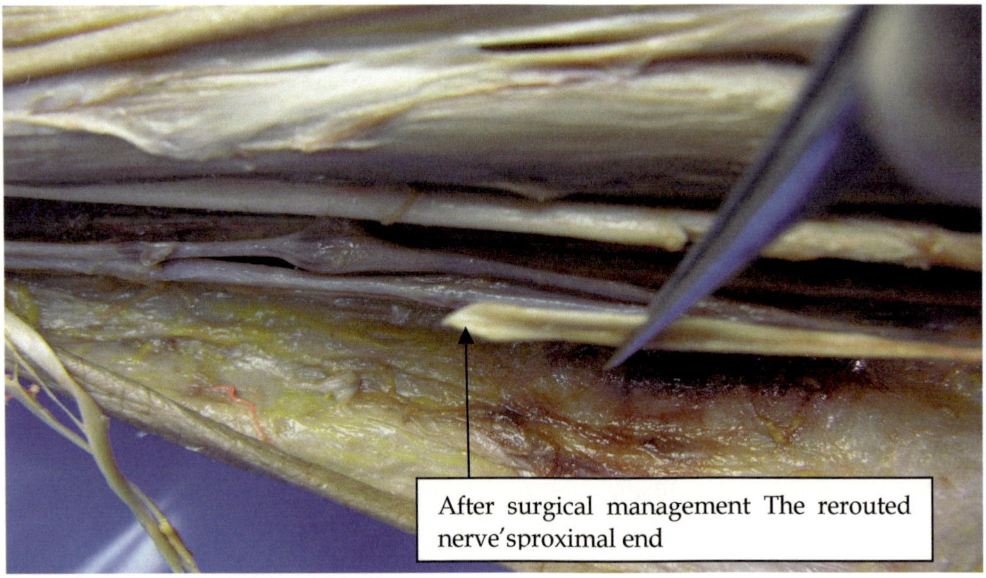

Fig. 1. Simulant procedures of Nerve rerouting ,insert grafting and selected suture interfascicular on cadaver specimen.

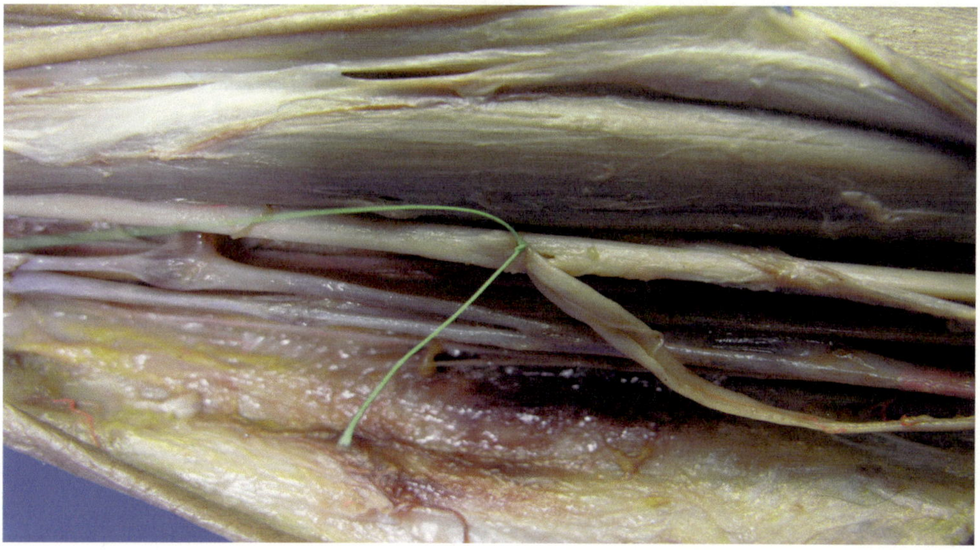

Fig. 2. Simulant procedures of Nerve rerouting ,insert grafting and selected suture interfascicular on cadaver specimen.

2. Patients with late incomplete rupture of spinal cord

2.1 Relief mini- incisions of the dura mater

This procedure was useful in incomplete paraplegic patients who showed early nerve function recovery 3 months after a traumatic injury in whom also there were no observed improvements after three additional months of physical therapy. CT scan and MRI images of these patients showed no severe spinal cord damages. For the procedure, under general anaesthesia, the patient was placed in a lateral or prone position prepped and draped. A midline lumbar skin incision was made and exposure done down to the level of the spinal canal. Impediments to functional recovery of the spinal cord such as bone compression, for some patients or unstable canales spinalis stenosis, in others were eliminated. The *endorhachis* of the involved segment of the spinal cord was exposed and found to be thickened, hardened, and without pulsation. We made about three to six 1cm longitudinal slit-like incisions on this layer with the assistance of a 4-6X forehead microscope in the thickened and hardened areas, leaving the arachnoid and pia mater spinalis intact (Figure 2.1).The pulsation of the dura mater recovered, which is obvious after complete release. We covered the spinal cord with artificial dura mater or sacrospinal muscle flap and closed the wound. We may conclude that the compression in the dural sac is the main obstacle to nerve function recovery, a condition which could not be relieved by the body itself. This microsurgical technique did promote functional nerve recovery in our patients.

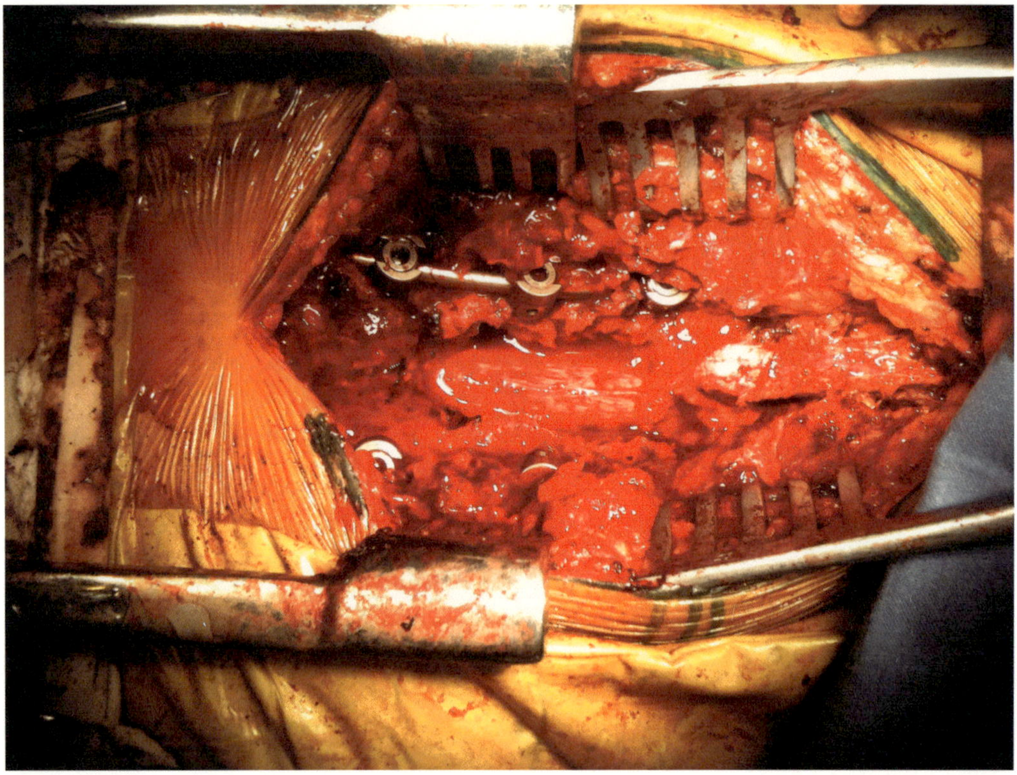

Fig. 3. Intra-op view showing mini incisions on the dura.

2.2 Intra-dural microlysis of the spinal cord and nerve roots

Similar to the procedure described in section 2.1, in some patients with late spinal cord injury, whose MRI pictures show that the injured spinal cord area is very close to the dura, or where the nerve roots are adherent to the dura by scar tissues, or where there are other strange shadows between the spinal cord and the dura, we may still open the *endorachis.* Since the fibrous band, strip, or scar were small and inconspicuous, careful and repeated observation to determine their presence and subsequent removal was necessary, as missing any of these would adversely affect the results (Figure 2.2). It was always observed intra-operatively that the initial parts of the nerve root were adherent to the spinal cord, and that a strip of fibrous tissues were seen between the anterior and posterior branches of the nerve root which dragged or pinched the spinal cord. We noted that the adhesions of the arachnoid and the pulling of the ligamenta denticulatum by these fibrous tissues made that affected segment of the spinal cord to appear structurally changed. The pia mater spinalis became thicker and adherent to the spinal cord, thus compressing it. The adhesion between the spinal cord and the arachnoid, compression by the pia mater spinalis, ligamenta denticulatum, nerve root, as well as the peripheral fibrous tissues were all completely relieved by the same microsurgical technique.

Finally, the *endorachis* and spinal canal were covered by a sacrospinal muscle pedicle flap. All the patients showed descend in their sensory planes and an increase in muscle force above grade one. The major muscle force of both lower extremities recovered above grade three and partial ability of walking was regained. Additional benefits were bowel and bladder functions improvement.

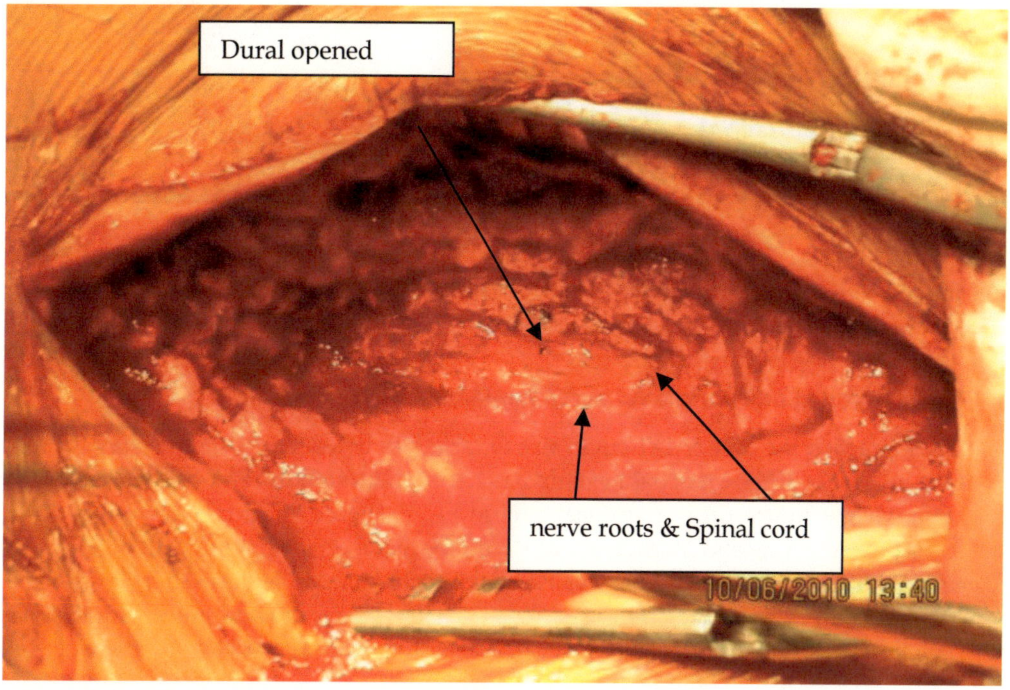

Fig. 4. Intra-op view of intradural microlysis.

2.3 Intradural lysis and peripheral nerve implantation

In some patients with late spinal cord injury, following decompression and lysis of the dura, the abnormal crimpled spinal cord was opened by making three to six incisions on its surfaces dorsally and laterally, each about 0.1 mm to 0.2 mm deep and extended beyond the abnormal part. Autogenous sural nerve segments were harvested corresponding to the length of the area of abnormality (Figure 2.3). After these peripheral nerve segments were microsurgically denuded of their epineuriums and perineuriums, making them resemble cauda equina-like tissues, they were aligned longitudinally with severed strips implanted into the spinal cord incisions.

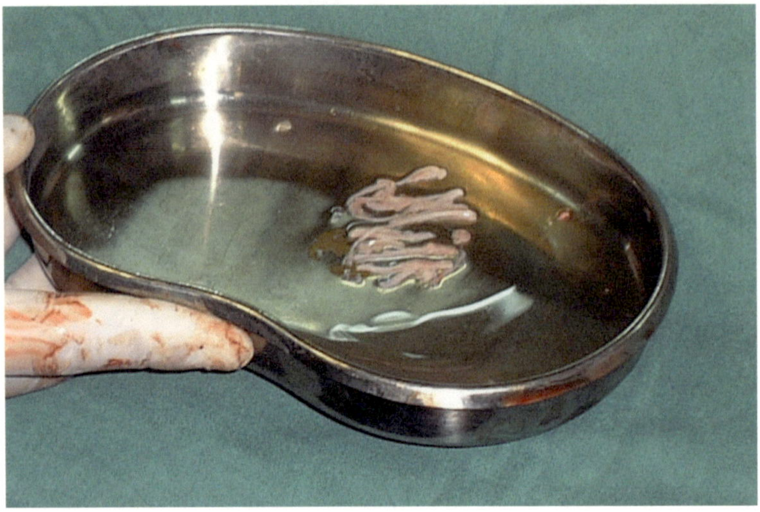

Fig. 5. Harvested autogenous sural-nerve segments.

Finally, the endorachis and spinal canal were covered by a sacrospinal muscle pedicle flap. All patients showed recovery of sensory, motor, as well as bowel and bladder functions.

2.4 Cyst aspiration and peripheral nerve implantation

In clinical practice, if a cyst of 1×1 cm in size or larger, as indicated by the pre-surgical MRI imaging review, or if the cyst could clearly be observed through its dark-colored, fluctuant, and thin-walled nature during surgical procedure, it should be punctured with a fine needle, aspirated a little and incision about < 3mm be made on the injured cord area, and its content drained out. The defect thus created by this technique can be covered with segments of peripheral nerve implants as described in section 2.3. This is done to prevent sudden sac wall collapse which might further complicate the existing spinal cord injury. Finally closure is done in layers. Such method can improve the function of sensory, motor nerves, and bowel and bladder activities.

3. Patients with late complete rupture of the spinal cord

3.1 Microlysis of proximal spinal cord and nerve roots

To present, there is still no convincing method of recovering spinal cord function in paraplegic and quadriplegic patients suffering from spinal cord injury. Meanwhile, it is well known that, due to its anatomic characteristics, there are always different degrees of injury to nerve root 1-3 segments above the ruptured spinal cord level (Figure 3.1). In clinical practice, these functions experienced complete loss in the acute period, and partially restore with regression of the acute traumatic reaction. Unfortunately, 1-3 months post-injury, in the proximal end of the spinal cord, particularly due to the reaction, scars formed and caused nerve roots adhesions such that the recovered function could not be conducted by nerve roots.

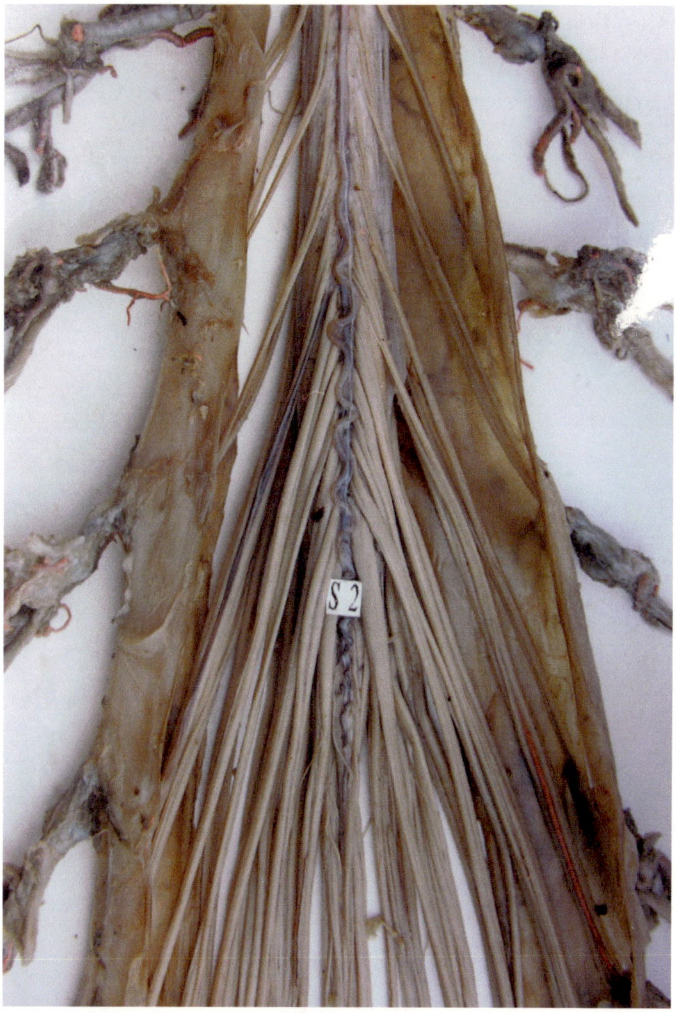

Fig. 6. Anatomy showing nerve roots in their original position.

To save the function of these nerve roots and improve the quality of life for patients with lower cervical and thoraco-lumbar region complete spinal cord injury, we perform another microsurgical technique. Under general anaesthesia, a dorsal midline incision is made on the skin and dissection made down to the spinal canal. After general epidural lysis of scars and decompression, the dura mater of the involved area was exposed and opened with the help of a 4-6X forehead microscope or a 6× to 40× operating microscope, where necessary. The proximal broken end of the spinal cord and corresponding nerve roots were exposed. These nerve roots with their relatively integrated continuity in anatomical morphology were thoroughly and sharply released from their initial parts to the intervertebral foramen area under the microscope. After lysis, the injured spinal cord area was covered with artificial dura mater or sacrospinal muscle flap. All patients who underwent this procedure showed recovery or improved partial sensory and motor functions of 1-2 nerve root segments.

3.2 Function restoration of chronic complete spinal cord injury by peripheral nerve rerouting and nerve insert grafting

Various nerve-rerouting surgeries are described below:

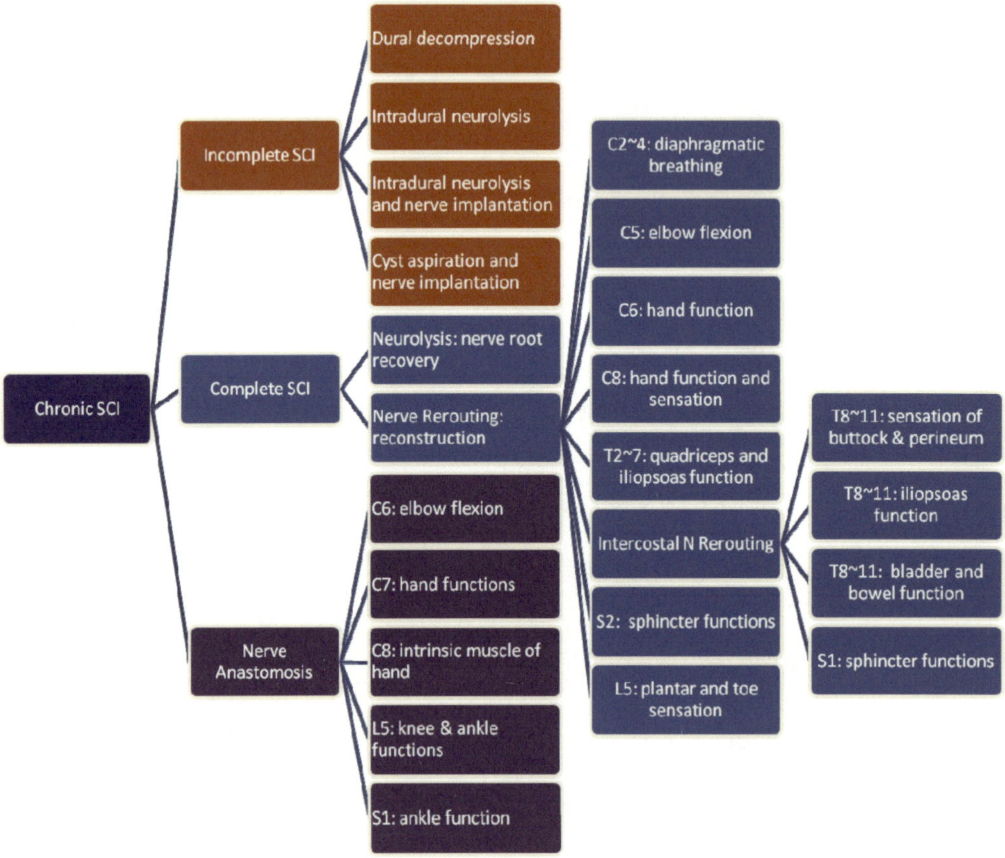

3.2.1 C2~4 Injuries: Connecting nerve branch of accessory nerve with phrenic nerve

Indications: C2~4 injured patients who show no spontaneous breathing and required ventilator support, and the strength of at least one side of the trapezius muscle. Surgical purposes: To restore part of diaphragmatic breathing function, which means breathing through the shrug movement without ventilator support in the awaken state. Anatomy: Accessory nerve is formed by cranial nerve root and spinal cord root (mainly C1 ~ 4), and cervical plexus nerves are composed of anterior branches of C1~4. So accessory nerve function was intact in spinal cord injury below C5 nerve level. Sternocleidomastoid and trapezius muscles were mainly dominated by accessory nerve, but most of the muscular branches were bifurcated in muscles, therefore cutting accessory nerve at supraclavicular level only affect partial strength of the trapezius muscle, with no loss of other important function. Surgical procedures: Accessory nerve was cut off proximally, and then rerouted and "grafted" into phrenic nerve in the relaxed state (Figure 7).

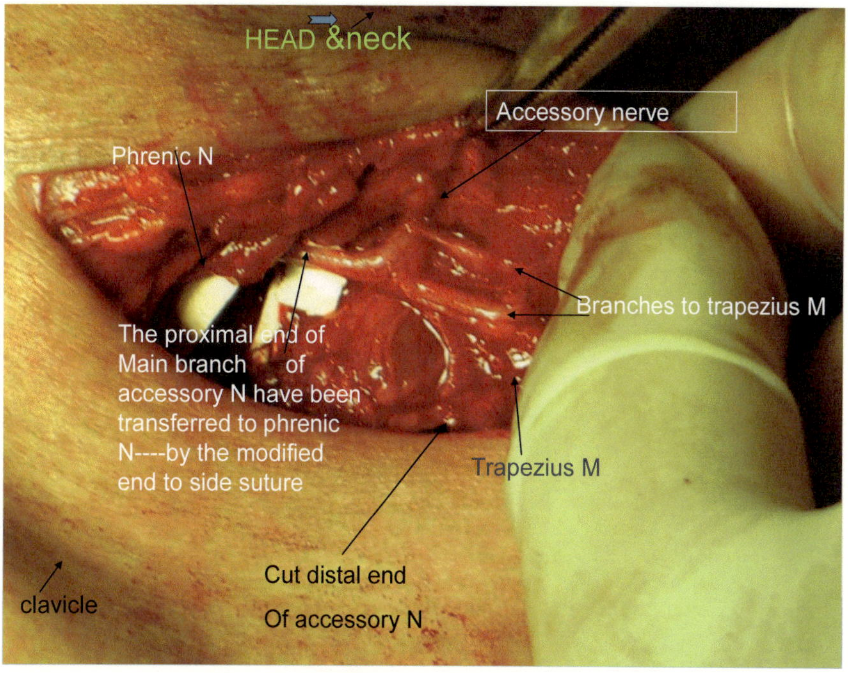

Fig. 7. Surgical procedure where accessory nerve is connected to phrenic nerve in the neck.

3.2.2 C5 Injury: Connecting nerve branches of accessory nerve and cervical plexus nerve with musculocutaneous nerve

Indications: C5 injured patients with quadriplegia for more than one year, no recovery of elbow flexion function, intact trapezius muscle function, and age <50-year-old.

Surgical purposes: To reconstruct elbow flexion.

Surgical procedures: A small transverse incision was made at the supraclavicula level, and then the main branch of accessory nerve was exposed and cut off. Musculocutaneous nerve was exposed below the clavicle and part of nerve fiber was cut off selectively. Get through an under-skin tunnel between the two incisions, then reroute and "graft" accessory nerve with musculocutaneous nerve.

3.2.3 C6 Injury: Connecting nerve branches of accessory nerve and cervical plexus with median nerve

Indications: Patients with no recovery of hand/wrist function.

Surgical purposes: To reconstruct some hand function.

Surgical procedures: Branches of accessory nerve and cervical plexus were cut off distally, then transferred to the supraclavicular level and "grafted" into the internal root or proximal segment of the median nerve (Figure 8).

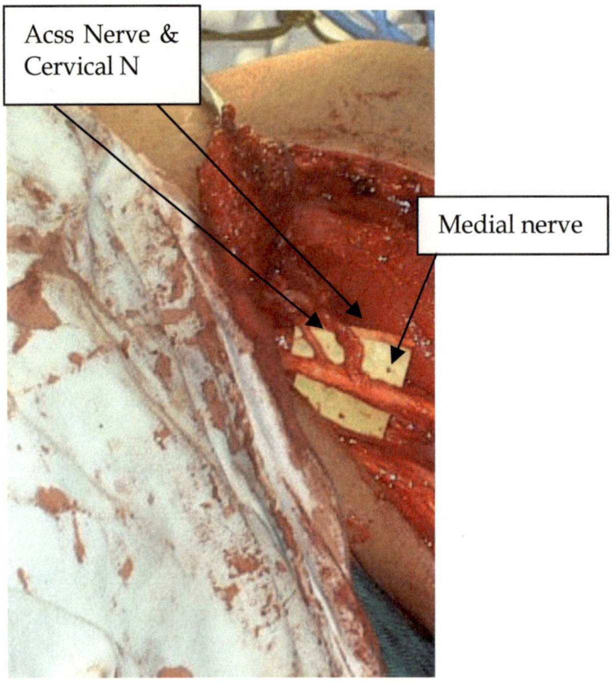

Fig. 8. Intra-op view of connections of accessory, cervical plexus and Median nerves in the supraclavicular region.

3.2.4 C8 Injury: Connecting pronator quadratus muscle branch of anterior interosseous nerve with deep branch of ulnar nerve, and superficial branch of radial nerve with superficial branch of ulnar nerve

Indications: loss of intrinsic muscles function, and sensitivity of little finger and ulnar part of ring finger. The strength of pronator quadratus muscle is of level 3 or more.

Surgical purposes: To rebuild part of motor functions of hand and sensitivity of ulnar part of hand.

Anatomy: Anterior interosseous nerve is composed of nerve fibers from C6 and C7. Thus there is no significant effect by cutting off pronator quadratus muscle branch.

Surgical procedures: Cut off pronator quadratus muscle branch of anterior interosseous nerve in the volar forearm, and then "graft" to the ulnar nerve. Superficial branch of radial nerve is connected to the superficial branch of ulnar nerve using conventional methods (Figure 9).

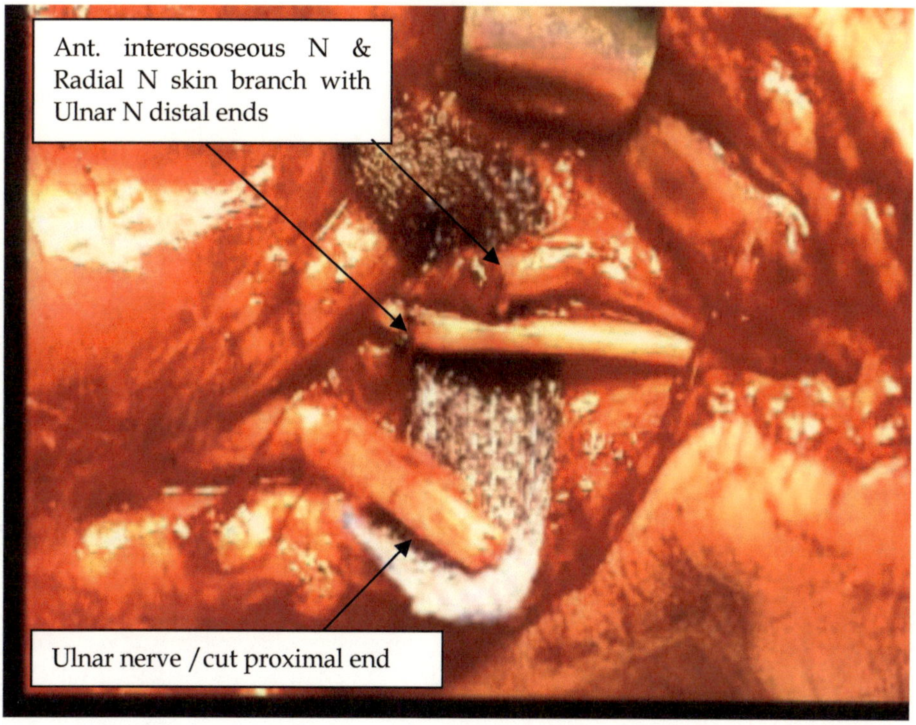

Fig. 9. Segments of Ant. Interosseous, and branches of radial and ulnar nerves.

3.2.5 T2~7 Injuries: Connecting vascularized ulnar nerve with femoral nerve

Indications: *Young patients who sustained T2~ 7 injuries want to have the operation; also to fully understand the functional damage in recipient nerve area.*

Surgical purposes: To rebuild partial motor function of quadriceps and iliopsoas muscles. This may improve walking ability with brace assistance.

Anatomy: Ulnar nerve is composed of nerve fibers from C7~ T1. Femoral nerve is composed of nerve fibers from L2~4, which dominate quadriceps and iliopsoas muscle innervations.

Surgical procedures: Ulnar nerve is transected from the wrist area. The remaining distal end of ulnar nerve is connected to the median nerve using conventional methods. Alternatively, this distal end may be connected to the anterior interosseous nerve or superficial branch of radial nerve to maintain some function of the ulnar nerve in the arm. The detached ulnar nerve is then separated *non-invasively*, together with the forearm portions of the ulnar artery and vein or superior ulnar collateral vessels, up to its beginning in the brachial plexus. Through subcutaneous tunnel in the trunk, the ulnar nerve is rerouted to the groin region (Figure 10). Separate and connect thoracodorsal artery and vein with the superior ulnar collateral artery and vein in the side of the chest wall, or connect ulnar artery and vein with deep iliac artery and vein or femoral artery and vein. Then the deep or superficial branches of ulnar nerve are connected to the femoral nerve, and the dorsal branch stitched to the ilioinguinal nerve.

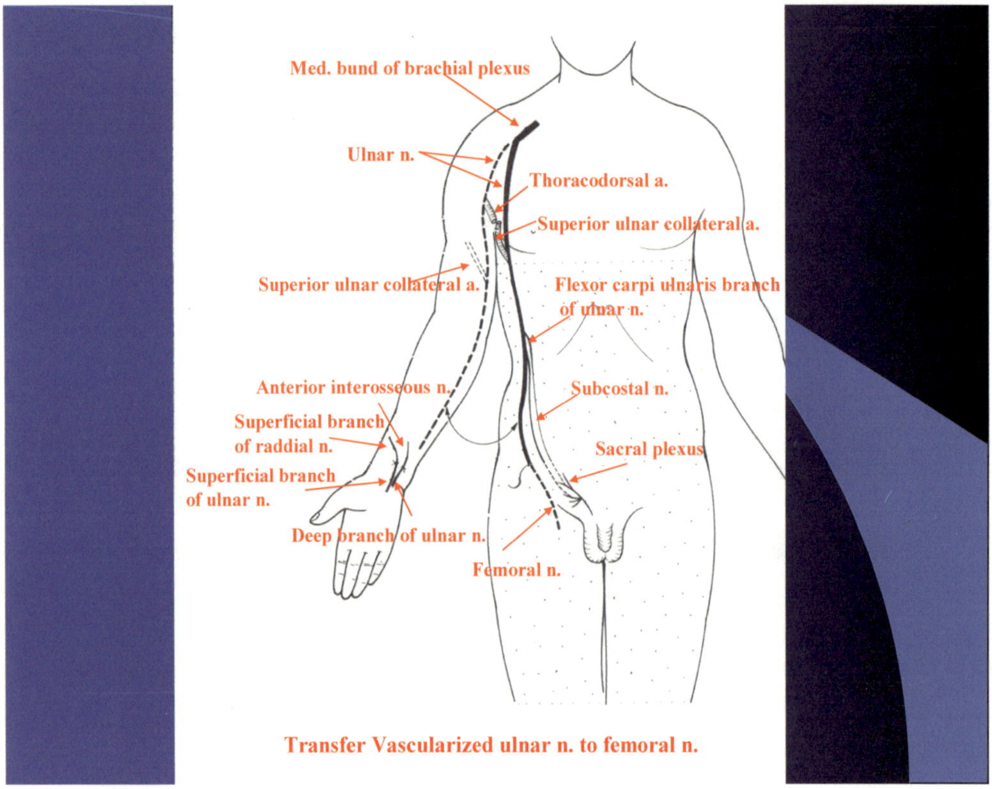

Fig. 10. Diagram of restoration of stepping-forward and ambulatory functions in individuals with paraplegia through rerouting of vascularized ulnar nerve to femoral nerve in the groin.

3.2.6 Vascularized intercostal nerve rerouting

Transferring intercostal nerve to the cauda equina or terminal nerve roots has been carried out for nearly a hundred years, but because of no significant effect comparing with high expectations; recently few doctors are willing to carry out such surgeries with hope of achieving better results. We have made some modifications: 1. Reroute intercostal nerve along with its vessels, to improve blood supply to nerve and decrease adhesion (Figure 11); 2. Only transect particular bundles of receptor nerve fibers, to maintain proper muscle tension and pathological reflex; 3. Stitching nerve in the epidural area is suggested, according to results from animal experiments and clinical trail; 4. Vascularize the nerve to be bridged, for example, arterialize the sural nerve by anastomosis of small saphenous vein with intercostal artery.

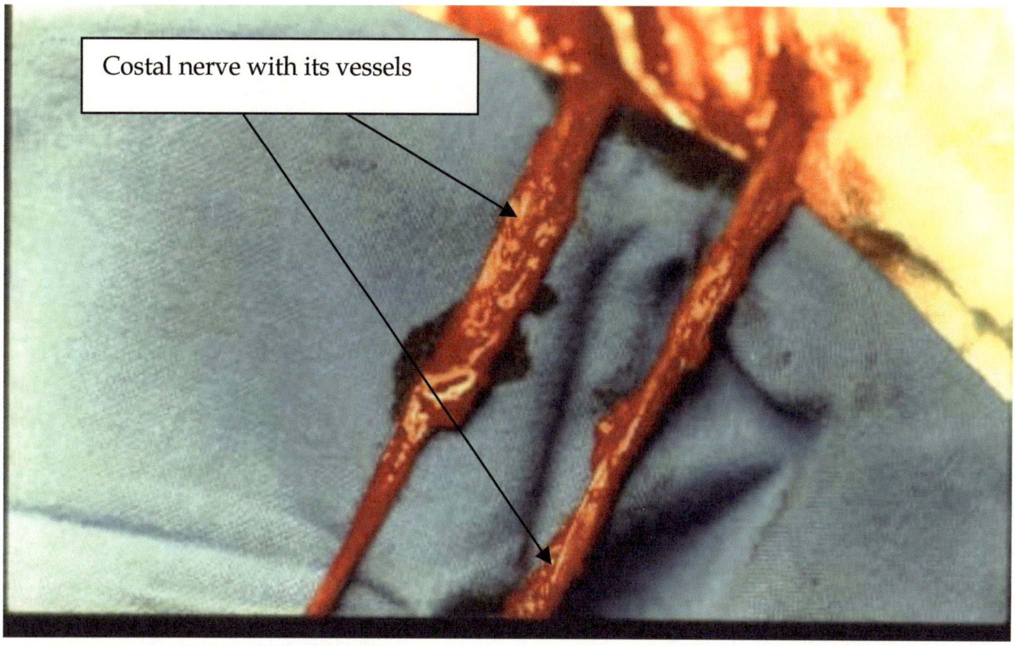

Fig. 11. Costal nerve with its vessels.

3.2.6.1 T8-T11 Injuries: Vascularized intercostal nerve rerouting to connect lateral femoral cutaneous nerve with ilioinguinal nerve to regain sensation of buttocks, lateral femoral and external genitalia regions

Indications: Male patients with complete injury to nerve roots T9~11 and show no recovery of sensory and motor functions, however, they do experience penile erection. It is also indicated for young women with strongly expressed desire to improve genital sensation.

Surgical purposes: To regain sensation of buttocks, the lateral femoral and external genitalia regions.

Anatomy: The intercostal nerve is formed by the anterior branch of the thoracic nerve while the lateral femoral cutaneous nerve is formed by L2~3 nerve fibers, which is divided into anterior and posterior branches in the groin. The anterior branch distributes to the skin of the anterolateral thigh, and the posterior branch distributes to the skin of the lateral thigh. Ilio-inguinal nerve is formed by T12~L2 nerve fibers, which distributes to the skin of upper and medial thigh, the penis and scrotum or labia.

Surgical procedures: Take separately the 8th and 9th intercostal nerves as example: separate intercostal nerves with their vessels, and reroute them to the ilio-inguinal and lateral femoral cutaneous nerves, and then connect them directly or bridge with sural nerve segment.

3.2.6.2 T8-T11 Complete Injuries: Connecting vascularized intercostal nerve with selective bundles of L1/2 nerve roots to reconstruct iliopsoas function (grafting technique)

Indications: Spastic paralysis of both lower extremities.

Surgical purposes: To reconstruct iliopsoas function (mobile with brace)

Anatomy: iliopsoas, quadriceps and vastus medialis are controlled by nerve fibers from L2~4 nerve roots. Patients with improved iliopsoas function could achieve hip flexing, and train quadriceps to contract synchronously to facilitate knee extension.

Surgical procedures: Isolate and transect two intercostal nerves above paraplegic plane with intercostal vessels, and connect them with selective bundles of L2 or L2/3 nerve roots. If the length of the intercostal nerve is not enough, then harvest sural nerve for bridging.(Fig 12)

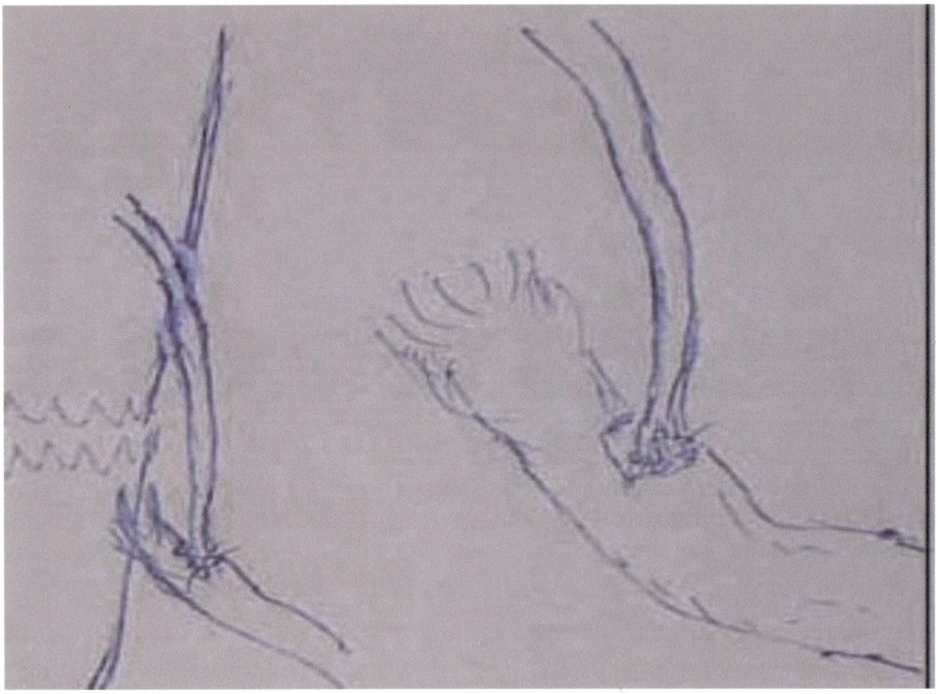

Fig. 12.

3.2.6.3 Connecting vascularized intercostal nerve with sacral nerve root to reconstruct partial bladder and bowel function (grafting technique)

Indications: T8-T11 injuries.

Surgical purposes: To reconstruct partial bladder and bowel functions.

Anatomy: S2~4 nerve roots innervate the anal and urethral sphincters. In patients with spinal cord injury above T12, lower central nervous system functions of defecation and urination are preserved and their low-level reflex arc remains intact, but lost contact with the high-level central nervous system. So, bladder and bowel functions could be improved as long as the establishment of such a neural pathway, which only needs a few nerve fibers to rebuild, exists. This approach allows part of the normal mixed nerve (intercostal nerve) fibers to connect with the sacral nerve roots and pelvic nerve plexus to establish urination reflex, and also rebuild partial sphincter and sensory function at the same time.

Surgical procedures: The procedures are the same as that of connecting L1/2 nerve roots, except that the receptor nerve is the sacral nerve not lumbar nerve. The number of receptor nerve root fibers to be transected depends on the severity of bladder and sphincter spasm (Figure 13a & Figure13b).

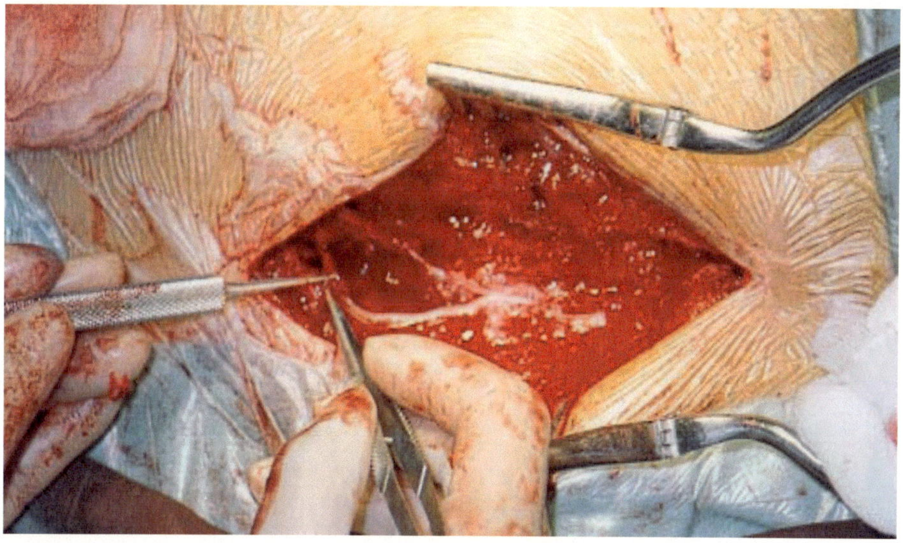

Fig. 13a.

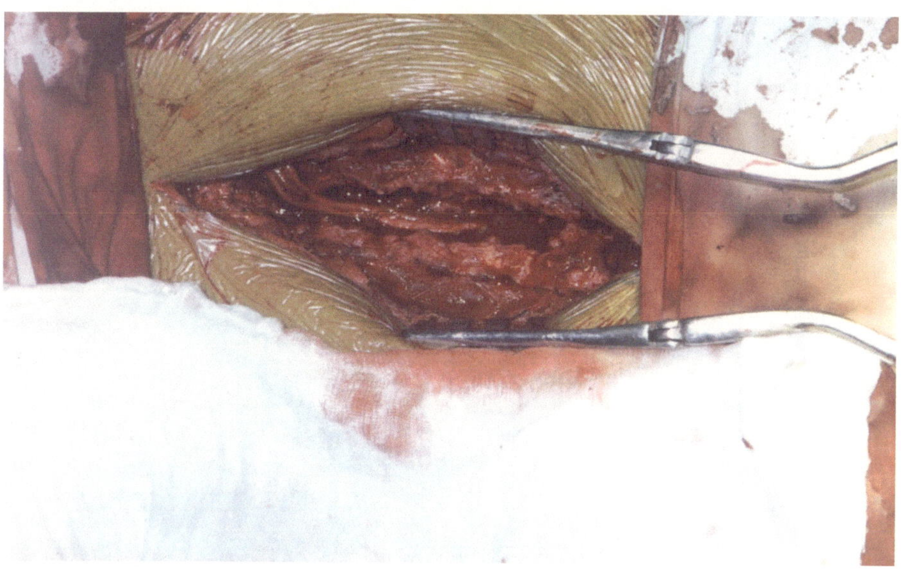

Fig. 13b.

3.2.6.4 Connecting vascularized intercostal nerve with ilio-inguinal nerve for sensation in the perineum

Surgical procedure: 0ne incision about 12cm long laterally on the chest wall along the 8th or 9th rib. Expose the underlying tissues and take the vascularized intercostals nerve. Make another incision about 8cm long laterally in the costo-iliac region of the abdominal wall; explore and identify the ilio-inguinal nerve. Make a subcutaneous tunnel connecting the two incisions (Figure 3.2.6.4a). Anastomose the intercostal nerve with the ilio-inguinal nerve in this tunnel by bridging sural nerve graft (Figure 14a/b).

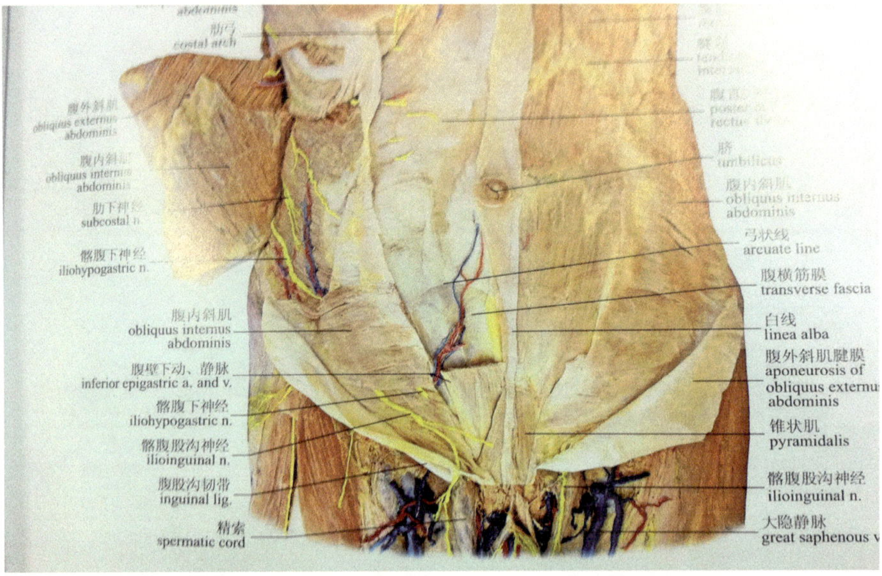

Fig. 14a. Anatomy Atlas illustrating musculo-cutaneous nerves and vessels ilioinguinal nerve.

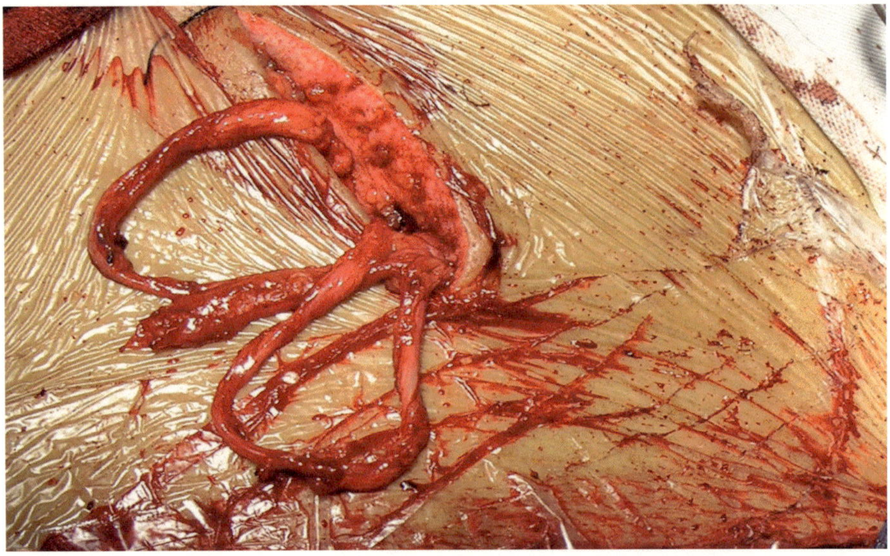

Fig. 14b. Intra-op demonstration of tunneling technique in the subcostal-iliac region.

3.2.6.5 S1 Injury: Connecting vascularized intercostal nerve to pudendal nerve

Indication: Incontinence after the injury with injury time <6 months

Surgical purpose: To restore the urethral anal sphincter functions, and improve stool and incontinence.

Surgical procedure: Locating and transecting the intercostal nerve as described in section 3.2.6. Locating the pudendal nerve, this can be found at the basin of a 1-2cm long incision in the hip, and connect it with intercostal nerve through a subcutaneous tunnel (Figure 15).

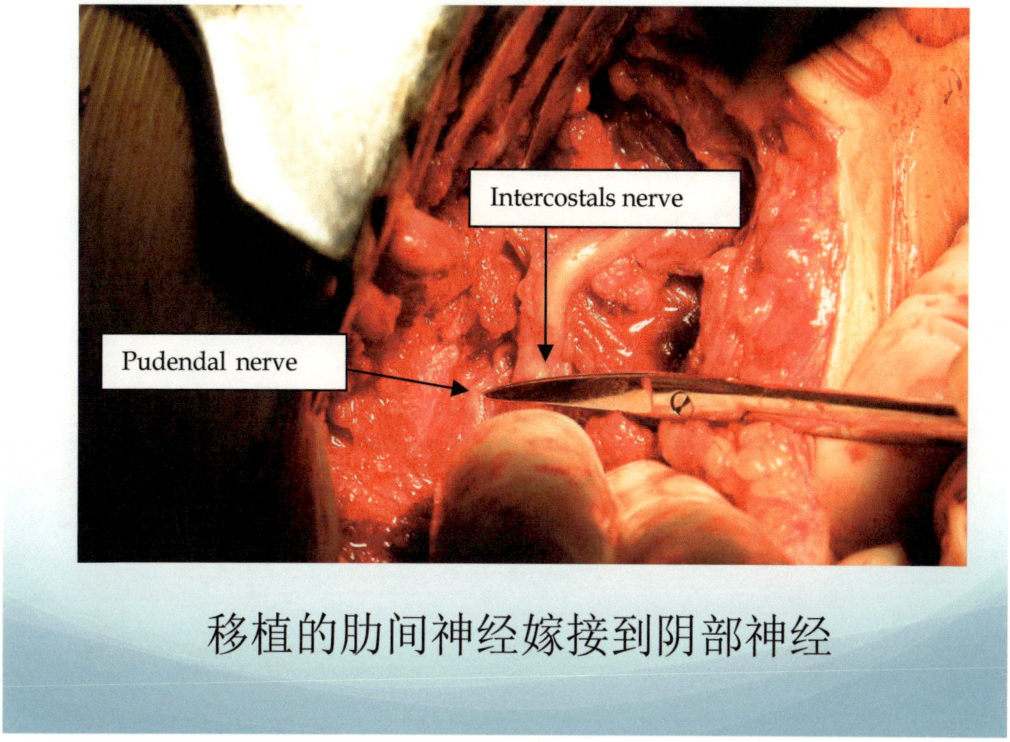

Fig. 15. Intercostal and pudendal nerves anastomosis.

3.2.6.6 S2 and below injuries: Connecting muscle branch of superior/ inferior gluteal nerve with pudendal nerve

Indications: Incontinence for >6 months and the strength of gluteus muscle > level 3.

Surgical purpose: To reconstruct part of the urethral and external anal sphincter function

Anatomy: superior/ inferior gluteal nerve is mainly composed by nerve fibers from L4~S1, with a trunk of about 2cm length, and then divided into multiple muscular branches into the gluteal muscle. Cutting one of these muscular branches would not cause significant gluteal dysfunction. Pudendal nerve is formed by nerve fibers from S2~4. The place where these two nerves go out of pelvis are very close to each other. And the muscular branches of superior/ inferior gluteal nerves are long enough to be connected with pudendal nerve directly.

Surgical procedure: In the incision in the hip, isolate superior/inferior gluteal nerve near piriformis muscle and find the pudendal nerve by the outer edge of the sacrum. Cut off one of the muscular branches of superior/inferior gluteal nerve, and connect it with pudendal nerve.

3.2.6.7 L5 or below injury: Connect sural nerve to tibial nerve to improve sensation of plantar surface and toe

Indications: *Restore the ability of walking and sense of lateral malleolus/ instep, but no sense of plantar and toe.*

Surgical purposes: To improve sensation of plantar surface and toe.

Anatomy: Sural nerve can be cut at the distal lateral malleolus and connected to the tibial nerve.

Surgical procedure: Separate sural nerve in the distal lateral incision on the leg, and connect it to the tibial nerve via a subcutaneous tunnel.

Injury	Method	'Donor'	'Receptor'	Function
C2~4	R	Branch of accessory nerve	Phrenic nerve	Diaphragmatic breathing function
C5	R	Branch of accessory nerve and cervical plexus nerve	Musculocutaneous nerve	Elbow flexion
C6	R	Branch of accessory nerve and cervical plexus	Median nerve	Hand function
C6	A	Axillary nerve	Musculocutaneous nerve	Elbow flexion
C7	A	Lateral root of median nerve	Medial root of median nerve	Hand function
	A	Posterior brachial plexux	Ulnar nerve	
C8	R	Pronator quadratus muscle branch of anterior interosseous nerve	Deep branch of ulnar nerve	Hand function and sensation
		Superficial branch of radial nerve	Superficial branch of ulnar nerve	
C8	A	Median nerve	Ulnar nerve	Hand intrinsic function
T2~7	R	Ulnar nerve	Femoral nerve	Walking
T8-T11	I	Lateral femoral cutaneous nerve	Ilioinguinal nerve	Sexual life
T8-T11	I	Intercostal nerve	Selective bundles of L1/2 nerve roots	Walking
T8-T11	I	Intercostal nerve	Sacral nerve root	Bladder and bowel function
L5	A	L3	L4	Knee and ankle function
L5 or below	R	Sural nerve	Tibial nerve	Plantar and toe sensation
S1	I	Intercostal nerve	Pudendal nerve	Bladder and bowel functions
S1	A	Peroneal nerve	Tibial nerve	Ankle function
S2 and below	R	Muscle branch of superior/ inferior gluteal nerve	Pudendal nerve	Bladder and bowel function

4. Peripheral nerve side- to- side interfascicular anastomosis

This operative technique involves several steps. First, the site of injury is explored and the injured nerve recovered and repaired by standard techniques. Second, a relatively normal nerve root, termed "donor nerve", is identified close to the injured nerve as possible. Third, this "donor" nerve is then drawn toward the injured nerve below the level of its site.

For example, if the L4 and L5 lumbar nerve roots had been injured, the nerve was chosen for side-to-side neurorrhaphy at the lower ventral thigh. If the lower trunk of the brachial plexus had been injured, the ulnar and median nerves were chosen for side-to-side neurorrhaphy which placed two nerves abreast closely at an appropriate segment. 1cm - 2cm longitudinal incision is made on the epineurium and partial perineurium were performed at the neighbor side. Then the incised epineurium and partial perineurium were sutured closely side-to-side with 9 to 11 monofilament nylon and microsurgical instruments. Fourth, the limb with the neurorrhaphy is immobilized with a cast for three to four weeks after surgery to avoid tension on the sutured nerves. *Finally, physical therapy is advised, and neurotrophy medication is administered in appropriate dosage.*

The methods for peripheral nerve side-to-side anastomosis are as follows:

The procedure, as described above, involves shifting of a normal peripheral (donor) nerve in the paralyzed region to a receptor nerve to the same site. This is accomplished by transposing the distal end of the donor nerve to the region of the receptor nerve where we wish to establish the anastomosis. The length of side-to- side segments of the two nerves is 1cm-2 cm. The perineurium and epineurium layers of the two nerves are carefully opened and the side of the donor nerve is inserted into the incision made on the side of the receptor nerve. The two nerves are then embedded and stitched to each other and their perineuriums and epineuriums closed in layers.(Fig.16) For instance, if the tibial nerve lacks function due to injury and the lateral popliteal nerve is normal, their neighboring segments, about 5 cm proximal to their bifurcations, would be drawn together and approximated as described above. (Fig.17,18,19)

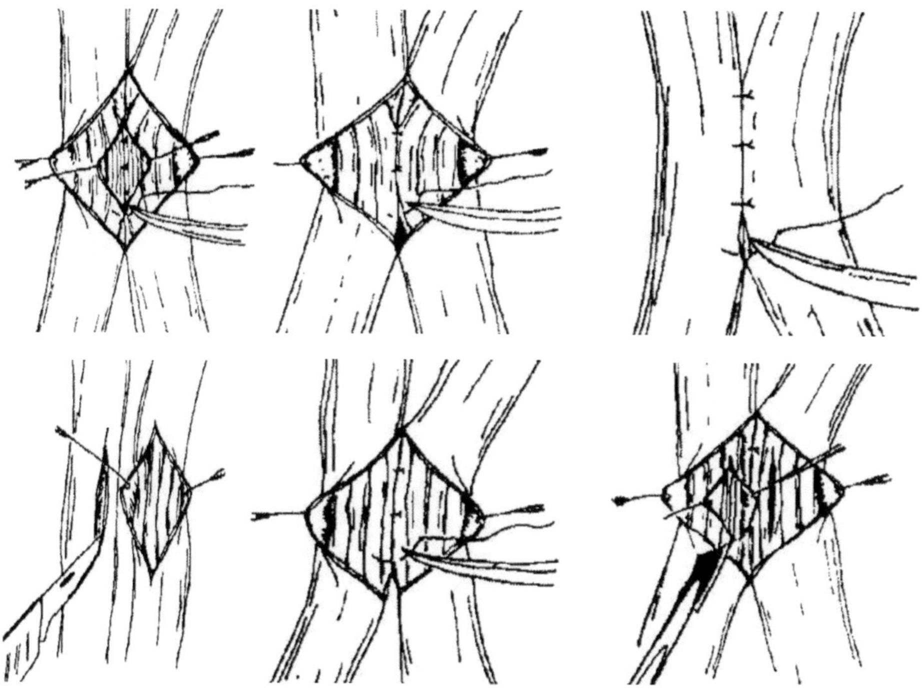

Fig. 16. Schematic Diagram of Side-to-side Neurorrhaphy: (*A*). Epineurium incision of the two neighboring nerves; (*B*). Suture on one side of the epineurium ;(*C*). Incision of the perineurium; (*D*). Suture one side of the perineurium ;(*E*). Suture another side of the perineurium ;(*F*). Suture another side of the epineurium.

Table 4.1 shows different types of donor-receptor nerve fiber anastomosis and their potential resultant benefits.

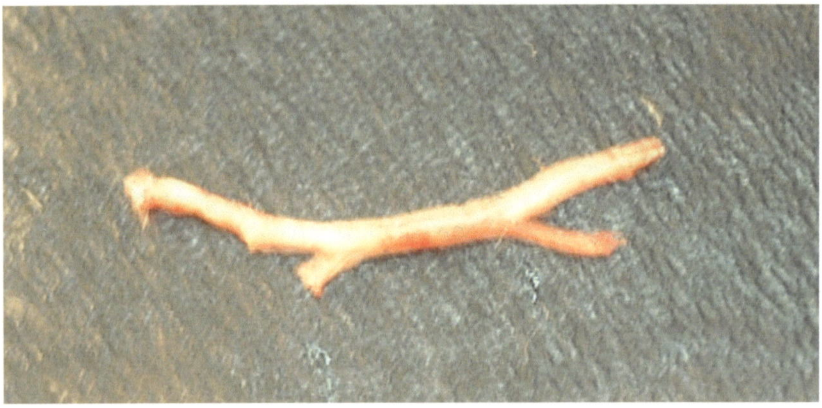

Fig. 17. Rat's tibia with fibular N side to side suture post operation 3 months ---looked as one nerve trunk).

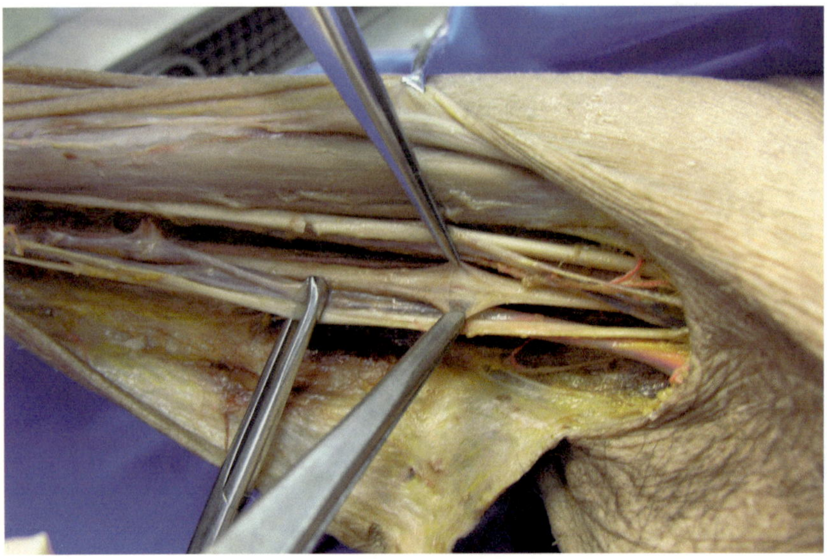

Fig. 18. Anatomy show.

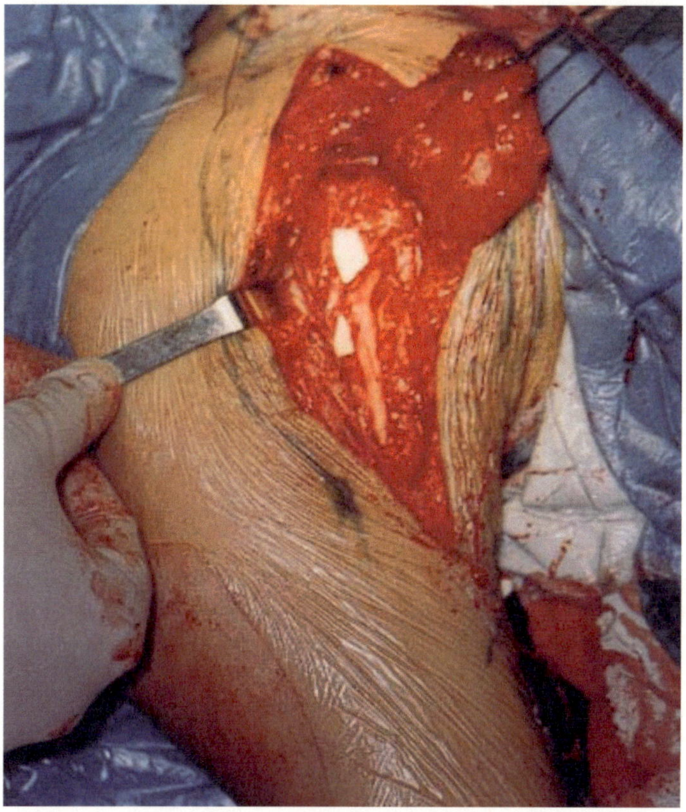

Fig. 19. Intra-op photo showing side-to-side suture of Lateral Cord with medial cord for restoration of hand function for a C7 level Spinal cord injured patient.

The level of spinal cord injury	Donor nerve	Receptor nerve	The anastomosis site	Functional reconstruction
C6	Axillary nerve	Musculocutaneous nerve	The anterior axillary region	The function of elbow flexion
C7	The lateral root of median nerve posterior plexus brachialis	The medial root of median nerve Ulnar nerve	The initial part of median nerve axilla	The function of hand
C8	Median nerve	Ulnar nerve	Upper arm in the lower 1 / 3	The function of Intrinsic muscle of the hand
L5	L3	L4	Pelvis	The functions of knee and ankle
S1	Peroneal nerve	Tibial nerve	The superior popliteal fossa region	The function of ankle

Table 4.1 The donor/receptor sites of side-to-side anastomosis in different levels of spinal cord injury.

5. Conclusion

The main objective of most current operations is to eliminate outside compression of the dural sac and stabilize the spine. Lacking the knowledge that the arrested functional recovery of the spinal cord can be due to scar formation on the inner dural sac, intradural sac lysis is often ignored, which influences the recovery of the spinal cord. Using microsurgical techniques, we completely loosened the scars and adhesions, and as for the scarring or a cystic spinal cord, the spinal cord was opened and autogenous peripheral tissues were implanted, so the functional recovery of a damaged spinal cord segment would be better improved, and the results be satisfactory by the time of initial clinical evaluation.

According to our clinical observation, most patients with chronic complete spinal cord injury received partial functional restoration by peripheral nerve rerouting and nerve grafting procedures. For complete paraplegic patients, even partial sensory, motor with additional bladder and bowel function restorations can bring much convenience, reduce complications and greatly improve their quality of life. As only a few nerves can be used for rerouting techniques, these series of microsurgical procedures can only restore limited and key functions. More training of muscle contraction caused by pathological reflex and

grafted nerve is necessary for effective motor function. In 226 cases follow-up between 3-28yaers, effect active movement functions (M3) were restored in 37%, sensation (S2-S3) in 76%, *refelection* in 81%. Therefore, patients who cannot receive standard rehabilitation training would not get a satisfactory result. It can be recommended not to treat older patients in poor general condition, or patients of difficult economic standard with such surgery.

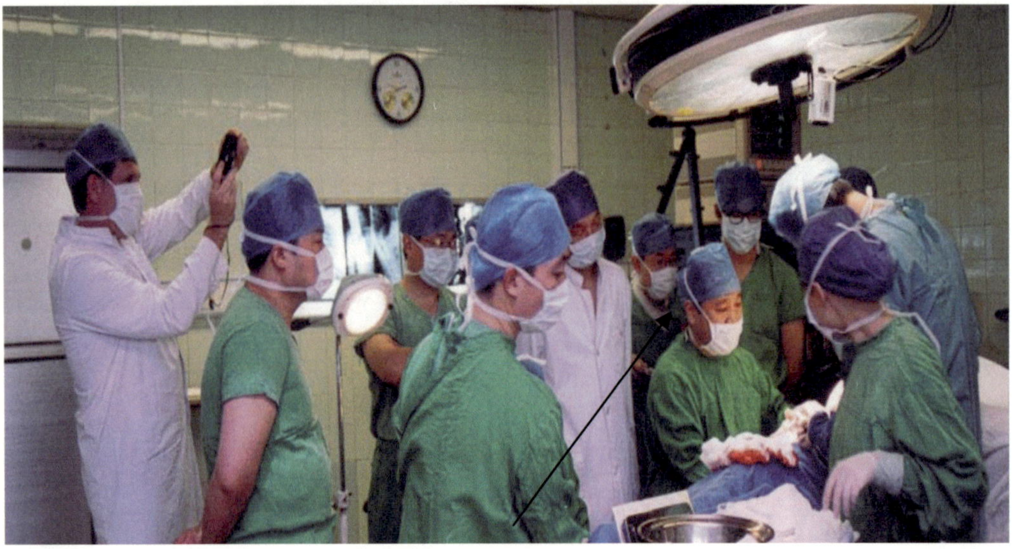

Fig. 20. Dr. Zhang Shaocheng M.D, the operator.

6. References

[1] Frankel HL. Traumatic paraplegia. Nurs Mirror Midwives J. 1975; 141(19); 48-52.

[2] McCormick PC. Spinal Cord Injury without Radiographic Abnormality. Neurosurg. Suppl. 2002; 50; 53:100.

[3] Dang R, Zhang S, Ji R, et al. Applied anatomy of lumbosacral nerve roots corresponding to the T12-L4 vertebra. Chinese J Anatomy. 1996; 19:381-4.
[4] Cigliano A, Scarano E, De Falco R, et al. The posterolateral approach in the treatment of post traumatic canal stenosis of the thoraco-lumber spine. J Neurosurg Sci. 1997; 41:387-93.
[5] Horvat JC. Spinal cord reconstruction and neural transplants. New therapeutic vectors. Bull Acad Natl Med. 1994; 178(3):455, dis. 464.
[6] Zompa EA, Cain LD, Everhart AV, et al. Transplant therapy: recovery of function after spinal cord injury. J Neurotrauma 1997;14(8):479-506.
[7] Giovanini MA, Reiter PJ, Eskin TA, et al. Characteristics of human fetal spinal cord grafts in the adult rat spinal cord: influences of lesion and grafting conditions. Exp Neurol. 1997; 148(2):523-43.
[8] Delamarter RB, Sherman J, Carr JB, et al. Pathophysiology of spinal cord injury: recovery after immediate and delayed decompression. J Bone Joint Surg (Am). 1995; 77: 1042-9.
[9] Zhang SC, Zhao J. Gatism treated with neuroanastamosis. J Neurol Orthop Med Surg. 1993; 14:37-8.
[10] Zhang SC, Ma Yuhai, Liu Huiren, et al. Intradural Lysis and Peripheral Nerve Implantation for Traumatic Obsolete Incomplete Paralysis. Orthopaedic Surgery. .Surgical Technology International, 2007; 15:321～24
[11] Shaocheng Zhang, Xuesong Zhang, Rongming Ji. Functional Reconstruction of Peripheral Nerves in Paraplegia. J Neurol Orthop Med Surg 2000 20(3):89～97
[12] Zhang SC, Zhao J. Gatism treated with neuroanatomosis.J Neurol Orthop Med Surg, 1993, 14(1):37～38
[13] Zhang SC. Ulnar nerve transfer to the sciatic and pudendal nerves in paraplegia. J Neurol Orthop Med Surg, 1993, 14(6):3～4
[14] Zhang SC, Laurence J, Zhang ZW. Restoration of stepping-forward and ambulatory function in patients with paraplegia: rerouting of vascularized intercostals nerves to lumbar nerve roots using selected interfascicular anastomosis. Surgical Technology International, 2003; 11:244～248
[15] Zheng MX, Xu WD, Qiu YQ, Xu JG, Gu YD. Phrenic nerve transfer for elbow flexion and intercostal nerve transfer for elbow extension. J Hand Surg Am. 2010 Aug; 35(8):1304-9. Epub 2010 Jul 8.
[16] Sullivan J, Spinal cord injury research: review and synthesis. Crit Care Nurs Q. 1999; 22(2):80-99.
[17] Prochazka A, Mushahwar VK. Spinal cord function and rehabilitation-an overview. J Physiol 2001; 533(Pt 1):3-4
[18] Pearson KG. Could enhanced reflex function contribute to improving locomotion after spinal cord repair? J Physiol. 2001; 533(Pt 1):75-81.
[19] Zhang SC. Paraplegia treatment by anastomosis of lateral cutaneous nerve of thigh and ilioinguinal nerve with vascularized intercostals nerve for sensation reconstruction. Acad J Sec Mil Med Univ 1998; 19(3):264-5.
[20] Zhang SC, Zang X. Functional reconstruction of peripheral nerves in paraplegia. J Neurol Orthop. Med Surg 2000; 20(3):89-97.
[21] Zhang SC, Xiu XL, Li QH, et al. Nerve degeneration of lower extremity after paraplegia. Acad J Sec Mil Med Univ. 1999; 20(9):684-5.

[22] Zhang Shao-cheng, Ma Yu-hai, Xu Shuo-gui, et al. Autoperipheral nerve implantation for the treatment of obsolete incomplete paralysis. Chinese Journal of Clinical Rehabilitation. 2006, 10(5): 161-163

[23] Zhang Shao-cheng, Ma Yu-hai, Johnson Laurence, et al. Reconstruction of bowel and bladder function in paraplegic patients by vascularized intercostal nerve transfer to sacral nerve roots with selected interfascicular anastomosis. Chinese Journal of Clinical Rehabilitation. 2006, 10(17): 190-192

[24] Zhang Shaocheng, Luo Chaoli, Zhao Yongjing, and YH Ma. The treatment of spastic cerebral palsy with side-to-side peripheral nerves anastomosis. AANOS, 2001, 21(3): 84-87.

2

Unilateral Minimally Invasive Posterior Lumbar Interbody Fusion (Unilateral Micro-PLIF) for Degenerative Spondylolisthesis: Surgical Technique

Shigeru Kobayashi
Department of Orthopaedics and Rehabilitation Medicine, Faculty of Medical Sciences, The University of Fukui, Fukui, Research and Education Program for Life Science The University of Fukui, Fukui Japan

1. Introduction

Degenerative spondylolisthesis has long been recognized as a cause of chronic low back pain and sciatica. Extensive anatonmical and embryological studies have not fully explained the cause of this painful condition. The mechanism of pain in degenerative spondylolisthesis has been confirmed by demonstrating the disc lesion pre-operatively by X-rays and MR imaging followed by surgical treatment in which the abnormal disc is totally removed and replaced with bone grafts to effect an interbody fusion. Ralph Cloward first performed the posterior lumbar interbody fusion (PLIF) in 1940 in Hawaii.(1952, 1953, 1981, 1985) . Over the last decade, PLIF has become a popular technique for achieving interbody fusion. The development of pedicle screw fixation system is significant in the history of PLIF. PLIF with pedicle screw systems have apperently improved the rate of arthrodesis (Bridwel et al., 1993, Zdeblick et al., 1993, Yvon et al., 1994, Fischgrund et al., 1997). However, the result of exposure technique can be ischemic necrosis induced by forceful retraction of the paraspinal muscles and postoperative low back pain. The first percutaneous screw placement technique was reported by Magerl (1982) and involved the use of external fixators. The development of technology for minimum invasive placement of rods and pedicle screws was driven by concerns over the amount of paraspinal muscle retraction required in the open approaches. Forley (2001) made a significant contribution to resolving this dilemma with his invention of instruments and a technique to pass rods in a minimally traumatic fashion using an arc-based system called Sextant (Medtronic). The percutaneous pedicle screw system have served as adjuvants in the development of minimally invasive PLIF. And also, interbody spacers have far more better results in term of disc height maintenance and in direct neural decompression than bone grafts alone. Various radiolucent interbody spacers, such as carbon cages (Brantigan & Steffee, 1993), and polyetheretherketone (PEEK) interbody spacers (Park & Foley, 2008), are wide and long and provide a large surface area for fusion and generous reconstruction of collapsed disc spacers on the use of interbody spacers for

PLIF. The graft bone material in the interbody spacers mainly consists of autologous bone which is harvested from the ilium, local bone acquired by posterior decompression and artificial bone, such as hydroxyapetite and β-tricalcium phosphate (β-TCP). The use of local bone and artificial bone has the advantage of avoiding the necessity to harvest from iliac bone, and this advantage is connected with less operating time, blood loss and no postoperative iliac pain. Interbody spacer far better results in term of disc height maintenance, preventing of collapse and indirect neural decompression than bone grafts alone. The first to report the unilateral approach for bilateral spinal canal decompression were Young et al. (1988). Development of this surgical corridor requires the removal of bone from the ipsilateral spinolaminar junction. Tubular access to the lumbar disc was first reported by Faubert and Caspar (1991) and this led the way for the development of tubular retractor systems. The microscope is then utilized to visualize across the midline, and access is achieved to the contralateral recess of the spinal canal (Takeno, et al., 2010). With advances in minimal access technology using operating microscope, PLIF can now be performed through a minimally invasive, unilateral approach, providing an adequate decompression and circumferential fusion, and avoid many of the disadvantages of the traditional posterior open approach. In this report the authors present a surgical technique and clinical outcomes of the unilateral minimally invasive posterior lumbar interbody fusion (unilateral micro-PLIF) for degenerative spondylolisthesis.

2. Surgical technique

Following induction of general anesthesia, the patients were positioned prone on a radiolucent table. Reduction of the abdominal pressure is necessary to decrease the blood loss. Before prepping the patient, lateral and anteroposterior C-arm fluoroscopic images were obtained to ensure that the pedicles could be adequately visualised prior to starting the operation.

2.1 Skin incision

Surgical access for interbody fusion was obtained under operating microscope using Casper retractor (Aesculap) and a self-retaining retractor of PLIF system (Codman). The approach of unilateral micro-PLIF can be performed from the side that was most symptomatic. An 3 cm. to 5 cm transverse or longitudinal skin incision is used for 1 level operation (Fig.1A). The subcutaneous fat is incised from lumbosacral fascia and performed the slightly arcuate fascial incision 1.5 cm from midline (Fig.1B). The median edge of the fascial incision is dissected, bluntly, back to the midline with the aid of surgical forceps and a small raspatory or scissors, and held back with two holding sutures. The midline structures can be shown more easily from the inside. It is important not to release the paravertbral muscles from spinous process subperiosteally and the periosteal membrane of lateral surface on the spinous process should carefully preserved to prevent the blood loss. The paramedian incision later makes uninterrupted suturing of the fascia easier. With a small raspatory, the musculature is detached bluntly from the midline structures up to the arches. In order to unintentionally not go beyond the midline, the detachment should always begin on the lateral surface of the cranial spinous process (in the lower one third) and should be carried out strictly vertically along the bone. The deep anatomical situation is palpated with the finger. Orientation on the position, course, with of the arches, position of the articular portions and width of the interlaminar space is thus provided (Fig.1C). At the same time, the distance between the skin surface and the upper edge of the arch is determined using the index finger, so that the appropriated Casper retractor is selected. The musculature is vigorously pulled away about 2 cm in the lateral direction with the fluted introducer. The Casper retractor is introduced via the surgical hook as near vertically as possible and the interlaminal space is exposed widely, enough to see the facet (Fig.1D). At this stage, X-ray control is taken to confirm the disc level. Under microscope, the ligamentum fluvum is cleared carefully of fat, connective tissue or muscle fiber residues which are still attached to it with a dissection swab by pushing away in the lateral direction. If necessary, these structures are coagulated bipolarly and removed with a rongeur to clearly expose the ligamentum fluvum prior to incision.

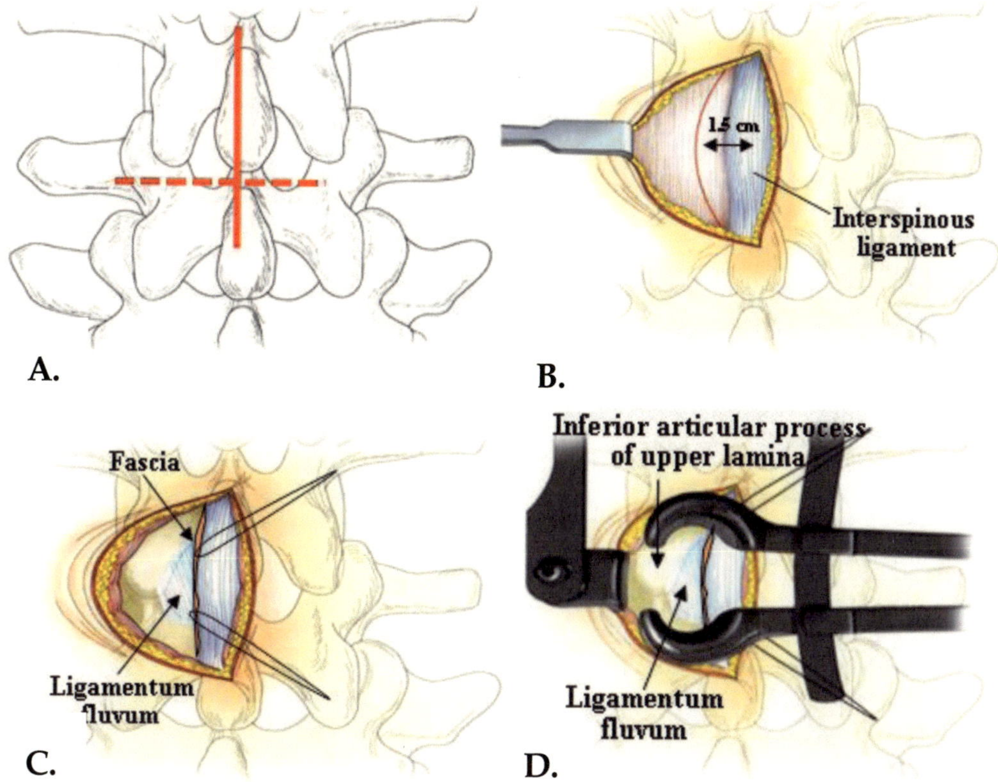

Fig. 1. A. Longitudinal or transverse incisions (3-5 cm) for exploration in one segment. B. Slightly arcuate fascial incision 1.5 cm from the midline. C. Exposure of ligamentun fluvum and facet. D. Setting of Casper retractor.

2.2 Ligamentum flavum, inferior and superior facet removal

A transverse cut is made along the lower margin of the upper laminae with a 6-10 mm osteotome (Fig.2A,B). The bone cut is continued laterally to remove the lower 1/3 of the facet joint. The osteotome is then placed at a 45° angle and the tip of the superior articular process of the lower lamina confirmed. The upper margin of the lower lamina is removed with a narrow osteotome from the base of the spinouts process to the facet. The resection of inferior articular process is safer than that of superior process, because the nerve tissue is protected by superior process. It is safer to break superior articular process just before it is cut completely. If necessary, we can use up-cutting punch, to remove the remnant. The lateral bone strip is removed with a narrow disc rongeur and bone bleeding controled with bone wax. The medial bone strips are then grasped with a disc rongeur and removed with a strong pull. Bleeding from veins in the epidural fat is immediately coagulated bipolarly and packed with Gelfoam and cottonoid patty. The ligamentum flavum is removed from the lower margin and under side of the upper laminae using a curved periosteal elevator (Fig.2C). Removal of medial half of the superior facet exposes 2 cm or more of the spinal canal lateral to the nerve root (Fig.2D,E), which is filled with epidural fat and veins. These are separated from the lateral margin of the nerve root and dural sac which are retracted medially with a flexible hand held retractor. The resection of inferior articular process is safer than that of superior process, because the nerve tissue is protected by superior process. It is safer to break superior articular process just before it is cut completely. If necessary, we can use upcutting punch, to remove the remnant.

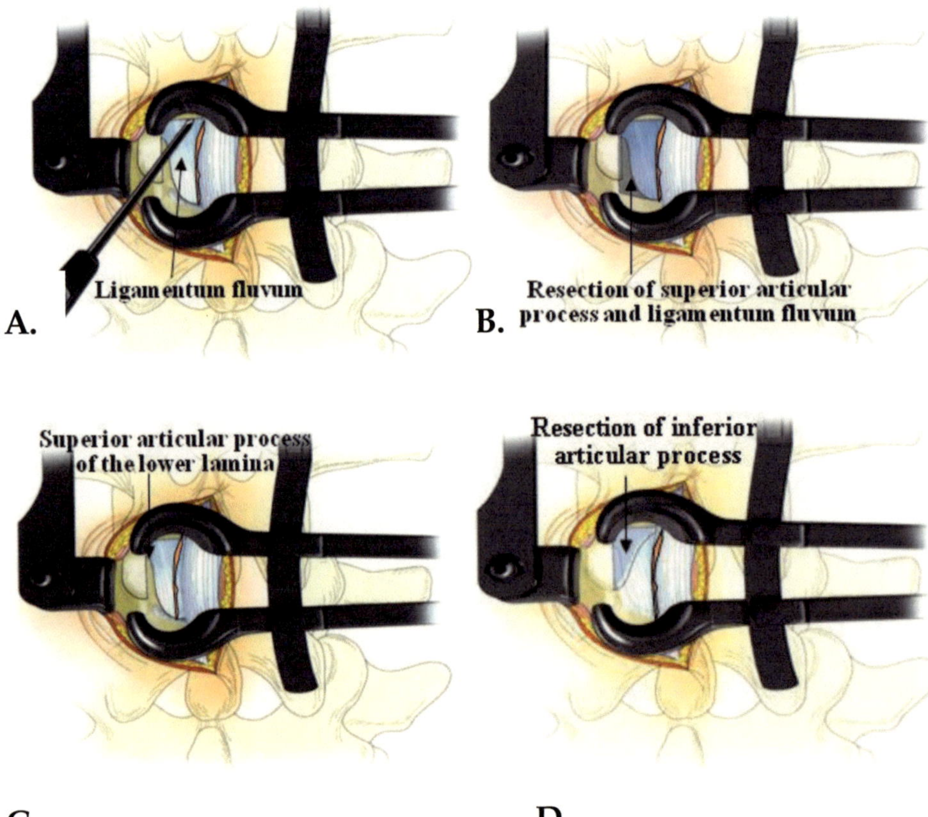

Fig. 2.

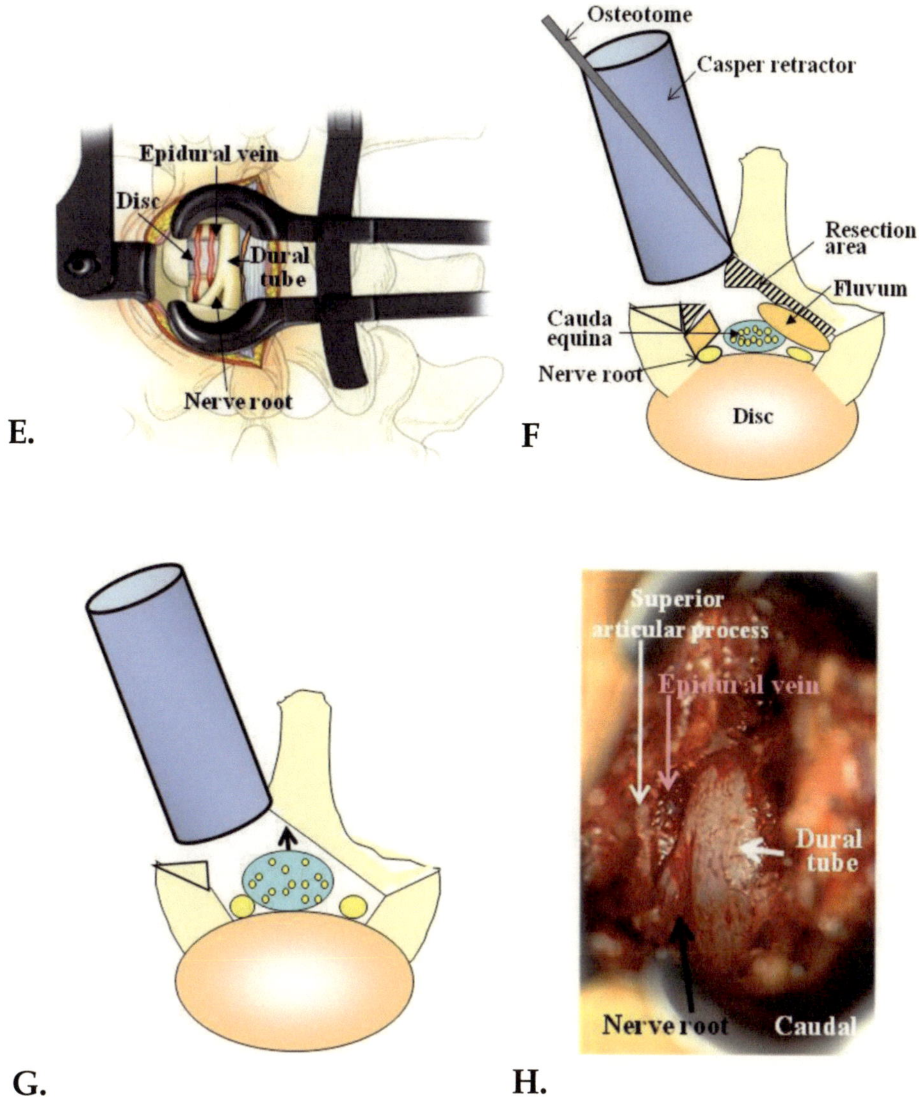

Fig. 2. Removal of the inferior (A,B), superior facet and ligamentum flavum (C,D) and exposure of the nerve tissue and disc surface (E). Then the microscope is tilted, and the cortex is excised from the base of the spinous process to the vertebral arch on the opposite side, exposing the ligamentum flavum on the dorsal aspect of the dura mater (F-H).

With an operating microscope tilted inwards, the area from the base of the spinouts process to the inner rim of the vertebral arch on the opposite side is resected with an osteotome to semi-circumferentially expose the cauda equina as well as expand the spinal canal (Fig.2F). The ligamentum flavum is identified as a yellow mass under microscope that is loosely contact to the dural sac and the dural sleeve. The ligamentum flavum can completely excised, and adequate decompression of the cauda equine and nerve roots can confirmed under microscope (Fig.2G, H).

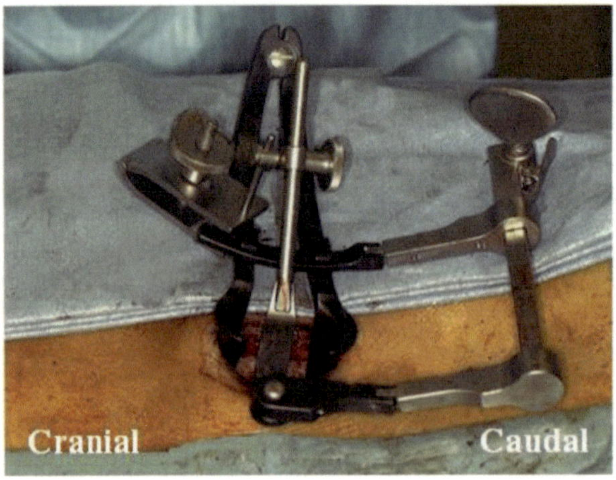

A.

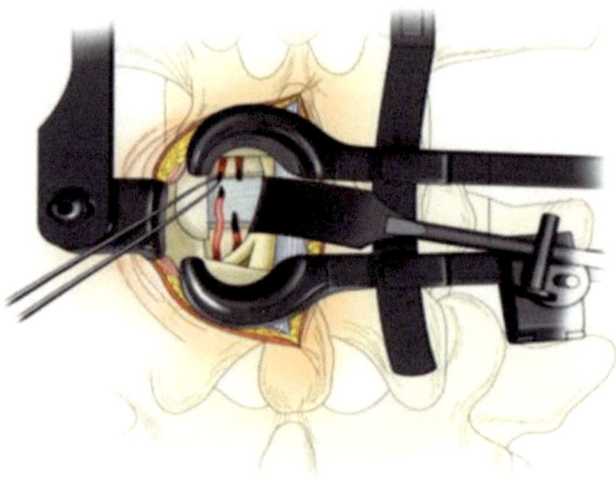

B.

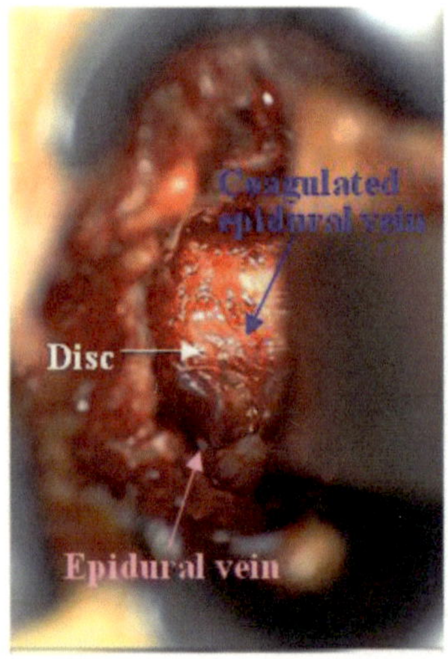

C.

Fig. 3. Setting of a self retaining nerve retractor (A) and treatment of epidural vein on the disc (B,C).

A self retaining nerve retractor can be used to fit the exposed nerve root and dural sac. The tip of a self-retaining retractor is placed beneath the nerve root and dural sac, gently retracted to the midline and secured to the clamp on the Casper retractor (Fig.3A). This eliminates strong manual retraction of the nerve root and gives wide exposure of the disc surface. It is very important to control the epidural hemorrhage using electric coagulator and coagulant like cottonoid patty. If it is possible, the epidural veins are immediately coagulated bipolarly before bleeding (Fig.3B,C) and cut with long pointed scissors. This may be a difficult part of the operation, but the disc surface must be widely exposed and completely dry as a bloodless field is essential for the operative attack on the intervertebral disc.

2.3 Disc removal and interbody fusion

The primary goal of this operation is to remove the entire disc and replace it with as much bone as can be inserted into the intervertebral space. A long handled scalpel with pointed blade is used to cut out the posterior half of the disc (Fig.4A). A deep vertical incision is made in the midline beneath the retracted dural sac and nerve root. Then horizontal insicions are made following the margins of the vertebral bodies as far lateral as the exposure will permit, usually beyond the pedicle of the lower vertebra. The incised annulus and disc material is removed enough in this side till the midline using surgical knife, pituitary rongeur, and curette. Next, the posterior edge of the vertebra (end plate) is cut off using an osteotome. An osteotome is hammered at an angle paralleling the disc space and to a depth of around 2 cm (Fig.4B) and the cartilage end-plates of the lower and upper vertebra removed with a large disc rongeur. This gives a wide opening into the interspace for total removal of the remaining disc tissue. The residual cartilage end plates may be stripped from the vertebral bodies with a long curved osteotome and a ring curette (Fig.4C,D). It is necessary to remove the cartilage end plate and part of the bone plate until enough bleeding comes from the vertebral body. Complete decortication of the surface of the adjacent vertebral bodies is mandatory to obtain blood supply for the interbody bone grafts.

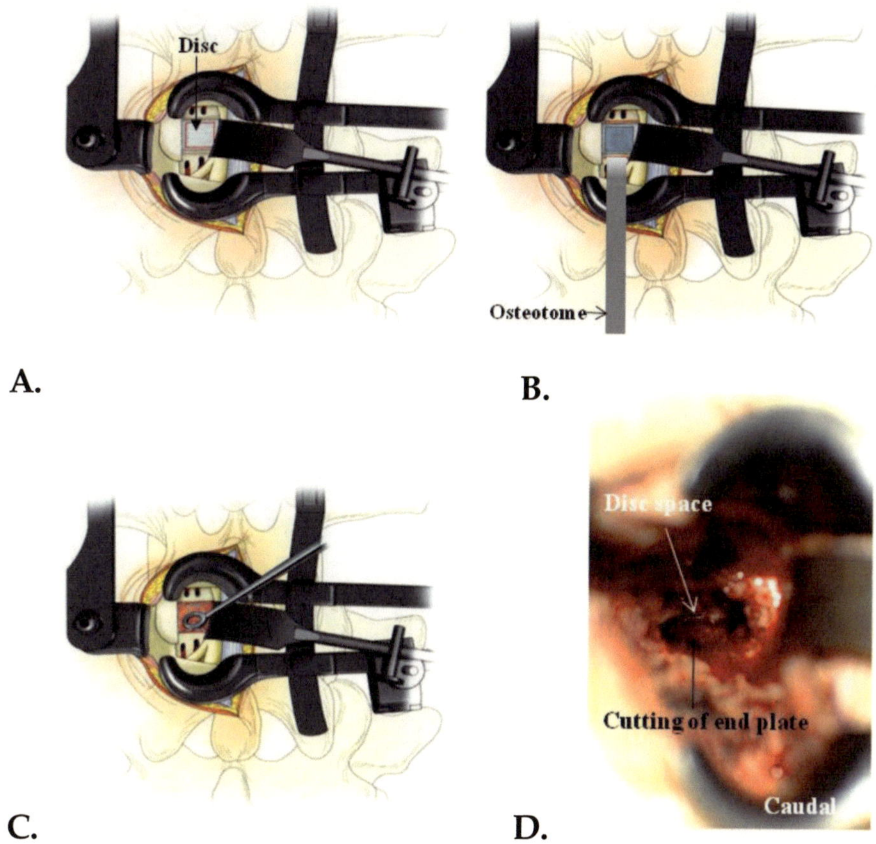

Fig. 4. Cut off end plate (A,B) and disc removal (C,D).

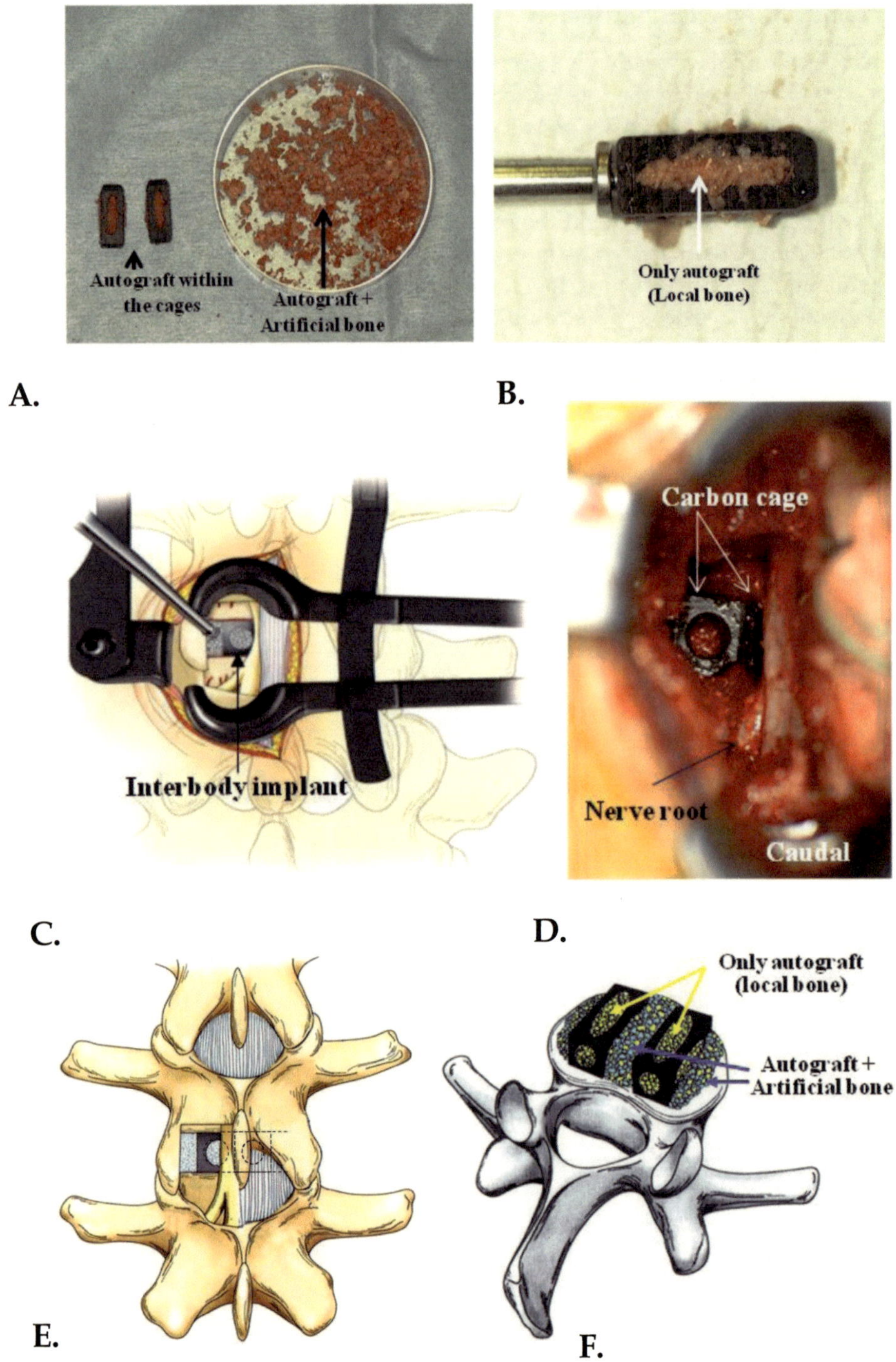

Fig. 5. Interbody fusion using interbody spacers (A-F).

Bone grafts for the interbody fusion can be obtained from the patient's lamina, inferior and superior facet (local bone tips) and artificial bone (Fig.5A). The graft in an interbody spacer (Branigan carbon cage or polyetheretherketone [PEEK] interbody implant) is only living local bone tips. Around 2g of local bone tips can graft in an interbody spacer(Fig.5B). The residual local bone tips (around 2-6 g) and the artificial bone (β-tricalcium phosphate [β-TCP], around 5g) is mixed and a half of this tips are packed into the anterior disc space. Then, two cages are inserted in the disc space and moved medially using Cloward's puka chisels(Fig.5C-F). Finally, the graft of the residual local bone tips with the artificial bone is inserted laterally(Fig.5D). It is important to spread the intervertebral space enough and to insert and move it. If it is impossible to insert two cages in one side, the same operation is down on the opposite side to insert an another one.

2.4 Pedicle screw fixation

Pedicle screws and rods were placed percutaneously (CD Horizon Sextant, Medtronic Sofamor Danek). The placement pf pervutaneous pedicle screws requires the surgeon to be able to accurately interpret antero-posterior and lateral fluoroscopic images to safety insert these devices. The Sextant technique involves placing guidewires through the pedicles passing between 50 and 75% of the sagittal length of the vertebral body. Standard tubular dilation techniques are performed over the wires. A cannulated tap is placed over them, screw holes are made, and the screws are placed. During percutaneous pedicle screw placement, care must be taken to ensure that the guidewire does not advance through the ventral wall of the vertebral body where it might cause vascular or visceral injury. The screw towers are then coupled together and an arc device with a perforating tip at its distal end is connected to them. The tip is then rotated down to meet the skin. A distal stab incision is then made and the arc is pushed through to make a subcutaneous tract to the aperture of the most proximal screw. A measuring device is then placed on the arc system to

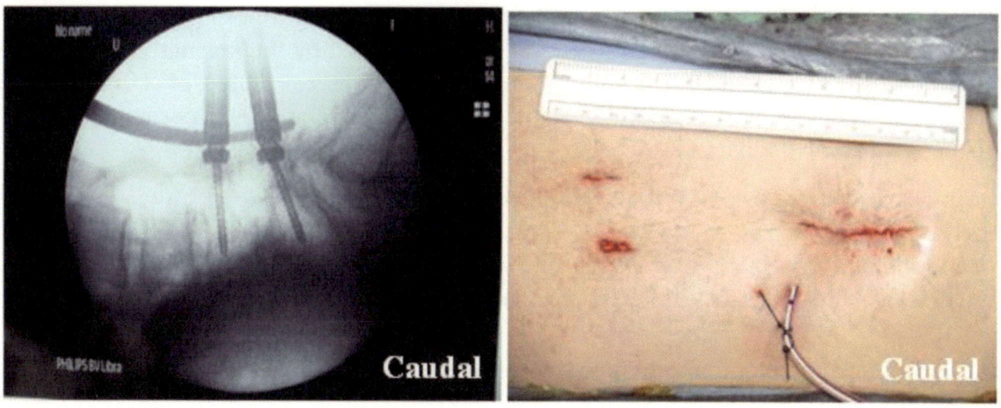

A. B.

Fig. 6. A. Intraoperative fluoroscopic images demonstrating left L4-5 PLIF procedures with percutaneous pedicle screw, rod and PEEK interbody spacer. B. Final skin wound after operation. Caudal wound made for the Casper retractor and bilateral pedicle screw system. Two 1 cm wound was needed in the cranial area for rod insertion.

calculate rod length. The arc is swung back and temporarily withdrawn, and the perforating tip is replaced with the premeasured rod. It is then passed through the priviously made tract that is typically in an ideal vector to engage both screw apertures (Fig.6A). After the position of interbody construct is confirmed under fluoroscope, the pedicle screws are attached to and compressed on the rod, thereby restoring lumbar lordosis while maintaining the restored disc height.

After washing with saline solution, it is possible to hervest subcutaneous fat as a covering and gliding layer for the dura and the root. This remains viable and serves to minimize adhesions formation. A drainage tube is inserted over the grafting fat tissue. After removal of the retractor, the musculature returns spontaneously to the midline. The tendency is further supported by suturing the paraspinally incised fascia. After the subcutaneous tissue are sutured, atraumatic subcuticular skin suture are performed using 5-0 Vicryl (Fig.6B).

3. Resuls of unilateral micro-PLIF

3.1 Patients and methods

Fifteen patients (5 men and 8 women) with Grade I and II degenerative spondylolisthesis (Meyerding, 1932) underwent unilateral micro-PLIF (Table 1). The mean age was 59.3 years (range, 42-76 years old). We used an arc-based system called Sextant (Medtronic) and interbody spacers (Branigun carbon cages or PEEK) were used in all. Presenting symptoms were low back pain with radiculopathy in all patients. All patients had a single-level interbody fusion. Simple PLIF was done at the L4-L5 level in 12 cases and the L3-4 level in one case. Follow-up ranged from 18-40 months (mean, 28.5 months). In these cases, clinical results, operating time, intraoperative blood loss, time for bone union and correction rate of the spondylolisthesis were analysed. Clinical results were evaluated by subjective symptoms (low back pain, 3 points; leg pain and/or tingling, 3 points; gait, 3 points) and clinical signs straight leg raising test, 2 points, sensory disturbance, 2 points, motor disturbance, 2 points) based on the scoring system advocated by the Japanese Orthopaedic Association (JOA) (Table 1). The rate of improvement was calculated by Hirabayashi's method as follows: [(postoperative points - preoperative points)/(normal points - preoperative points)] x 100 (%).

Percent of slip was measured following Taillard W (1954) (Fig.7). Bone union was evaluated based on criteria by Yamamoto et al (1990). as follows: (1) a diminished line between the bone grafts and vertebrae, (2) a change in the obtuse angle between the bone grafts and vertebrae, and (3) an increase in the trabeculae of the bone grafts.

3.2 Clinical and radiological outcomes

In the cases of degenerative spondylolisthesis treated by unilateral micro-PLIF, blood loss was 384.1 ± 134.7 ml and operating time was 219.6 ± 31.7 minutes **(Table 2).** The pre- and postoperative JOA score is 14.5± 4.0 points and 24.4 ± 2.0 points, respectively **(Table 3)**. The improvement rate of JOA score was 67.6 ± 11.1%. Percent slip before and after operation is 18.3± 5.2 % and 11.5 ± 4.4 %, respectively (Fig.7). The correction of the spondylolisthesis was spontaneously perfomed by prone position on a table withiout the reduction screw. The time for bone union was 7.5 ± 2.3 months. All patients presenting with preoperative low back pain and sciatica had resolution of symptoms postoperatively and had solid fusions radiographically at lastest follow-up.

I. Subjective Symptoms	(9 points)
A. Low-back pain	
a. None	3
b. Occasional mild pain	2
c. Frequent mild or occasional severe pain	1
d. Frequent or continuous severe pain	0
B. Leg pain and/or tingling	
a. None	3
b. Occasional slight symptom	2
c. Frequent slight or occasional severe symptom	1
d. Frequent or continuous severe symptom	0
C. Gait	
a. Normal	3
b. Able to walk farther than 500 m although resulting in pain, tingling, and/or muscle weakness	2
c. Unable to walk farther than 500 m owing to leg pain, tingling, and/or muscle weakness	1
d. Unable to walk farther than 100 m because of leg pain, tingling, and/or muscle weakness	0
IV. Urinary bladder function	(-6 Points)
a. Normal	0
b. Mild dysuria	-3
c. Severe dysuria (incontinence, urinary retention)	-6

II. Clinical Signs			(6 points)
A. Straight-leg-raising test (including tight hamstrings)			
a. Normal			2
b. 30–70°			1
c. Less than 30°			0
B. Sensory disturbance			
a. None			2
b. Slight disturbance (not subjective)			1
c. Marked disturbance			0
C. Motor disturbance (MMT)			
a. Normal (Grade 5)			2
b. Slight weakness (Grade 4)			1
c. Marked weakness (Grade 3–0)			0
III. Restriction of Activities of Daily Living (ADL) (14 Points)			
a. Turning over while	0	1	2
b. Standing	0	1	2
c. Washing	0	1	2
d. Leaning forward	0	1	2
e. Sitting (about 1 hour)	0	1	2
f. Lifting or holding	0	1	2
heavy objects	0	1	2
g. Walking	0	1	2

Table 1. Score rating system of the Japanese orthopaedic association (JOA score).

Case No.	Age	Sex	Follow-up Period	Operated Levels	Interbody Spacer	Autograft(g) [Local bone]	Artificial Bone(g)	Blood Loss(g)	Operation Time(min.)
1	70	F	40	L4-5	CC	5	6	460	331
2	44	F	39	L4-5	CC	7	5	300	235
3	65	F	38	L4-5	PEEK	6	5	360	272
4	55	F	38	L3-4	PEEK	7	5	460	195
5	71	M	35	L4-5	PEEK	8	4	420	250
6	76	M	34	L4-5	PEEK	6	5	515	210
7	44	F	30	L4-5	PEEK	5	5	330	165
8	62	M	30	L4-5	PEEK	6	5	250	235
9	53	F	28	L4-5	PEEK	6	5	270	255
10	57	M	24	L4-5	PEEK	8	4	280	220
11	53	F	20	L4-5	PEEK	4	6	550	190
12	47	F	18	L4-5	PEEK	8	5	190	222
13	69	M	18	L4-5	PEEK	6	5	600	202
Average	59.3		28.5			6.4	4.9	384.1	219.6
S.E.M.	10.2		7.6			1.3	0.5	134.7	31.7

CC: Branigan carbon cage, PEEK: polyetheretherketone interbody implant)
β-TCP: β-tricalcium phosphate

Table 2. Summary of patients treated by unilateral micro-PLIF.

Case No.	JOA score	JOA score	Rate of Improvement	%-Slip (Pre-ope)	%-Slip (Post-	Periods for Bone Union
1	9	23	70.0	30.0	23.3	12.0
2	15	25	71.4	24.0	9.5	6.0
3	18	25	63.6	29.6	8.7	6.0
4	17	25	66.7	17.4	13.0	6.0
5	13	22	56.3	20.0	16.0	12.0
6	15	23	57.1	21.7	19.2	9.0
7	9	22	65.0	10.0	8.0	6.0
8	10	22	63.2	15.4	11.5	9.0
9	19	27	80.0	16.7	8.7	5.0
10	21	26	62.5	13.0	4.3	5.0
11	15	23	57.1	20.8	16.7	9.0
12	13	27	87.5	15.8	10.8	6.0
13	10	26	84.2	20.8	9.5	9.0
Average	14.5	24.4	67.6	18.3	11.5	7.5
S.E.M.	4.0	2.0	11.1	5.2	4.4	2.3

Table 3. Clinical and radiological outcome before and after surgery.

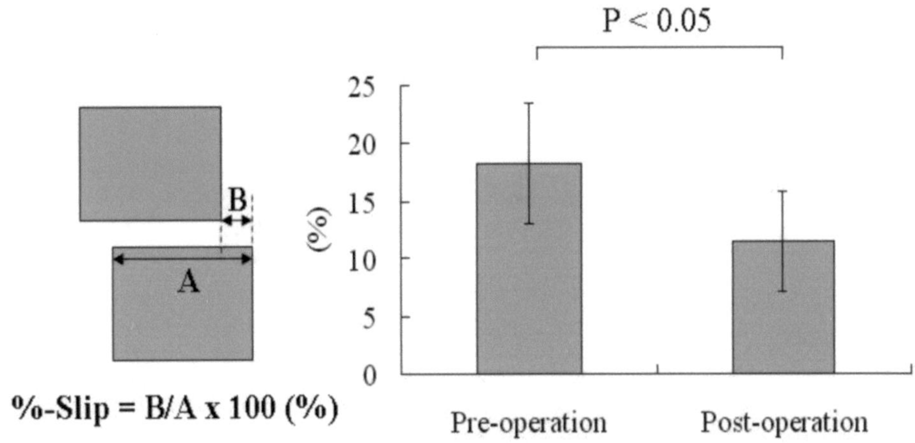

Fig. 7. Measurement of slip percent before and after surgery.

4. Case report

A 65-year-old woman (Case 3) presented with a long history of severe low back pain and left leg pain. This patient had numbness and hypesthesia of L5 root area on her left leg. Straight leg raising test is negative on both sides. Leg muscles are powerful. JOA score was 18 points. Preoperative plain films showed evidence of degenerative Grade II spondylolisthesis at L4–L5 (Fig.8A-C). She failed all attempts at nonoperative therapy, including nonsteroid anti-inflammatory drugs, epidural steroid injections and physical therapy. In the preoperative imaging study, extension and flexion plain film revealed a mobile spondylolisthesis at L4–L5. MR imaging showed the circumferential cauda equina and nerve root compression at L4-L5 disc level (Fig.9A,B).

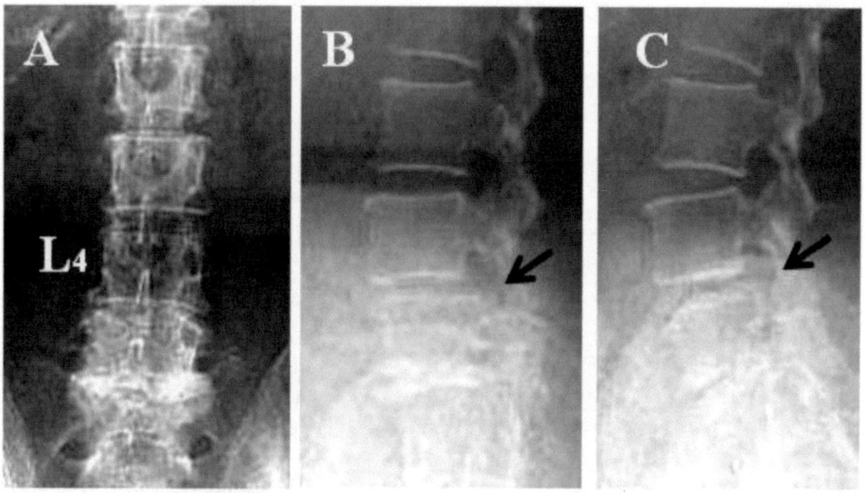

Fig. 8. Pre-operative anteroposterior (A) and lateral (B, flexion position, C, extension position) plain radiographs. Flexion and extension plain film revealed a mobile spondylolisthesis (arrows).

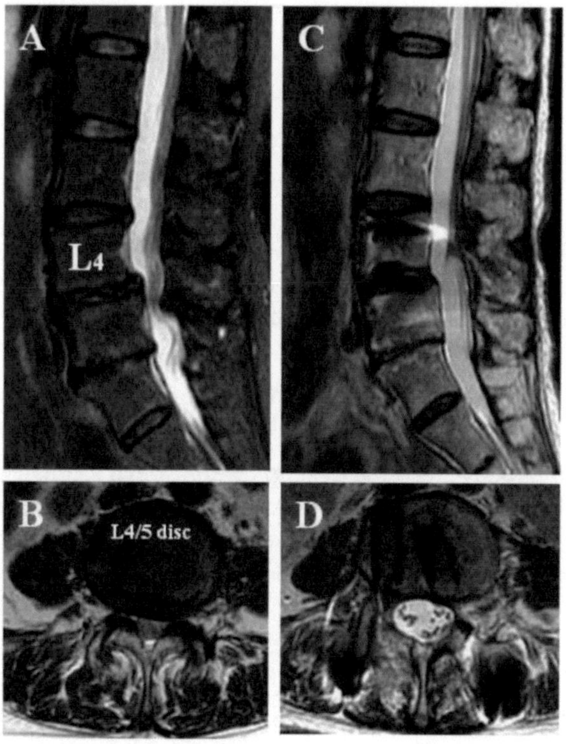

Fig. 9. Pre- (A,B) and Post- (C,D) operative T2 weighted MR imaging. A,C. Sagittal view, B,D. Axial view.

Preoperative MR imaging demonstrated mild central canal stenosis secondary to degenerative spondylolisthesis L4-L5 (A,B). Postoperative MR imaging did not show cauda equina compression 2 year after surgery (C,D). Restration of disc hight and lordosis also demonstrated .

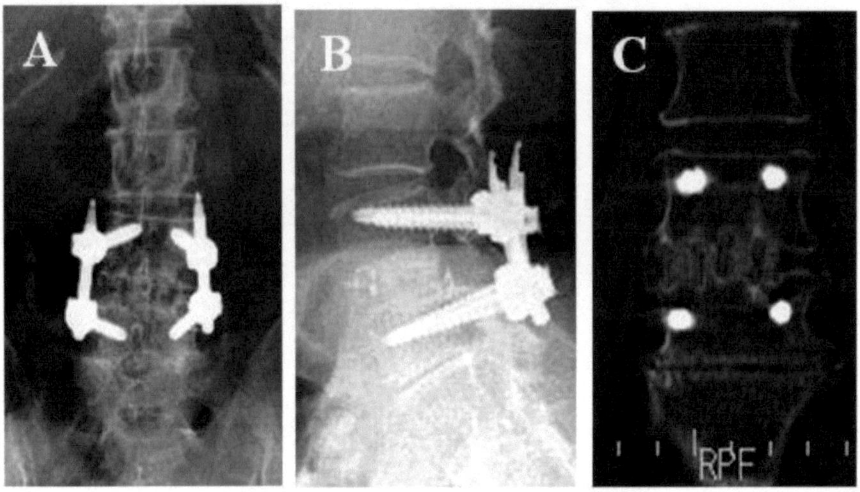

Fig. 10. Post-operative plain radiographs [anteroposterior view (A) ,lateral view(B)] and coronal reformatted CT (C).

This patient underwent a minimally invasive PLIF via a Casper retractor placed from a left-sided approach. The interbody fusion was supplemented with percutaneous pedicle screw and rods. The patient's surgery was uneventful. She was discharged on postoperative day 14 and returned to her previous job in 3 months after this operation. After 24 months of follow-up, she had no evidence of low back pain but slightly numbness requiring no medication persisted. The X-ray showed the bone union of PLIF without collapse at 2 years after operation. Frontal view (Fig.10A) and coronal CT scan (Fig.10C) showed bone union in PEEK interbody spacers. Lateral view showed solid fusion (Fig.10B). MR imaging did not show cauda equine compression (Fig9C,D).

5. Complications of minimally invasive arthrodesis procedure

The goal of lumbar interbody fusion is to stabilize the spinal segment and decompress the neural elements. PLIF can completely remove the pathological focus by the naked-eye or using an operating microscope. However, the PLIF requires significant retraction on the dural sac and nerve roots. As a result, it is associated with higher risks of cerebrospinal fluid leakage, dysesthetic nerve root pain syndrome, nerve root injury, and epidural fibrosis (Lin, 1985, Fritzell, et al., 2002, Scaduto, et al., 2003). These complications can be avoided by microscope visualization of the working space during surgery.

Transforaminal lumbar interbody fusion (TILF) is originally described by Blume and Rojas (1981) and Harms and Rolinger (1982). The TILF approach was popularized by Harms et al (1997). TILF was reported to be an effective surgical technique for the treatment of various degenerative lumbar diseases because it allows lateral access to the neural canal. This incision is two fingerbreadths off of the midline and allows for a paraspinal muscle splitting (Wiltse) approach to be performed (Wiltse & Spencer, 1988). The procedure involves less retraction of the dural sac and nerve roots resulting in low complication rate, and produces clinical outcomes and fusion rates similar to those of other techniques. However, the ideal indication for a TILF is a grade 1 or grade 2 spondylolisthesis without neurologic deficit or with a deficit on one side only (Moskowitz, 2002). This approach cannot completely remove the pathological focus with central canal stenosis. Although offering certain advantages, minimally invasive arthrodesis procedure has several limitations and potential complications. There is a learning curve associated with the development of technical skills necessary to perform these procedure.

6. Conclusions

Minimal invasive spinal surgery is an expanding technique and percutaneous pedicle screws are often used to minimize muscle injuries. However, there is no proof that spinal outcomes are better with minimally invasive spinal surgery than with conventional spinal surgery, which remains the gold standard against which new techniqus should be evaluated. The PLIF procedure has come into a fair amount of disfavor because of perceived and actual complications related to the procedure. These complication include bleeding, dural laceration, nerve root injuries, graft migration and pseudarthrosis. High fusion rates with good clinical outcomes can be achieved with few complications using microscope and minimal invasive technique. Our clinical experience using the microscope has showed excellent visualization, appropriate safety control, and low complication rate. Skilled surgeons familiar with the technique, anatomy, and instrumentation involved in minimally invasive approaches can achieve good-to-excellent clinical results..

7. References

Blume,H.G. & Rojas, C.H. (1981). Unilateral lumbar interbody fusion (posterior approach) utilizing dowel graft. *J Neurol Ortop Surg*, 2, 171-175.

Brantigan, J.W.& Steffee, A.D. (1993). A carbon fiber implant to aid interbody lumbar fusion two-year clinical results in the first 26 patients. *Spine*, 18, 2106-2117.

Bridwel, K.H.; Sedgewick, T.A.; O'Brien, M.F., et al. (1993). The role of fusion and instrumentation in the treatment of degenerative spondylolisthesis with spinal stenosis. *J Spinal Disord*, 6,461-472

Cloward, R.B. (1952). The treatment of ruptured lumbar intervertebral disc by vertebral body fusion. III. Methods and use of banked bone. *Ann Surg*, 136, 987–992

Cloward, R.B. (1953). The treatment of ruptured lumbar intervertebraldiscs by vertebral body fusion. I. Indications, operative technique,after care. *J Neurosurg*,10, 154-168.

Cloward, R.B. (1981). Spondylolisthesis, treatment by laminectomy and PLIF. Clin Orthop. 154, 74-82.

Cloward, R.B. (1985). The treatment of ruptured lumbar intervertebral disk by vertebral body fusion. *Clin Orthop*, 193, 5-154.

Faubert, C. & Caspar, W. (1991). Lumbar percxtaneous discectomy. Initial experience in 28 cases. Neuroradiology, 33, 407–410.

Fischgrund, J.S.; MacKay, M.; Herkowitz, H.N., et al. (1997). Degenerative lumbar spondylolisthesis with spinal stenosis: A prospective, randomized study comparing decompressive and arthrodesis with and without spinal instrumentation. *Spine*, 22, 2807-2812.

Foley KT, Gupta SK, Justis JR, et al. (2001). Percutaneous pedicle screw fixation of the lumbar spine. *Neurosurg Focus*, 10, E10

Fritzell, P.; Hagg, O.; Wessberg, P., et al. (2002). Chronic low back pain and fusion. A comparison of three surgical techniques: a prospective multicenter randomized study from the Swedish Lumbar Spine Group. *Spine*, 27, 1131-1141.

Harms, J. & Rolinger, H. (1982). A one-stage procedure in operative treatment of spondylolisthesis: dorsal traction-reposition and anterior fusion. *Z Orthop Ihre Grenzgeb*, 120, 343–347

Harms, J.; Jeszenszky, D.; Stolze, D., et al. (1997). True spondylolisthesis reduction and more segmental fusion in spondylolisyjesis. In: *The Textbook of Spinal Surgery*. 2nd Ed. Philadelphia: lipponcott-raven, 1337-1347.

Lin,P.M. (1985). Posterior lumbar interbody fusion technique: complications and pitfalls. *Clin Orthop*, 193, 90-102.

Magerl, F. (1982) External skeletal fixation of the lower thoracic and lumbar spine, in Uhthoff, H.K. & Stahl, E. (eds.): Current Concepts of External Fixation of Fractures. New York: Springer-Verlag, pp 353–366.

Meyerding, H.W. (1932). Spondylolisthesis: surgical treatment and results. *Surg Gynecol Obstet* 54:371–377.

Moskowitz, A. (2002). Transforaminal lumbar interbody fusion. Orthop Clin North Am, 33, 359–366.

Park, P. & Foley, K.T. (2008) Minimally invasive transforaminal interbody fusion with reduction of spondylolisthesis: technique and outcomes after a minimum of 2 years' follow-up. *Neurosurg Focus*, 25,E16.

Scaduto, A.A.; Gamradt, S.C.; Yu,W.D., et al. (2003). Perioperative complications of tgreaded cylindrical lumbar interbody fusion devices: anterior versus posterior approach. *J Spinal Disord Tech*, 16, 502-507.

Takeno, K., Kobayashi, S., Miyazaki, S., et al. (2010). Microsurgical excision of hematoma of the lumbar ligamentum flavum. *Joint Bone Spine*, 77, 351-354.

Taillard, W. (1954). Le spondylolisthesis chez l' enfant et l'adolescent (Etude de 50 cas). *Acta Orthop Scand*,24, 115-144.

Wiltse, L.L. & Spencer, C.W. (1988). New uses and refinements of the paraspinal approach to the lumbar spine. *Spine*, 13, 696–706.

Yamamoto, M.; Kadowaki, T.; Ota, N. et al. (1990). PLIF for lumbar degenerative spondylolisthesis. *Rinsho Seikeigeka*, 25, 487-494.

Young, S.; Veerapen, R.; O'Laoire, S.A.. (1988.): Relief of lumbar canal stenosis using multilevel subarticular fenestrations as an alternative to wide laminectomy: preliminary report.. *Neurosurgery*, 23, 628–633.

Yvon, H.A.; Garfin, S.R.; Dickman, C.A. et al. (1994). A historical comfort study of pedicle screw fixation in thoracic, lumbar and sacral spinal fusions. *Spine*, 19(Suppl), 2279S-2296S.

Zdeblick, T.A. (1993). A prospective, randomized study of lumbar fusion. Spine, 18, 983-991.

Part 2

Upper Extremity

3

The Distal Forearm Region – Ultrasonographic Anatomy in Children and Adolescents

Johannes M. Mayr[1,*], Wolfgang Grechenig[2], Ursula Seebacher[3], Andreas Fette[3], Andreas H. Weiglein[4] and Sergio Sesia[1]
[1]*Department of Pediatric Surgery, University Children's Hospital Basel, Basel,*
[2]*Medical University of Graz, Graz,*
Department of Traumatology
[3]*Medical University of Graz,*
Department of Pediatric Surgery
[4]*Department of Anatomy, Medical University of Graz, Graz*
[1]*Switzerland*
[2,3,4]*Austria*

1. Introduction

The distal forearm, particularly the distal radius, the radio-carpal joint and surrounding soft tissues are commonly affected by acute and chronic disorders. Ultrasonography has gained increasing importance in both the evaluation of acute injuries and chronic disorders in adults and in the diagnosis and follow-up of fractures in children and adolescents[1-4]. In children, the use of ultrasonography allows the chondral parts of the epiphyseal region to be better evaluated without exposure to radiation than using standard radiographic techniques.

The main advantage of sonography over CT and MRI is the possibility of performing dynamic examinations, resulting in exact clinical functional evaluation of the muscles, tendons and joints in question[3,5,6]. Furthermore, the contralateral limb can be examined in direct comparison when initial findings are uncertain.

It is the aim of this study, to demonstrate the normal ultrasonographic findings in the distal forearm region in children and adolescents, as this area is frequently involved in injuries.

2. Probands and methods

We studied 100 children and adolescents 2 months - 18 years old (mean ± standard deviation [SD] = 7.1 ± 4.5 years) and 25 healthy adults aged between 20 and 60 years. Children were recruited from our institution's paediatric surgical outpatient clinics. The patients had been admitted for unrelated disorders, requiring surgery, and the ultrasound study of the distal forearm was obtained together with the ultrasound study of the abdomen, urinary tract or soft tissue small parts. The area of the distal forearm was used first to demonstrate the painlessness

*Corresponding Author

of the ultrasound examination to the child and the parents. Thereafter the linear ultrasound scanning probe was adjusted at the beginning of the ultrasound study, and the sonography of the distal forearm together with the ultrasound examination of the abdomen, retroperitoneum or small part region of interest was carried out. Consent was obtained from the parents, or in the case of older children, from both the children and parents. Patients with a history of forearm trauma or pathology were excluded from this investigation. However, a limited number of these patients are shown to demonstrate different pathological ultrasound findings (like fractures and osteomyelitis) in a separate chapter.

A 12-5 MHz linear probe (Philips-ATL®, HDI 5000, Philips®, Bothell, WA, USA) and high frequency probes (7.5 - 12 MHz) (Siemens® Acuson® and Elegra®, Siemens®, Erlangen, FRG) were used for static and dynamic examination of the distal forearm region concentrating on the distal radius, the radiocarpal joint and surrounding soft tissues.

All 100 children and adolescents were examined in 3 longitudinal and 2 transverse standard planes and Doppler colour sonography was used to demonstrate vessels running within the cartilage of the distal radius supplying the epiphysis of the distal radius(Fig. 1). The wrist joint was examined in neutral position with the child sitting in front of a table either on a chair or on a parent's lap.

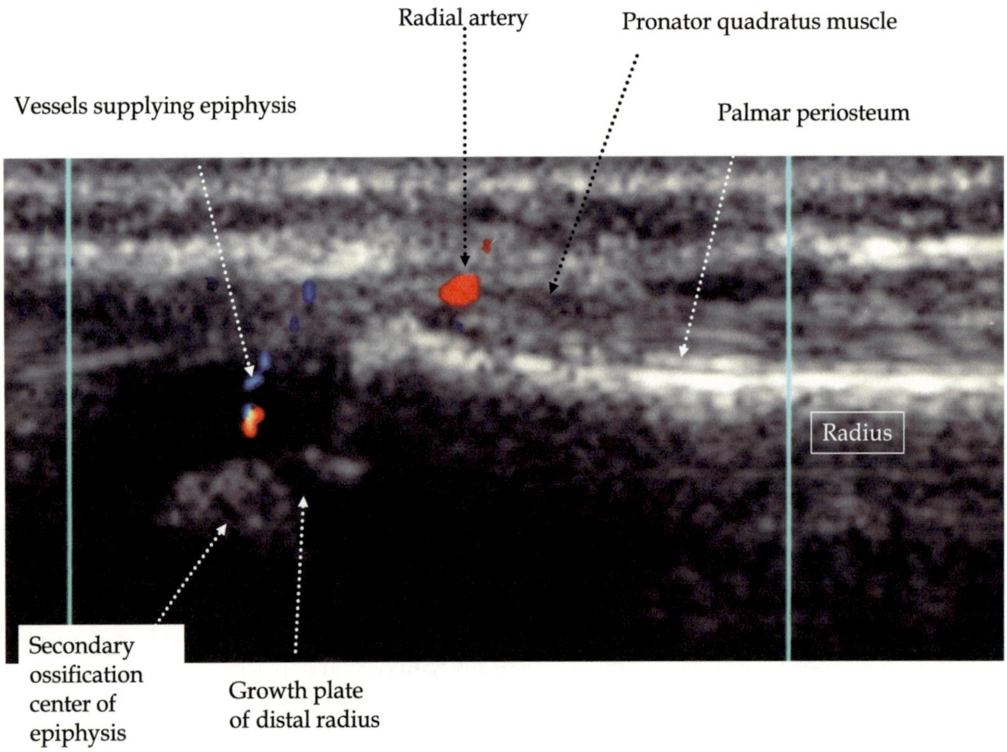

Fig. 1. Palmar-radial longitudinal colour coded duplex sonography scan in a boy aged 3 years showing the radial artery and an epiphyseal vessel. The ossification centre shows an echogenic reflex with dorsal acoustic shadow; the pronator quadratus muscle is visualised transversely beneath the radial artery.

The median nerve was visualized during static and dynamic ultrasound investigation. No standoff pad was used. Instead, a liberal amount of coupling gel was applied. For young children pre-warmed contact gel was used. The contra-lateral limb was also investigated to allow comparison.

For evaluation of age-related changes, the patients were divided into 4 groups (25 children per group). Group 1 included infant and toddler children from 2 months - 3 years old; group 2, young children 4 - 6 years old; group 3, pre-adolescent children 7 - 11 years old; and group 4, adolescent and teenage children 12 - 18 years old.

3. Technique of examination / standard planes

A dorsal, radial and volar longitudinal plane and corresponding transverse sections were investigated. The radius was defined as the leading structure for longitudinal scans. By moving the probe distally, the cavity of the radiocarpal joint was localised and positioned in the centre of the image. From this standard position, the probe was moved in both a radial and ulnar direction, maintaining an "orthograde" probe position to avoid hypo-echogenicity of tendons caused by a non-orthograde transducer position[7].

In the dorsal transverse plane, the scan began in the distal forearm region, identifying the radius and ulna as osseous leading structures.

The dorsal longitudinal scans were used to measure the width and investigate the echogenicity of the epiphyseal growth plate cartilage and to document the ossification of the secondary ossification centre of the distal epiphysis of the radius. From the dorsal radio-ulnar position, the probe was moved distally along the distal forearm, the wrist joint and the carpus.

The musculo-tendinous junction of the dorsal forearm muscles and the course of the extensor tendons was examined.

In order to evaluate the tendons, the probe was placed in an orthograde position and slow active and/or passive movement of the tendons and muscles was performed to demonstrate the function of the forearm muscles and their tendons.

The volar region of the distal forearm and wrist was examined using a similar technique.

To identify the median nerve the probe was placed in the transverse volar position and the focus was adjusted to a position just beneath the level of the skin. The median nerve was identified in its course running between the palmaris longus tendon and the flexor carpi radialis tendon.

The volar longitudinal scans were used to search for branches of the radial artery supplying the distal epiphysis of the radius.

4. Ultrasonographic findings in adult probands (n = 25)

In all planes, the osseous structures were shown as bright echogenic lines with dorsal acoustic shadows, due to the difference in impedance of bone when compared to the surrounding soft tissue. The radiocarpal joint was identified as an echo-free gap between the radius and the carpal bones. The proportion of articular cartilage of the carpal bones that could be visualized was dependent on the functional position of the hand. This should be considered when anechoic formations or structures (e.g. ganglia; intraarticular effusions) are evaluated.

Dynamic examination in a dorsal radio-ulnar plane allows the course of the extensor tendons to be accurately evaluated. Special attention has to be paid to the course of the extensor pollicis longus tendon in the region of Lister's tubercle, as the tendon crosses the underlying tendons of the extensor carpi radialis longus and brevis muscles. In the region of the musculo-tendinous junctions of the forearm extensor muscles, the tendons are occasionally surrounded by a thin hypoechoic muscular layer. Ultrasonographically, this small hypoechoic area must not be confused with extensor tenosynovitis[3].

The radial neurovascular bundle on the volar aspect of the distal forearm was identified by its pulsation by grey-scale ultrasound and confirmed by its flow characteristics by colour Doppler sonography in all probands. The course of the radial artery and its distribution can be depicted by distal movement of the probe. Due to the width of the soft tissue coverage on the volar aspect, identification of a single tendon is easier when compared to the dorsal distal forearm region. By functional evaluation, the superficial and deep flexor tendons were depicted in the longitudinal plane. Both the carpal joint and the median nerve were clearly identified. The flexor retinaculum is difficult to separate from the surrounding tissue[8]. The flexor retinaculum was identified in 13 of 25 patients (52%), suspected in 3 patients (12%) and not seen in 9 patients (36%). The main problem encountered with the identification of the flexor retinaculum was its hypoechogenicity, which was similar to the echogenicity of the overlying subcutaneous fat. The median nerve is characterised by its lower echogenicity when compared to its neighbouring tendons and its course between the superficial and deep flexor tendons is easily followed in a proximal direction[3,4,6]. Whilst the proband is moving his or her fingers, a characteristic transposition and change in the transverse shape of the median nerve can be noted. The median nerve is easily detected as it runs between the tendons of the flexor sublimis and flexor carpi radialis, and rather towards the radial side of the tendon of the palmaris longus. The palmaris longus tendon shows no longitudinal displacement during finger movements. The interosseous membrane and the pronator quadratus muscle on the volar aspect were identified easily in the transverse plane in all patients.

5. Ultrasonographic findings in children

Depending on the age of children various sonographic findings of the distal forearm region were observed.

In group 1 children (2 months - 3 years old), no ossification of the distal radial ossification centre was seen in 5 infants (aged up to 6 months). The echogenicity of the cartilage at the region of the distal radial growth plate was either anechoic with weak reticular echogenic pattern (5 children, aged from 0 - 3 months) or anechoic with weak echogenic spots (10 children). In 8 of 25 children (32 %) colour Doppler identified at least one small vessel within the cartilage of the volar distal radial epiphysis (Fig.1). Due to investigator problems (like coupling problems, more frequent forearm movements of infants, and very small structures) the median nerve was documented by ultrasound in only 18 of 25 children (72 %). Other sonographic characteristics of the distal forearm region are presented in Table 1.

	Group 1 (2 months - 3 years)	Group 2 (4 - 6 years)	Group 3 (7 - 11 years)	Group 4 (12 - 18 years)
Proximodistal diameter of the distal radial growth plate; mm[1]	4.16 ± 1.16 (2.8 - 6.0) (n = 20 / 25)	2.65 ± 0.49 (1.8 - 3.8)	2.19 ± 0.47 (1.4 - 3.5)	1.39 ± 0.86 (0.1 - 3.0) (growth plate fused in 5 children)
Absent ossification of the secondary ossification centre of the distal radius	5/25 (20 %)	0/25	0/25	0/25
Sonographic characteristics of the distal radius growth plate and epiphyseal cartilage				
- Anechoic	10/25 (40 %)	2/25 (8 %)	1/25 (4 %)	4/25 (16 %)
- Mixed type (echogenic spots / bands / reticular pattern) within anechoic cartilage	15/25 (60 %)	23/25 (92 %)	24/25 (96 %)	16/25 (64 %)
- Epiphyseal growth plate fused	0/25	0/25	0/25	5/25 (20 %)
Presence of vessels within the epiphyseal cartilage	8/25 (32 %)	0/25	1/25(4%)	0/25
Visualisation of the median nerve	18/25 (72 %)	25/25 (100 %)	25/25 (100 %)	25/25 (100 %)
Identification of the radial neurovascular bundle (grey scale and Doppler sonography)	25/25 (100 %)	25/25 (100 %)	25/25 (100 %)	25/25 (100 %)

* data are for n = 100 children (25 per group)

[1] mean ± standard deviation; range are shown in parenthesis.

Table 1. Sonographic characteristics of the distal forearm region in children and adolescents according to age groups*.

The majority of children in group 2 (4 - 6 years old) showed weak punctuated echoes (76 %) or weak echogenic bands (16 %) within an anechoic growth plate cartilage(Fig.2). The median nerve was seen in all children on grey scale sonography. On colour Doppler sonography, no vascularisation was noted in the cartilage of the distal radial epiphysis or growth plate.

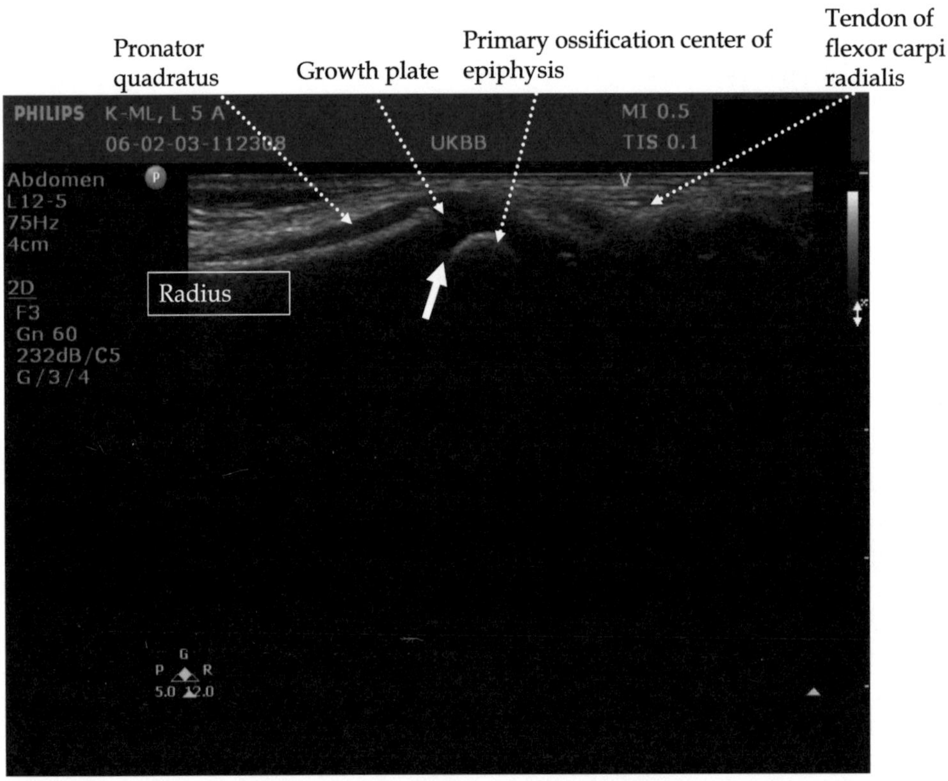

Palmar longitudinal transducer position along the distal radius

Fig. 2. Boy, 5 years of age; palmar longitudinal transducer position. Linear 12-5 MHz probe is placed along the distal radius. Anechoic cartilage of the growth plate and epiphysis of the radius shows small hypoechoic band-like spot within the growth plate cartilage (solid arrow).

In group 3 children the proximal-distal diameter of the distal radial growth plate was smaller when compared to group 2 (mean values 2,19 mm; 2,65 mm respectively). The appearance of the distal radial growth plate cartilage and epiphyseal cartilage in group 3 children (7 - 11 years old) resembled the appearance in group 2 children (4 - 6 years old)(Fig. 3-8). No problems were encountered during visualisation of the median nerve in group 3 children. On colour Doppler sonography, no vascularization was found in the cartilage of the growth plate. However, in one of these children a vessel was visualized entering the cartilage of the epiphysis from the palmar aspect of the epiphysis of the distal radius(Fig. 4).

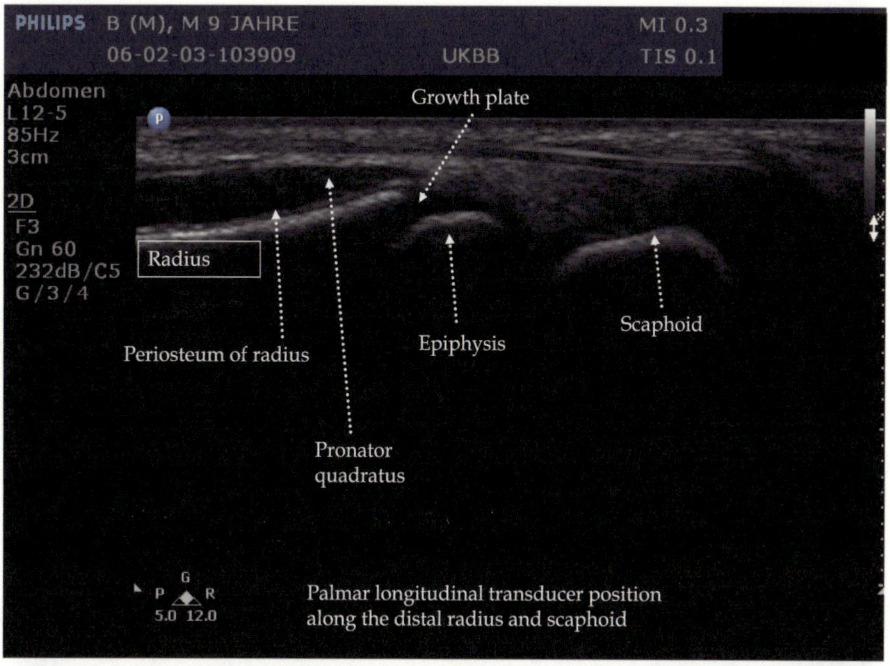

Fig. 3. Boy, 9 years of age; palmar longitudinal transducer position. The linear 12-5 MHz probe is placed along the distal radius.

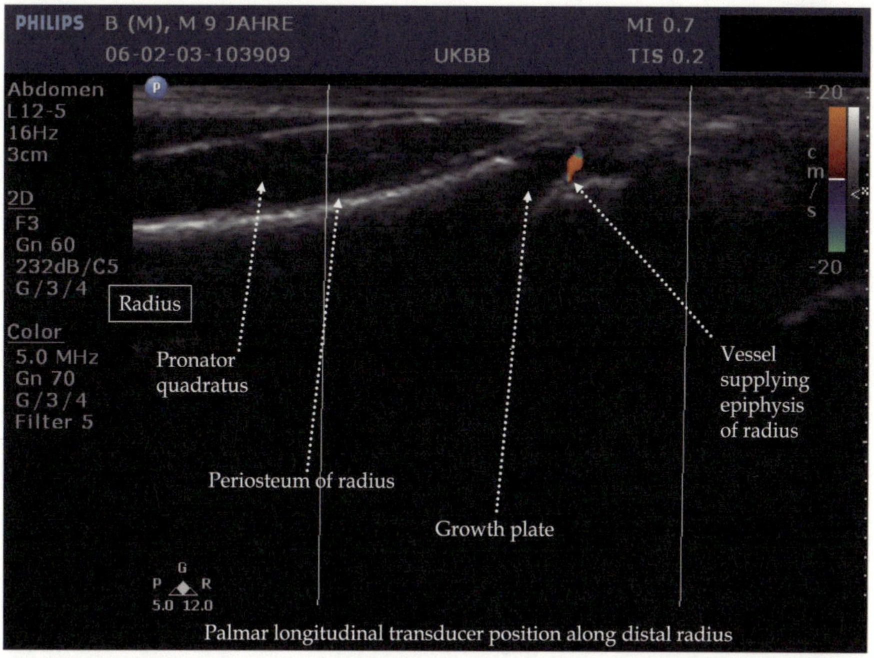

Fig. 4. Boy, 9 years of age; palmar longitudinal transducer position. Linear 12-5 MHz probe is placed along the distal end of the radius. Colour coded duplex ultrasound study shows vessel supplying the secondary ossification centre of the epiphysis.

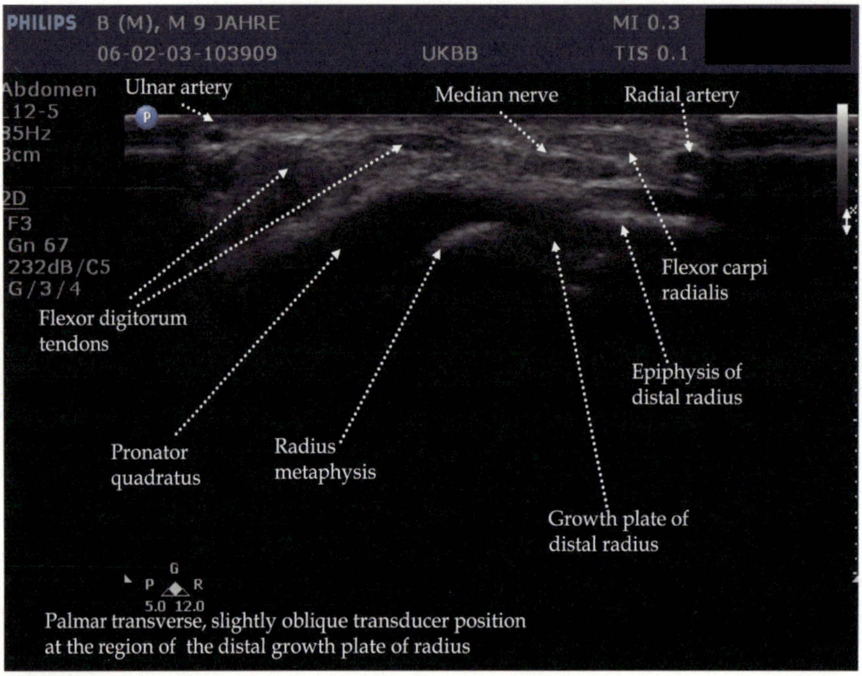

Fig. 5. Boy, 9 years of age; palmar transverse, slightly oblique transducer position. Linear 12-5 MHz probe is placed across the region of the growth plate of the distal radius. The cartilage of the growth plate of the radius appears anechoic.

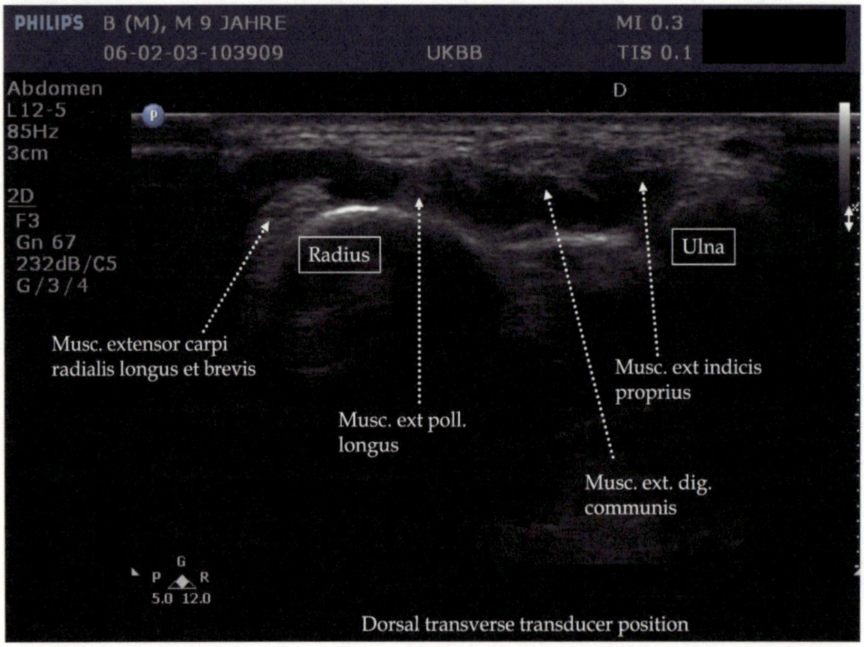

Fig. 6. Boy, 9 years of age; dorsal transverse transducer position. Linear 12-5 MHz probe is placed across the metaphyseal area of the distal forearm. The extensor tendons are shown.

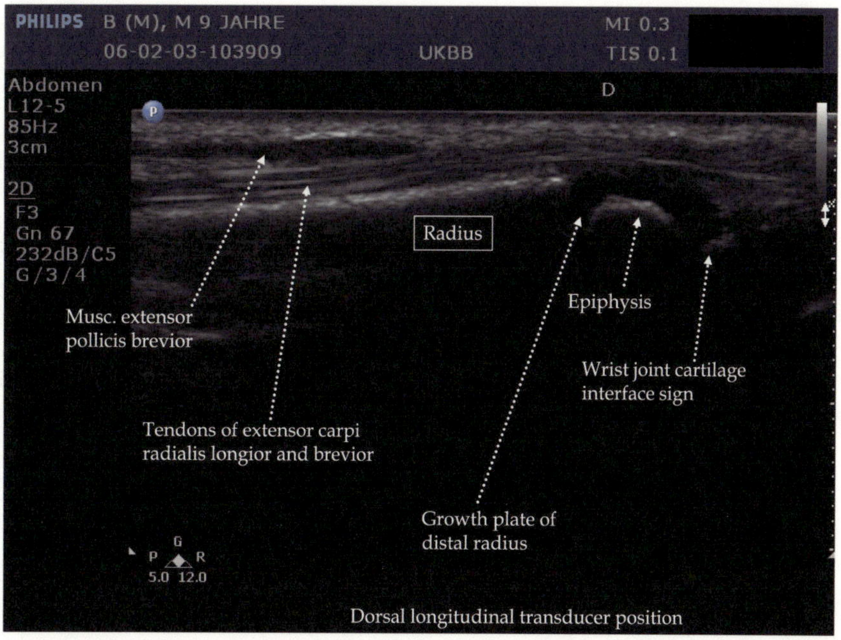

Fig. 7. Boy, 9 years of age; dorsal longitudinal transducer position. Linear 12-5 MHz probe is placed along the distal radius. The epiphyseal and growth plate cartilage of the distal epiphysis of the radius appears anechoic. Extensor tendons are overlying the dorsal contour of the distal radius.

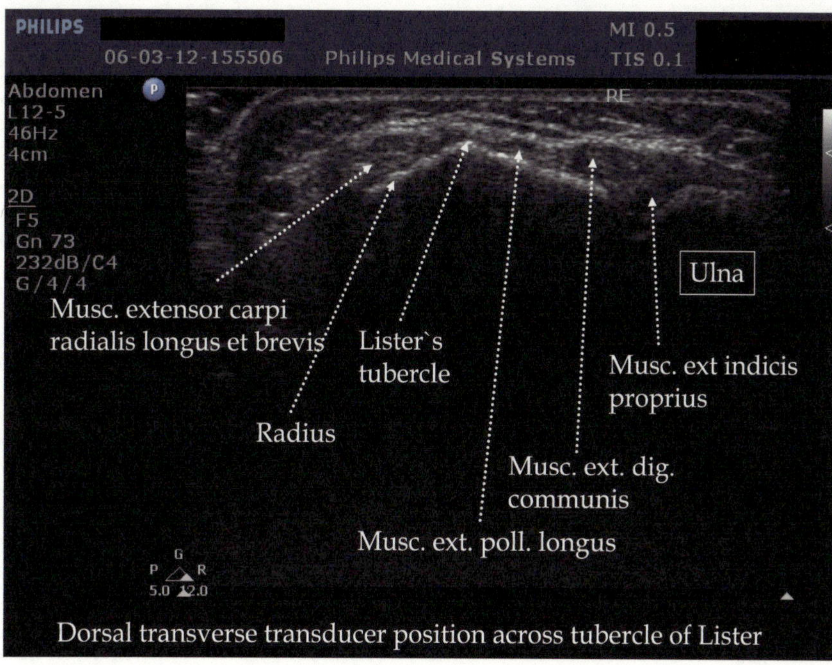

Fig. 8. Boy, 10 years of age; dorsal transverse transducer position. Linear 12-5 MHz probe is placed across Lister`s tubercle. The extensor tendons are shown.

In 5 children of group 4 (12 - 18 years old) the distal radial epiphyseal growth plate was fused (20 %). In the remaining children, the epiphyseal growth plate cartilage was either anechoic (16 %)(Fig. 9) or anechoic with weak echogenic spots within the cartilage (64 %). The median nerve was identified by ultrasound in all children of group 4(Fig. 10). No vessels were noted penetrating the epiphyseal or growth plate cartilage at colour Doppler sonography.

During the growth period, characteristic morphologic changes occur within the distal part of the radius which can be sonographically observed. The secondary ossification centre within the distal radial epiphysis appears on plain x-ray images as late as three to eighteen months post partum. However, morphologic changes during ossification are clearly visible: firstly, towards the end of the first trimester, the epiphyseal centre shows an increasing echogenicity. Subsequently, a small epiphyseal area with high echogenity and dorsal ultrasound extinction develops.

Using colour coded duplex sonography, vessels supplying the epiphyseal cartilage during the first and second year of life can be visualised frequently(Fig.1). Ultrasonographically, the periosteum is visible as a hyperechoic thin band-like structure, separated from the cortical reflex by a thin hypoechoic line.

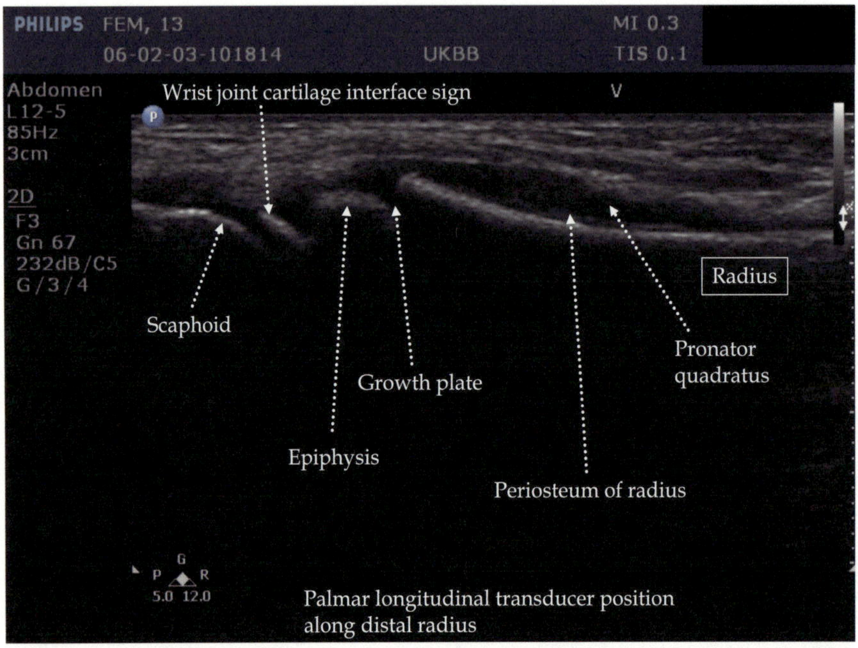

Fig. 9. Girl, 13 years of age; palmar longitudinal transducer position. Linear 12-5 MHz probe is placed along the distal radius. The cartilage interface sign is visible between the distal radius and the scaphoid articular cartilage.

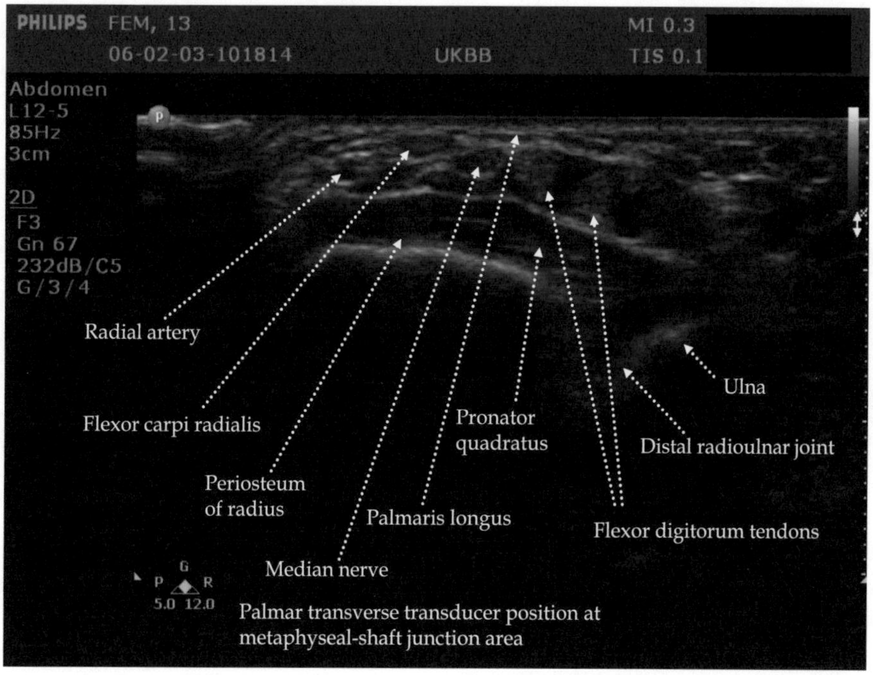

Fig. 10. Girl, 13 years of age; palmar transverse transducer position. Linear 12-5 MHz probe is placed across the distal metaphyseal-shaft junction of the forearm. Note the transverse muscle fibers of the pronator quadratus muscle. The median nerve and the flexor tendons are visualized.

The distal growth plate of the radius can not be differentiated from the cartilage of the epiphysis ultrasonographically, unless the secondary ossification centre is already discernable within the distal radial epiphysis (Fig. 1). The sonomorphologic characteristics of the distal radial growth plate are shown in Table 1. Its width gradually decreases during further development (Tab.1). With increasing age of the child, the chondro-osseous junction bends towards the epiphysis or appears slightly interdentated. Approaching the age of fusion of the distal radial epiphysis, it is represented by a narrow gap in the cortical bone and repetitive echoes can be seen posterior to the surface of the growth plate (Fig. 11).

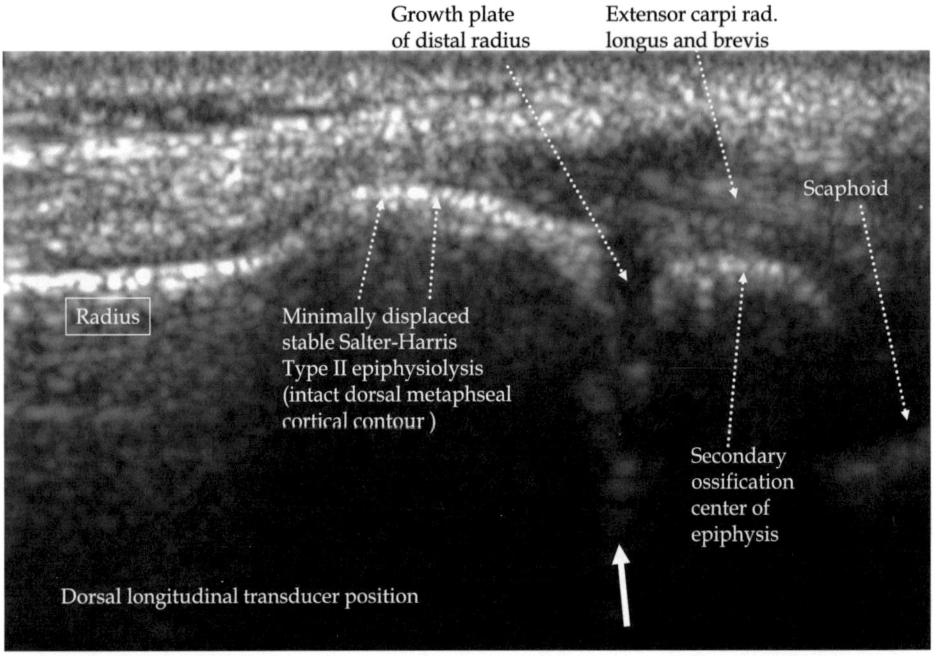

Fig. 11. Girl, 13 years of age; undisplaced Salter-Harris type II epiphysiolysis; This fracture is considered stable because there is no break in the dorsal metaphyseal corticalis of the radius. Longitudinal dorsal transducer position. Repetitive echoes are visible within the central part of the growth plate(marked by solid arrow).

Depending mainly on the gender of the individual, fusion of the distal radial epiphysis occurs between 15 and 18 years of age. During fusion of the distal radial physis towards the end of skeletal growth the gap like anechoic remnant of the physis was found to be wider on the dorsal side when compared to the palmar side of the radius.

General findings: At dynamic investigation using limited, slow movements of the wrist joint a characteristic change in shape and position of the median nerve was noted, whereas the palmaris longus tendon and flexor carpi radialis tendon showed longitudinal movements and nearly no change in shape. In contrast to the fine reticular fibrillary pattern of the flexor tendons the median nerve showed a coarse-grained fibrillary pattern.

After the occurrence of the hyperechoic secondary ossification centre of the distal radius the width of the dorsal epiphyseal cartilage was 1 - 2 mm wider when compared to the width of the volar epiphyseal cartilage (measurements taken between the dorsal contour of the secondary ossification centre and dorsal boarder of the epiphyseal cartilage); and the volar contour of the secondary ossification centre and volar contour of the epiphyseal cartilage (respectively).

6. Ultrasound applications in the region of the distal forearm

In the hands of an experienced clinician using high frequency linear probes (more than 7 MHz), and adequate equipment, ultrasonography is a suitable technique for the investigation of cortical structures and surrounding soft tissues[3-6]. Furthermore, there is the substantial advantage of dynamic examination, direct comparison to the contralateral limb and the lack of exposure to radiation[5-7]. As in most joints, the use of linear probes is also preferable in the distal radius region[7]. As the soft tissue coverage is relatively thin, high resolution and low penetration is preferable for this examination. Depending on the resolution capacity, the use of an echo-free standoff pad to increase the distance to the tissue can be helpful[7].

In the longitudinal plane, tendons are depicted as longitudinal structures of high echogenicity with parallel echos[3,5-7]. In the horizontal plane, a punctuated reticular, hyperechoic tendon fibre structure is seen[3,5-7]. The examiner must take into account that the probe is aligned parallel to the tendon and the sonographic impulse is directed orthograde to the tendon[7]. When high frequency probes are used, deviations of 15° from the orthograde transducer position can change the echogenicity of tendons and nerves. Because of these physical phenomena, smooth circular surfaces of small dimension create a reflex only in that area, where the sound impulse arrives perpendicularly. Furthermore, if there is no "orthograde" alignment, the whole tendon diameter shows lower echogenicity[7]. Thus, not all tendons are clearly depicted in a transverse plane and areas of low echogenicity are found. These artefacts have to be kept in mind especially in the evaluation of pathologic changes of the peritendinous tissue and fluid accumulation within the tendon sheaths and the carpal canal, respectively[7]. However, even tendon aplasia in children can be accurately diagnosed using this ultrasonographic technique[9].

Furthermore, it is very important to use an "orthograde" position of the probe towards the evaluated structure (bone, tendon) (Fig. 5,7). In most cases, it is impossible to find this position both for tendons and bones within one singular plane.

Ultrasonography can be considered as the gold standard for evaluation of tendinous disorders[3,5-7], localization and differentiation of fluid accumulations (possibility of sonographically guided punction)[3], diagnosis of intraarticular effusions[10], diagnosis of soft tissue tumors (ganglia, cysts, neuromas)[3,4,11] and foreign bodies[5,12,13].

It is especially important in children to consider the radiation exposure during radiographic diagnosis and follow-up of fractures. At ultrasonography the metaphyseal cortex is easily identified as a marked hyperechoic line with a dorsal acoustic shadow. Subsequently, fractures can be clearly evaluated, as well(Fig.11). So, ultrasonography is a reliable tool for the follow-up of distal fractures of the radius in children. In addition to the evaluation of the fracture gap, the course of fracture consolidation supplemented by stability tests and dynamic examination can also be evaluated and estimated[14]. So the follow-up of fractures could be a special field of interest for ultrasonography in the children in the future. However, primary radiologic diagnosis will not be replaced by sonography, especially in fractures of the distal forearm region. It must be kept in mind, that obtaining an ultrasound study is more time consuming compared to obtaining X-rays. Ultrasonography is especially suitable for the follow-up of fractures in children and adolescents, when there is no closed plaster cast applied. The examiner has to pay special attention to the investigation of the periosteum, as the width of the hypoechoic line between the periosteum and bone surface is of outstanding clinical relevance in the diagnosis of subperiosteal fluid accumulation, for example in acute osteomyelitis(Fig. 12). Therefore, it should only be evaluated in comparison to the contralateral limb. Due to the stable affixation of periosteum / perichondrium at the region of the growth plate, compared to the diaphyseal and metaphyseal region, subperiosteal fluid accumulations are only found in the metaphyseal and diaphyseal region (Fig. 12).

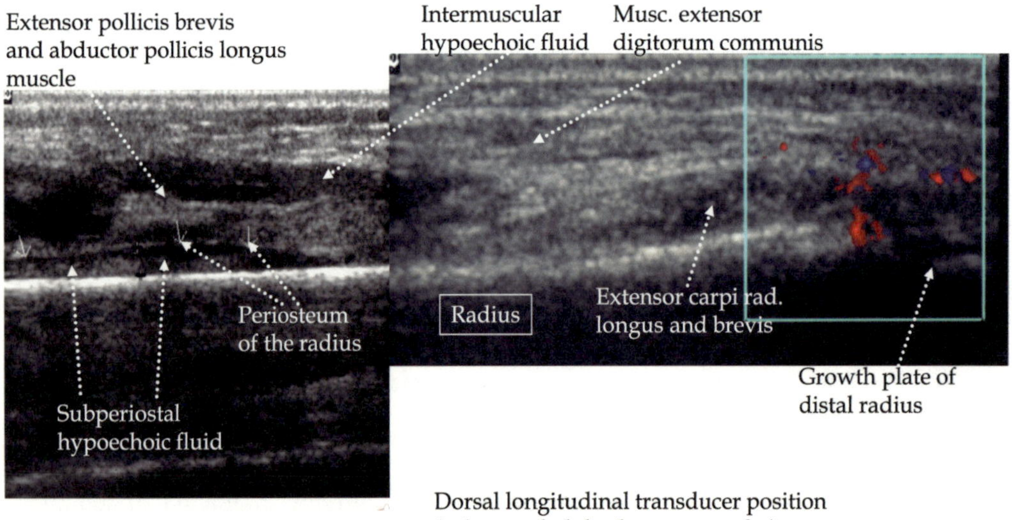

Fig. 12. Longitudinal distal dorsal-radial ultrasound scan in a boy aged 9 years suffering from acute osteomyelitis of the distal radius. The periosteum is detached from the corticalis of the distal radius, there is subperiosteal hypoechoic fluid accumulation with some low level echos. At operation acute purulent osteomyelitis of the distal radius complicated by subperiostal abscess formation and phlegmonous infiltration of the intermuscular spaces between the forearm extensor muscles was confirmed.

However, difficulties might arise during investigation of intra- and extraarticular pathologic changes of low echogenicity. For example, the differentiation of purely chondral articulating surfaces is facilitated only by the depiction of the "cartilage interface sign", a smooth, hypoechoic borderline reflex at the region of the articular gap(Fig.9).

7. Conclusion

High frequency ultrasonography can yield reliable information about the distal radial epiphysis and growth plate, the median nerve and the forearm tendons. The sonographic features of the normal distal forearm during growth described herein may hopefully contribute to a more widespread use of ultrasound in this anatomic region.

8. Acknowledgement

The authors want to thank Mrs. Helen Parker, Nottingham, GB for assistance in the translation of the manuscript.

No financial support for this investigation was given to any of the authors or their institutions.

9. References

[1] Cohen E, Blankstein A, Rosenstock M, Atou D. Greenstick fractures of distal radius followed-up by ultrasound - a prospective study. Akt Traumatol 2000; 30:227-229

[2] Hübner U, Schlicht W, Outzen S, Barthel M, Halsband H. Ultrasound in the diagnosis of fractures in children. JBJS 2000; 82B:1170 -3

[3] Ferrara Ma, Marcelis S. Ultrasound of the wrist. J Belge Radiol 1997;80:78-80

[4] Fornage BD. Peripheral nerves of the extremities: imaging with US. Radiology 1988;167:179-18

[5] Fornage BD, Schernberg FL, Rifkin MD. Ultrasound of the hand. Radiology 1985;155:785-8

[6] Fornage BD, Rifkin MD. Ultrasound examination of the hand and foot. Radiol Clin North Am 1988;26:109-29

[7] Fornage BD: The hypoechoic normal tendon – a pitfall. J Ultrasound Med 1987;6:19-22

[8] Nakamichi K, Tachibana S. Transverse sliding of the median nerve beneath the flexor retinaculum. J Hand Surg 1992; 17B: 213-216

[9] Grechenig W, Mayr J, Clement H, Peicha G. Aplasia of the flexor tendon of the fifth finger in a new born child – sonographic diagnosis. Eur Surg 2002; Suppl. 184 : 114-115.

[10] Fornage BD. Soft-tissue changes in the hand in rheumatoid arthritis: evaluation with US. Radiology 1989; 173: 735-737

[11] Cardinal E, Buckwalter KA, Braunstein EM, Mik AD. Occult dorsal carpal ganglion: comparison of ultrasound and MR imaging. Radiology 1994;193: 259-262

[12] Jacobson JA, Powell A, Craig J, Bouffard J, Van Holsbeeck M. Wooden foreign bodies in soft-tissue: detection at US. Radiology 1998; 206: 45-48

[13] Fornage BD, Schernberg FL. Sonographic preoperative localization of a foreign body in the hand. J Ultrasound Med 1987;6:217-9

[14] Dias JJ, Hui ACW, Lamont AC. Real time ultrasonography in the assessment of movement at the site of a scaphoid fracture non-union. J Hand Surg 1994;19B: 498-504

4

Limited Hand Surgery in Epidermolysis Bullosa

Bartlomiej Noszczyk and Joanna Jutkiewicz-Sypniewska
Medical Center for Postgraduate Education
Poland

1. Introduction

Epidermolysis bullosa (EB) is the name given to a group of rare congenital diseases with similar clinical symptoms. Their common feature is the susceptibility of the epithelia and skin to injury. Even minor shear forces from the sideways stretching of the skin contribute to epidermal tearing with blister formation. These blisters turn into wounds. In the most severe forms of the disease, wounds dominate on the skin and mucosa, leading to early death or deformations from scars and contractures.

1.1 Types of EB

Four main types of EB are distinguished based on the level of the ultrastructural defect in the area of the basement membrane zone (BMZ) (Fine, 2010). In epidermolysis bullosa simplex (EBS), the epithelium separates at the level of the basal cells, most commonly as a result of damage to keratin 5 and 14. In junctional epidermolysis bullosa (JEB), the level of the epithelial separation is in the lamina lucida and results from laminin -332, collagen XVII or integrin $\alpha6\beta4$ defects. In dystrophic epidermolysis bullosa (DEB), the epithelium is damaged below the lamina densa as a result of an incorrectly structured collagen VII building the anchoring fibrils. In Kindler syndrome, protein damage may affect several layers simultaneously. Apart from the epidermis, any basement membrane epithelia may become damaged. Most typically affected are the oral cavity and the esophageal and upper respiratory tract mucosa. The disease may also affect the tissues not covered with epithelium, such as tooth enamel, which is damaged in all the JEB forms.

The extent of symptoms involving the skin is varied and not completely characteristic. In the localized EBS form (EBS - loc) they manifest mainly as blisters on the hands and feet. In both generalized forms of EBS the blisters are located throughout the whole body. The risk of pseudosyndactyly in Dowling - Meara (EBS-DM) is estimated at 3% at or after the age of 3 (Fine et al., 2005). In the, non-Dowling-Meara (EBS-nDM), the blisters, although generalized, tend to spare the hands and feet (Fine, 2010).

Among the several different subtypes of junctional epidermolysis bullosa (JEB), two are generalized. The highest risk of death accompanies the Herlitz (JEB-H) form. In these patients, death stems from severe infectious complications or multi-organ failure. The predominating symptoms in this type are non-healing wounds covered with granulation tissue. It appears in the first months of life and can involve the upper respiratory tract. In the more common non-Herlitz (JEB-nH) form, the blisters are generalized and occur on the hands as well, often accompanied by atrophic scars and atrophic nails. The risk of pseudosyndactyly increases with advanced age.

The dystrophic type of epidermolysis bullosa (DEB) is divided into two main subtypes, depending on the mode of inheritance. In both, the generalized blisters lead to the formation of wounds, which typically heal and scar. The autosomal dominant form (generalized dominant dystrophic - DDEB) is characterized by symptoms of a slightly lower intensity. The risk of pseudosyndactyly is just 3% by the age of 40 (Fine et al., 2005). The forms with autosomal recessive inheritance have a more severe course. The most severe one, described as generalized recessive dystrophic epidermolysis bullosa (RDEB), occurs in 2 out of one million births (Pfendner et al., 2001). The disease activity in RDEB is extremely high in nearly every anatomic site (Devries et al., 2004).

1.2 Hand deformations in RDEB

The characteristic features of generalized RDEB are intensifying contractures and pseudosyndactyly affecting the hands and feet. Their risk by the age of 20 is estimated at 98% (Fine et al., 2005). In time, they lead the hands to contract into a cocoon. If such a severe disability appears in early childhood, it may hinder or preclude normal development. The mechanism of pseudosyndactyly, finger contractures and the development of the characteristic mitten deformities is not completely clear. The gradual web creep in children not undergoing surgery is probably facilitated by fine blisters and recurrent epidermal injuries. In the early postoperative period in operated patients, this complication typically stems from the adhesion of contacting wound surfaces. However, in all patients, this process also develops on the hands and feet under the influence of unknown causes. Observations suggest that the epithelium has a natural tendency towards migration "with shortcuts". It gradually retreats from the indented web spaces, leaving non-separated surfaces of the dermis. As a result, this retreat leads the dermal layers to stick under the surface of the forming cocoon. The contacting layers usually do not fully adhere. Hence, the pseudosyndactyly results. Initially, despite the adhesions, the fingers remain extended. During this period, the epithelium forming the cocoon continues to overgrow, forming a thick stratum corneum. Its structure at this time resembles paper, and it quickly becomes too rigid to allow movement. This rigidity leads to habitual finger bending and further cocoon overgrowth, which soon involves the entire hand.

1.3 Other complications of RDEB

Effective intervention for RDEB patients requires multidisciplinary treatment. Apart from dermatological care, the majority of patients require pediatric care due to multifactorial anemia and malnutrition. In some patients, kidney failure and cardiomyopathy develop, both of which may increase the risk of death. Among the other symptoms of note are corneal injuries requiring ophthalmologic treatment and esophageal stenosis, which can develop in early childhood. Sometimes, these are accompanied by microstomy and ankyloglossia. Difficulties with swallowing quickly contribute to malnutrition and growth retardation. The treatment requires esophageal dilation or gastrostomy. Some RDEB patients are diagnosed with squamous cell carcinoma by the age of 20. This cancer is a common cause of death in adults. The risk of this neoplasm is estimated at 7.5% by the age of 20 and 67.8% after the age of 35 (Fine & Mellerio, 2009a).

1.4 Repeated hand surgery – The problem in RDEB

Despite many attempts to use modern technology or to change surgical techniques, the recurrence of deformation is unavoidable and commonplace. Because every epidermal cell in the body has the same genetic defect, local therapy may result in only temporary improvement. Hand procedures may become necessary in 61% of RDEB patients. In this group, 5 or more operations are presumed to be the norm (Fine et al., 2005). It is estimated that recurrences appear, on average, every 2.4 years (1 to 5 years) (Terrill et al., 1992). In the experience of many surgeons, this time interval is even shorter. Furthermore, the time required for full wound healing after surgery for advanced deformations may reach 6 to 8 weeks (Fivenson et al., 2003). It is frequently observed, therefore, that patients spend a considerable period of potentially good hand efficiency in the hospital receiving dressing replacements. Most of these procedures require general anesthesia.

In order to support patients' independence and psychomotoric development, operations could be recommended early, when deformations may no longer be prevented by physiotherapy and splinting. In practice, however, patients typically present to the hospital when they or their parents are aware that surgery may no longer be postponed. If the deformations are advanced, the extent of the needed surgery influences the postoperative course. Patients then become discouraged by repeated hospitalizations and less likely to cooperate in the future.

1.5 Common methods in RDEB surgery

Removal of the thick epidermis that creates the cocoon is ineffective. In the beginning of the operation however, the hand may be "de-cocooned" using epidermal degloving technique. It outlines the area where direct force may be applied and saves intact epidermis beyond surgical manipulation (Ladd et al., 1996). This maneuver helps to apply manual traction to the tips of the affected fingers, which may be extended after a sharp release on the palmar side of the contracted joints. Other authors prefer to dispense with degloving, emphasizing however the need to apply some force in order to extend the contracted digits (Ciccarelli et al., 1995). Although such forceful manipulation destroys epidermis, the same principle applies to the first web space, where pseudosyndactyly often involves the adductor fascia and the first dorsal interosseous muscles (Ladd et al. 1996). The abduction and extension of the fingers is then maintained by Kirshner wires. Others have suggested the continuous use of acrylic gloves for three months following surgery (Terrill et al., 1992). Today modern splints from thermplastic materials are recommended, that may be easily remodeled or discarded after they become polluted.

The most thorough review and practical evaluation of surgical methods in RDEB was presented recently (Bernardis & Box, 2010). Currently, most authors prefer to avoid using force during joint extension to prevent neurovascular bundle injury and subluxation. It has also been suggested that the full release of contractures may be not useful or necessary. This procedure creates extensive defects, leaving a bare dermal surface and uncovered neurovascular bundles, which require grafting. Full thickness skin grafts (FTSGs) are often used in deeper defects. The amount of full-thickness dermis suitable for harvesting is limited, however. Therefore, other solutions have been proposed for the remaining surface of superficial defects. Various opinions exist over the use of split skin grafts (SSGs). The harvesting of SSGs is associated with the creation of dermal defects in the donor area that often become difficult-to-heal wounds. In addition, the use of dermatome can deepithelize the skin adjacent to the planned donor site and can destroy the graft epidermis, usually rendering it useless (Bernardis & Box, 2010). In such cases, leaving the wounds on the lateral surfaces of the fingers and on the palmar surface of the hand without any biological dressings may be an equally good solution. Some authors claim that this technique does not prolong the healing time similarly compared with any other methods (Ciccarelli et al., 1995).

Attempts to use allogeneic dermal substitutes have not produced clear results. Allogeneic culture skin substitutes (Eisenberg & Lleewelyn, 1998) and Apligraf (Fivenson et al., 2003) have been used. Although the time to recurrence was increased in allogeneic skin patients, the results for Apligraf were unclear. Some modern dressings were also used, but these did not reduce the duration of healing or the number of weekly dressing changes performed under general anesthesia (Jutkiewicz et al., 2010). All these methods, however, enabled the avoidance of dermatome use on the fragile epidermal surface.

2. Limited hand surgery in RDEB

2.1 Preparation for surgery

2.1.1 Basic recommendations

In the modern treatment of EB, a great degree of significance is placed on the establishment of centers that enable contact with a team of specialists experienced in managing this rare disease (Pohla-Gubo & Hintner, 2010). Pediatric surgeons unfamiliar with EB may make errors stemming from a lack of knowledge of basic care principles. The following recommendations are designed to help practitioners avoid iatrogenic skin injuries:

- Children should not be lifted up independently. In particular, grabbing by the armpits easily causes wounds. Patient transfers should be assisted by the parents. Heavier children should be transferred on a blanket.
- In the case of disposable cloths, any elastics or belts should be removed from. Also, buttons or zippers in the bedclothes may cause blisters, particularly in anesthetized patients. Disposable clothes or wristbands should not adhere to skin when moist.
- Do not pull by the naked skin. In particular, do not restrain a child who has broken free. Grabbing by the wrists or by the fingers when attempting to stretch them causes epidermal tearing. When swabbing the skin before an injection, do not rub it with the swab.
- Band-aids should not be applied to the skin. Wounds may be caused by a band-aid used for fixing the vein needle or the intubation tube. Remember not to affix disposable electrodes to the skin during the preparation for surgery, particularly ECG and diathermy or self-adhesive draping in the operating field.
- Ensure that information on the proper procedure is provided at level of the department and the operating suite.

2.1.2 Metabolic disorders

Metabolic disorders in RDEB may require treatment in the preparation for surgery. These stem from increased energy expenditure, impaired absorption due to defects of the small intestinal epithelium, and insufficient food supply caused by blisters in the mouth and esophageal stenosis. The progressing stenosis hinders the intake of liquids and the swallowing of saliva. Attempts to insert gastric tubes are often associated with skin and mucosal injuries. Confirmed stenosis should rather be an indication for esophageal dilation. The recommended method is contrast X-ray or fluoroscopic guidance balloon dilation. In the population of patients with RDEB, approximately one-third require at least one such procedure. In many patients, the stenosis recurs. The mean time between subsequent dilations is estimated at 1 to 2 years (Fine & Mellerio, 2009b).

In greater deficiencies or independently of esophageal dilation, gastrostomy should be considered. In particular, during the preoperative period, it enables easy supplementation of food taken orally. It should be emphasized that attempts to insert percutaneous endoscopic gastrostomy (PEG) tubes. These expose the patient to unnecessary risk. In the authors' center, laparotomy is performed under general anesthesia, without intubation. Such a choice also rules out laparoscopic gastrostomy.

Apart from food deficiencies, anemia also requires management. Many patients with RDEB are hospitalized with very low hemoglobin values. This is, to a large extent, caused by iron deficiency, associated with both insufficient supply in food and poor absorption in the intestine. Anemia in these patients also results from chronic inflammation associated with healing (Fine & Mellerio, 2009a). In a large portion of patients, despite the treatment with oral preparations, the hemoglobin level remains below 8 g/dl. With these levels, modern intravenous preparations are believed to be more effective. In the authors' center, Venofer is administered. This substitute has, thus far, prevented the need for treatment with blood, even at hemoglobin values below 6 g/dl. However, it should be emphasized that such a low hemoglobin is recognized as an indication for transfusion. Recently, erythropoietin has also been used, although there have yet been no studies indicating its clear advantage.

2.1.3 Skin infections

In preparation for surgery, local infections accompanying the non-healing wounds should also be considered for treatment. The patients admitted for hand surgery often have old wounds in other body regions. It is emphasized that the distinction between the colonization of such wounds and infection should be made based on the clinical picture and not the culture results. Systemic treatment is rarely required. However, the presence of group A streptococcus may constitute an indication for antibiotic use (Brandling-Bennett & Morel, 2010). The growth of beta - hemolytic streptococcus is also a contraindication for hand surgery (Bernardis & Box, 2010). The majority of the other microorganisms present in non-healing wounds do not affect the planning of surgery. Fungal infections in the mouth do not constitute a contraindication either. *Candida albicans* and *Candida parapsilosis* are both common florae of non-healing wounds in patients with EB (Brandling-Bennett & Morel, 2010).

2.2 Preparation for anesthesia

Before elective surgery, it is important to assess comorbid conditions. In over 75% of patients with RDEB, gastroesophageal reflux disease (GERD) is observed (Fine & Mellerio, 2009b). This condition increases the risk of choking during intubation. In the majority of children, continued treatment with proton pump inhibitors should be considered. Of note, the risk of cardiomyopathy may also constitute a relative contraindication for surgery. In patients with RDEB, this risk stands at 4.5% by the age of 20 (Fine & Mellerio, 2009a). To rule out the disease, echocardiography is required. The integrity of the respiratory tract should also be assessed. In view of the possibility of microstomy, ankyloglossia, and fixation of the epiglottis, intubation may prove difficult.

During the immediate preparation, the operating room should be supplied with appropriate dressings, and the operating table should be adapted. Adhesives should be removed from all needles and electrodes affixed to the skin. A good alternative for band-aids are silicone tapes with limited adhesiveness that are recommended for patients with EB (e.g. Mepitac). Fixing the intubation tube requires the use of a bandage or silicone tape. For the closing of the eyelids, moisturizing gels with methylcellulose are used. Petroleum-based products are difficult to rinse off post surgery and cause instinctive rubbing of the eyes (Goldschneider et al., 2010).

Two techniques for the safe use of anesthesiological masks are recommended. The first consists of the intensive moisturizing of the skin and mask edge with a moisturizing agent. The second uses silicone tapes such as Mepitac. After either product is affixed, it protects the facial skin while at the same time maintaining air-tightness with the mask (Goldschneider et al., 2010). In patients with RDEB, anesthesia may be considered without intubation, using a mask alone. The common finding of ankyloglossia hinders the tongue from falling back, protecting against the closure of the airway. In the authors' center, anesthesia without intubation is primarily used. The mask is secured with a common cotton swab or a hydrogel wound dressing. However, the depth of such anesthesia is harder to control. Therefore, the method requires an experienced team and good communication between the surgeon and anesthesiologist.

2.3 Indications for surgery

The long-term skin symptoms of RDEB in the hands, including pseudosyndactyly and scars, lead to the establishment of contractures in the joints. Some authors introduce precise angle measurements, describing the extension and flexion deficits in the metacarpophalangeal (MCP) and interphalangeal (IP) joints (Terrill et al., 1992). Based on similar criteria, precise indications for surgery have been proposed (Ciccarelli et al., 1995). These were the following: (1) palmar contracture, (2) contracture of the proximal interphalangeal (PIP) joint greater than 30 degrees, (3) significant involvement of the small finger, (4) pseudosyndactyly extending to the PIP joint, or (5) impairment of activities of daily living.

Many authors emphasize, however, that irrespectively of deformity grade lesions should be treated early enough to prevent irreversible consequences (Azizkhan et al., 2007). Surgery is typically thought to be indicated when the loss of function compromises the patient's independence and impairs his/her appearance (Bernardis & Box, 2010). Because thumb mobility contributes to 50% of hand functionality, the release of the first web space alone results in a significant improvement. Therefore the aim of surgery is to provide simple pinch grip and grasp, by releasing the first web space and flexion contractures; independent finger movement, by releasing pseudosyndactyly; and improved appearance of the hand (Bernardis & Box, 2010).

The treatment of early lesions is also beneficial in view of the higher probability of maintaining long-term hand function. Postponing the decision about the next surgery and delaying the treatment reduces the total duration of functionality. In the authors' center, the following assumptions have recently been made: (1) the treatment of early lesions permits the reduction of the scope of the surgery, (2) the reduction of the scope of the surgery lowers the number of dressing changes, and (3) giving up the aim of full finger extension may have little effect on the time to recurrence. These assumptions have enabled the formulation of the surgery objectives as pinch grip and grasp and independent finger movement. Therefore, indications for surgery may be defined as follows:

- Pseudosyndactyly of the first web space reaching the IP joint,
- Pseudosyndactyly of fingers II-V

Assuming that the patients present for regular visits, it is possible to adequately notice the progression of lesions early and make a timely decision with regards to surgery. With less frequent visits, the patients often present with palmar finger contractures secondary to pseudosyndactyly (Fig. 1a, 1b). Indications for surgery had occurred in those patients prior to presentation. Isolated flexion contractures without advanced pseudosyndactyly are less common. These are only a relative indication for treatment because they may be extended and maintained in such a state only for short periods.

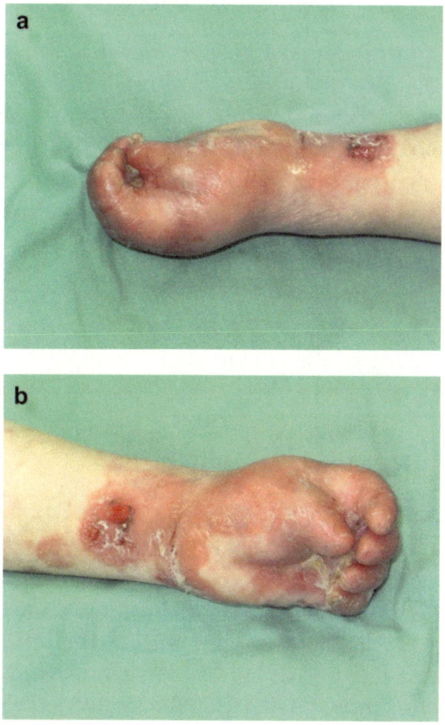

Fig. 1. (a) Pseudosyndactyly of the first web space. (b) Palmar contracture and pseudosyndactyly of fingers II-V. Explanation in the text. Patient AA.

Sometimes, discouraged by previous experiences with protracted healing, patients do not return for years. This avoidance leads to total deformations of the mitten type (Fig. 2a). This situation is still an indication for surgery, although the patients have to be aware of the poor prognosis concerning mobility in the IP joints. Such advanced lesions prolong healing and reduce the efficacy of subsequent rehabilitation.

2.4 Surgical treatment

2.4.1 Features of a limited approach

An important principle and advantage of the presented treatment is the possibility of avoiding direct contact with the patient's skin. This protection minimizes the extent of iatrogenic epidermal injury and, consequently, facilitates healing. The disadvantage of this treatment is that it eliminates the possibility of full forced extension of the fingers during surgery. Both factors differentiate the suggested approach from other methods.

2.4.2 Hand preparation in the operating room

Only one hand is operated on during each hospital admission. This does not hinder the patient's functioning and reduces the associated stress and discomfort of healing. Half an hour before the patient is brought into the operating suite, the hand may be soaked in a bowl with Betadine solution. Washing at the suite, immediately before the surgery, is limited to patting with a web swab. Energetic rubbing would lead to epidermal injuries.

The authors do not use a tourniquet. We believe that it is not necessary in the described technique. However, the majority of surgeons feel comfortable operating without a blood supply. If a tourniquet is used, it should be placed on an arm wrapped with a thick layer of cotton wool. Prior to pumping, the limb is raised for 2 minutes. It must not be wrapped with an elastic bandage or a rubber band to remove the blood. Prior to placing the limb on the table, a thick pad of sterile cotton wool should be placed under the elbow.

Before starting the dissection, thick sutures, e.g. Vicryl 3.0 or 4.0, are placed on the fingertips. Their ends are left long and are tightened with an instrument. They are then used to pull away the fingers during the contracture release. The assistant holds the sutures during the surgery, which avoids the direct handling of the patient skin. The surgeon holds in his/her left hand only the suture of the finger that is currently extended. As a result, the right hand is free.

2.4.3 Separation of pseudosyndactyly and contractures

In cases where the hand is curled in a complete cocoon (Fig. 2a), the fingertips are difficult to release without an initial dissection. A small, circular incision around the fingertips enables them to be detached and lever with blunt scissors. Only then can the suture be placed. In such advanced deformities, the epidermis is retained only on the dorsal surfaces of the fingers. Therefore, the surgery is continued by cutting the epidermis on the dorsal side. During cutting, it is clear that the dermal layers between the fingers remain "glued" rather than grown together into one whole (Fig. 2b). It is easy to find the web space by parting it with scissors. Separation of the fingers may be made easier by pulling them slightly sideways. On the dorsal side, the epidermis is cut to the MP joints level. On the palmar side, the fingers are separated to only half the length of the proximal phalanges. However, to reach this level, the fingers must be simultaneously released from contractures (Fig. 2c). This release usually requires sharp dissection. Particularly on the palmar side of the PIP joints, the use of scissors or a scalpel is necessary. Attention should be paid to the neurovascular bundles. If possible, they should not be exposed, and flexor sheaths should not be reached.

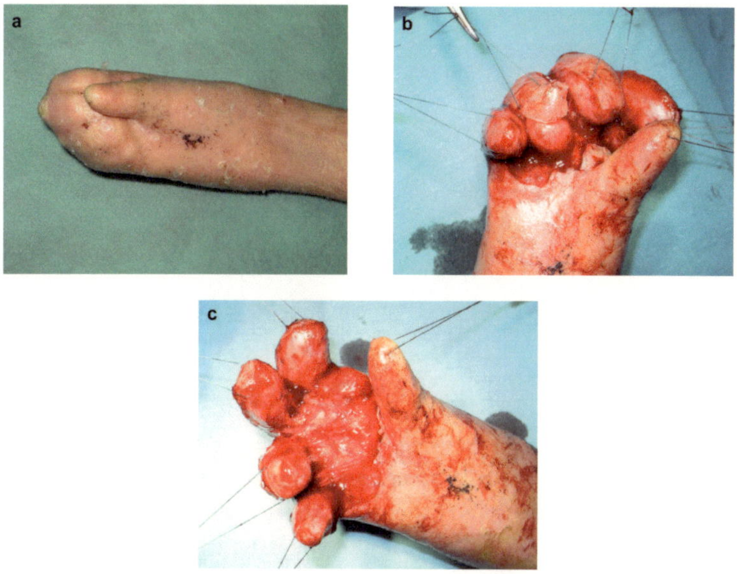

Fig. 2. (a) Mitten hand deformation, (b) Separated pseudosyndactyly. (c) Released contracture. Explanation in the text. Patient BB.

In most cases, the extension in the PIP joints does not have to exceed a right angle (Fig. 3a). Further extension would require the grabbing of the finger by the surgeon's hand and its forced pulling. Such a maneuver is used in more invasive surgical techniques; however, it leads to extensive epidermal injuries and complete exposure of the flexor sheaths.

The thumb is separated in a similar manner. The epidermis is cut on the dorsal side (Fig. 3a). Next, the surgeon moves to the palmar side, dissecting to the depth of the muscle fibers. Both the dermal contractures and some of the adductor pollicis fibers may require sharp separation. However, if possible, it is better to stretch the muscle and joints, gently pulling the suture on the thumb tip (Fig. 3b). This facilitates the protection of the neurovascular bundles near the flexor muscle sheath.

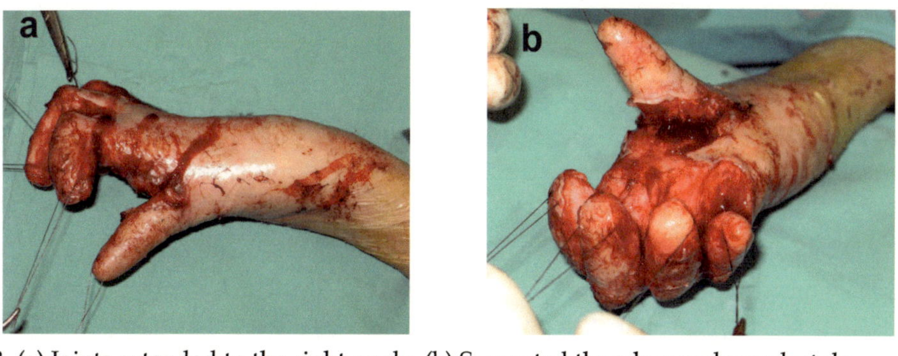

Fig. 3. (a) Joints extended to the right angle, (b) Separated thumb pseudosyndactyly. Explanation in the text. Patient BB.

In less advanced contractures (Fig. 1a, 1b), the described method allows for the nearly complete preservation of the thumb (Fig. 4a) and palmar epidermis (Fig. 4b). It also facilitates healing and limits the dressing changes to one or two subsequent hospitalizations.

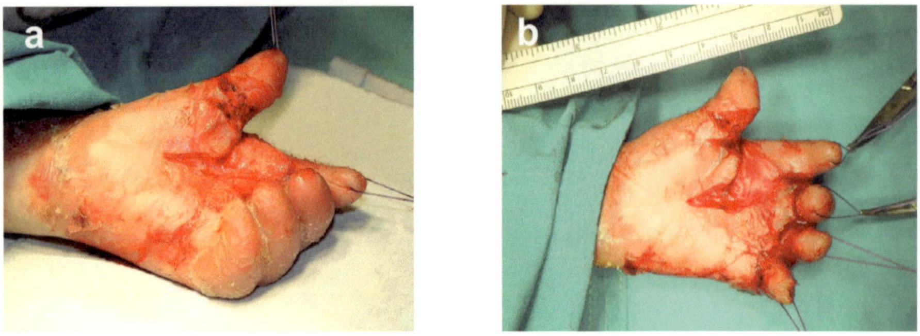

Fig. 4. (a) Minor palmar wound, (b) Epidermis on the fingers is preserved. Explanation in the text. Patient AA.

In some patients, the need for the release of contractures of fingers II-V should be carefully considered. This question concerns especially those whose multiple prior operations deterred from surgery (Fig 5a). The reduction of the extent of subsequent surgeries for the separation of the first web space (Fig. 5b) may sufficiently improve hand functionality.

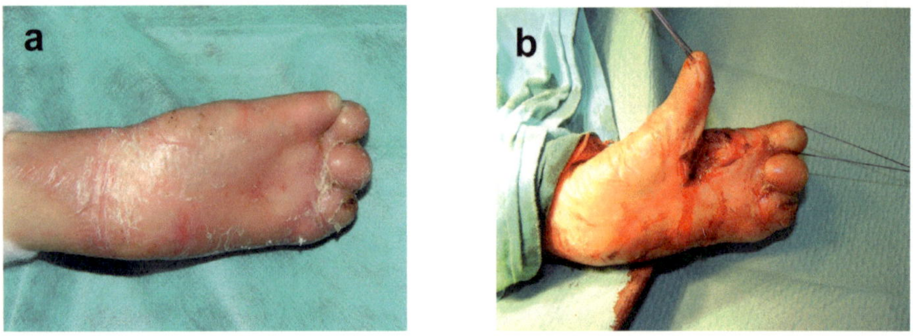

Fig. 5. (a) Recurrent mitten deformation, (b) Isolated thumb release. Explanation in the text. Patient CC.

2.4.4 Skin grafts

At sites where flexor muscle sheaths or neurovascular bundles are exposed covering with FTSGs may be required. These grafts usually undergo epidermal separation during manipulation associated with the defatting of the undersurface and placing. Despite the above, they usually heal well. On the other hand, it is not known whether FTSGs tendency to resist contracture delays the recurrence in patients with EB.

Due to the limited supply of FTSGs and the instability of SSGs, an intermediate solution was suggested over 30 years ago (Cuono & Finsteth, 1978). Since this technique facilitates healing, it is particularly suitable for surgeries of limited scope. It involves the acquisition of isolated epidermis in a technique called the "split-off". The graft is acquired from the thighs or from another surface on which blisters are not found. It should be collected with excess to ensure the thorough covering of all wounds. Bleeding from the collection site is minimal. Thus, the area does not require prompt compression dressing. If necessary the next graft can be harvested in immediate vicinity.

The graft margins should be marked with a felt-tip pen and cut superficially with a lancet (Fig.6a). Next, using the elevator, the epidermal edge is slipped off. Gently, it may be separated from the skin without any damage (Fig.6b). After complete layer separation, the outer surface of the graft is covered with a greased tulle, which facilitates the transfer of the epidermal layer (Fig.6c) and its splitting into appropriate fragments (Fig.6d). At the donor site, a typical tulle dressing is applied.

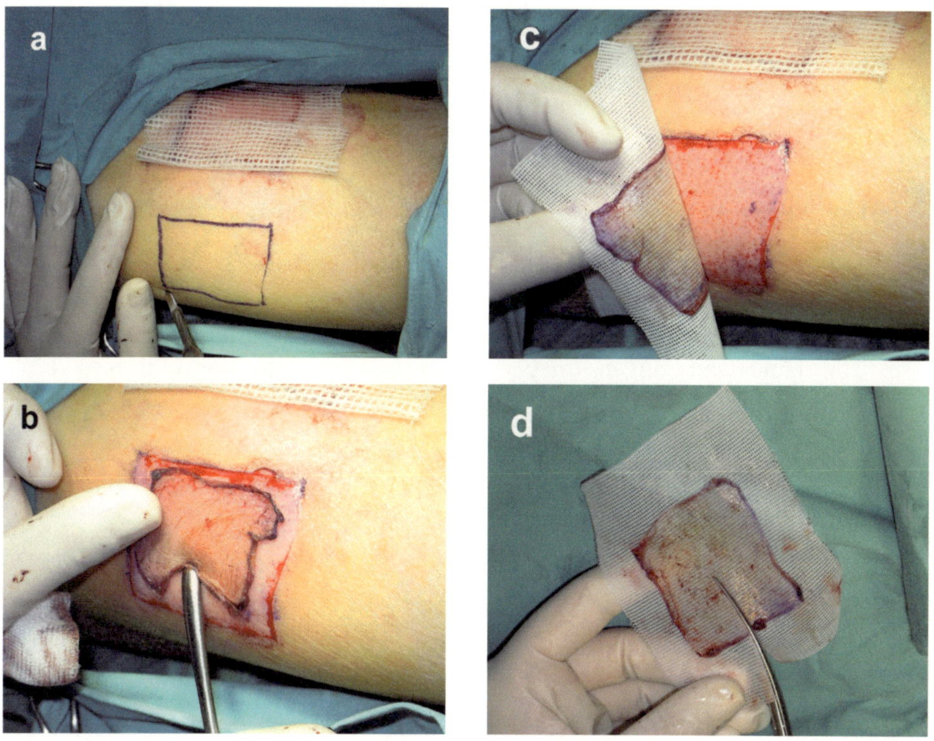

Fig. 6. (a) Markings on the thigh. (b) Harvesting the split-off graft. (c) Graft transfer. (d) Graft splitting. Explanation in the text.

The grafts, transferred to the recipient site may be implanted and fixed with sutures or applied to the wound with the transportation tulle, which then constitutes a part of the dressing (Fig.7a). The "split-off" epidermis may be combined, if necessary, with full-thickness grafts (Fig.7b).

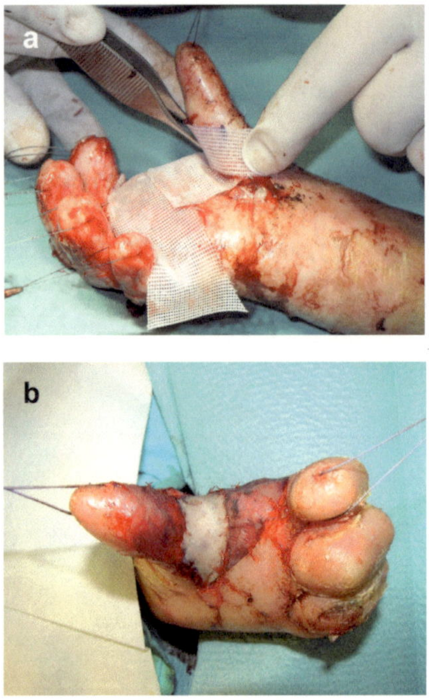

Fig. 7. (a) Grafts left with tulle. (b) Grafts sutured to their beds. Explanation in the text. Patients BB and CC respectively.

Prior to the application of further dressings, a polyurethane sponge is wrapped around the wrist (Fig. 8a). The subsequent dressings inserted into the web spaces are sutured to it (Fig.8b). The hand and fingers may be immobilized with an additional layer of thermoplastic splint applied on the palmar side.

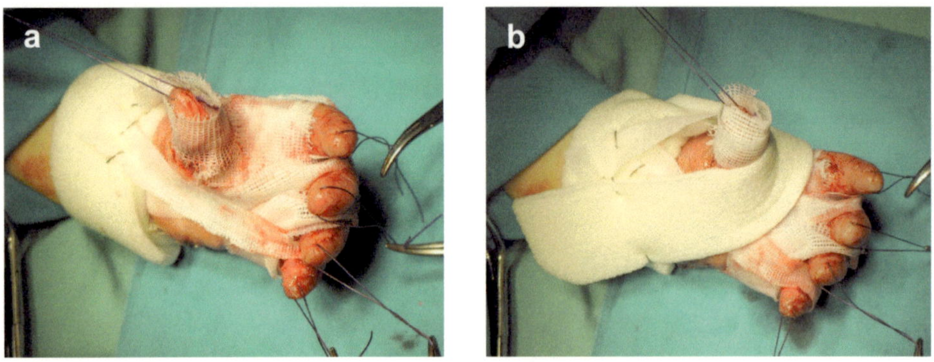

Fig. 8. (a) A sponge band wrapped around a wrist. (b) Dressings fixed to wrist band. Explanation in the text. Patient AA.

2.4.5 Postoperative dressings

The first dressing change after a week, requires the reservation of the operating room and general anesthesia. Before the removal of each dressing layer, it should be thoroughly soaked in Betadine solution. The non-healed, and in some areas, macerated epidermis separates easily from its base (Fig. 9a). Only after it dries up does it adhere fully to the wound (Fig. 9b). The spot bleeding appearing locally may be blocked by touching with a moist swab with 40% solution of silver nitrate (Fig. 9c). The donor area of the collected "split-off" graft does not heal during this time (Fig. 9d).

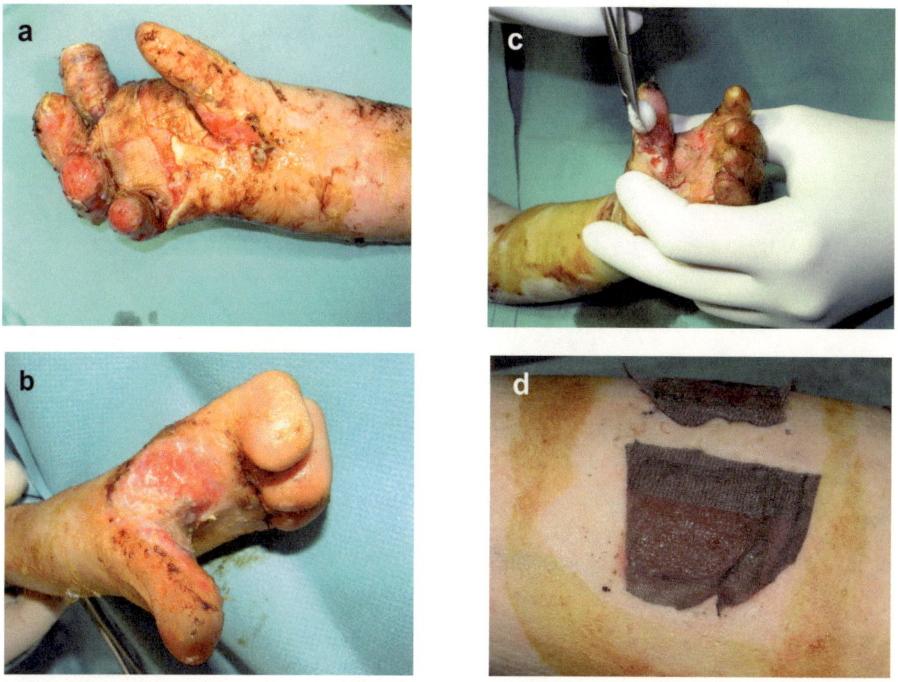

Fig. 9. One week after the operation. (a) Macerated epidermis. (b) Healing epidermis, (c) Minor bleeding, (d) Healing donor area. Explanation in the text. Patients BB, CC and AA respectively.

Both the donor area and the hand require new dressings that are made as described previously, using the greased (Fig. 10a) or silver impregnated tulles (Fig. 10b).

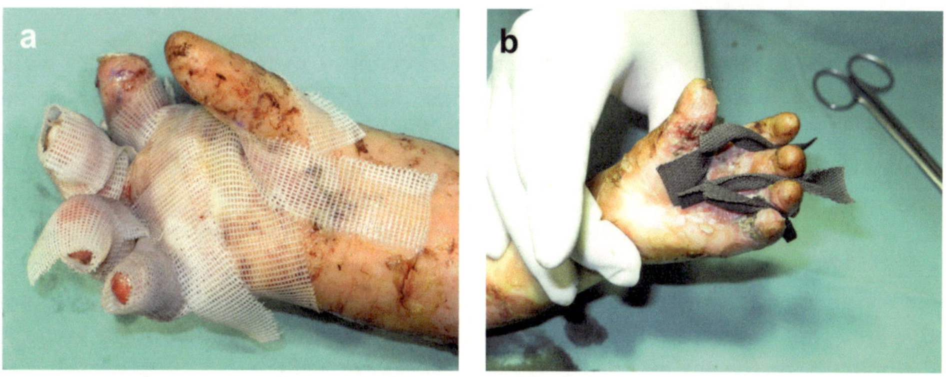

Fig. 10. One week after the operation. (a) Tulle dressing. (b) Silver tulle. Explanation in the text. Patients BB and AA respectively.

The dressing procedures at two weeks also require anesthesia in the operating room. The grafts, despite local maceration, are already clearly healed (Fig.11a). The dried up and macerated epidermis is not removed to avoid bleeding (Fig. 11b). Upon the application of new dressings, the hand is immobilized on the palmar side, with the use of a splint with thumb support (Fig. 11c). A properly adjusted thermoplastic splint further supports the extension of the fingers, even if they were left partly flexed during the operation (Fig. 11b). The "split-off" graft donor area is, by this time, already healed and does not require any dressing (Fig. 11d).

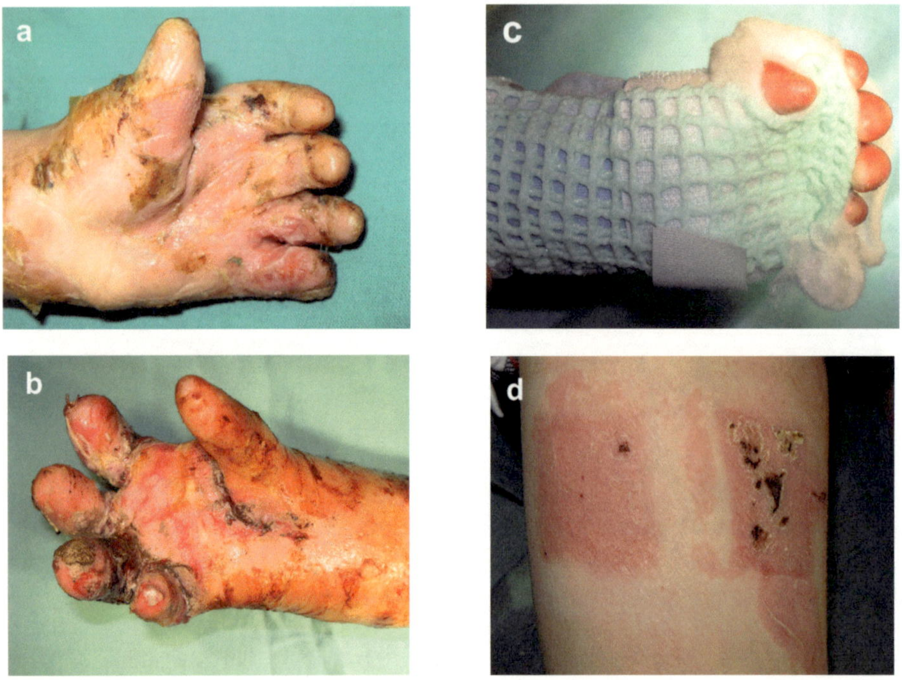

Fig. 11. Dressings at two weeks. (a) Local maceration. (b) Minor wounds. (c) Splint. (d) Healed donor area. Explanation in the text. Patients AA, BB and AA respectively.

After three weeks, most of the dressings may be changed in the dressing room without anesthesia. Minor wounds are present at that time only in patients in whom a decision was made to undertake a more extensive approach. These wounds are often associated with secondary injuries occurring during the removal of old dressings (Fig. 12a). The removal of subsequent dressing layers should therefore be preceded by the soaking of the hand in Betadine solution. From the third week post surgery, despite the presence of minor wounds (Fig. 12b - 12d), daily hygiene procedures should be performed in a home setting. Parents should continuously collaborate with the rehabilitation specialist. The dorsal thermoplastic hand splints with bands on the fingers are used from the third week until the end of the third month during the day and night. The daily application of the thermoplastic splint after dressing replacement may require an ongoing adjustment of its setting. Without parental cooperation, this adjustment would be impossible.

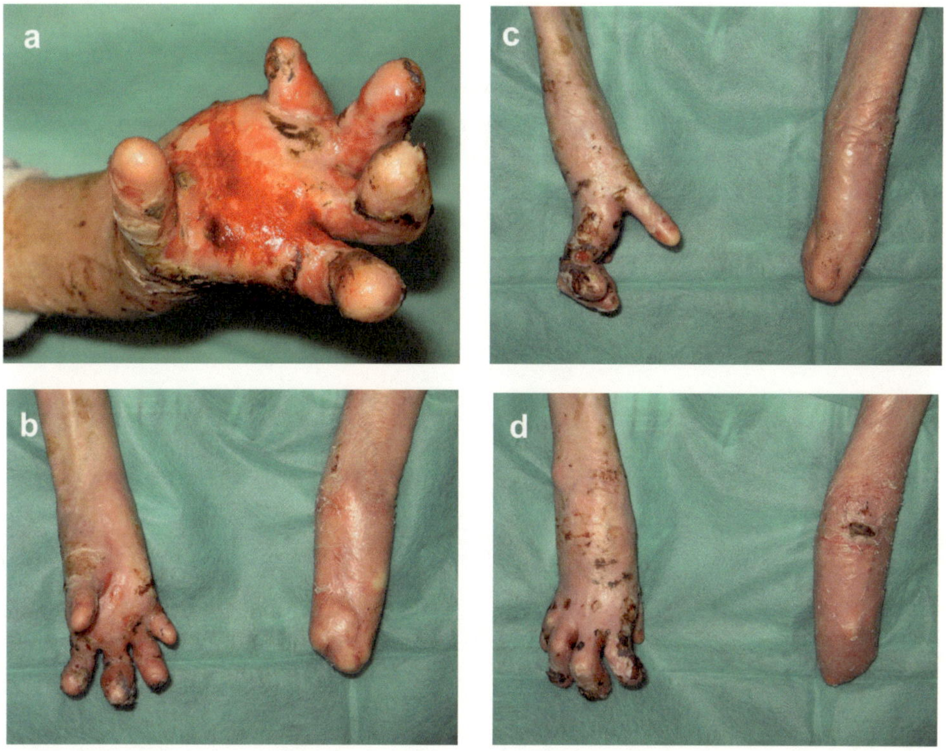

Fig. 12. Twenty one and twenty four days after the operation. (a) Accidental trauma. (b - d) Wounds healed. Explanation in the text. Patients BB.

In the authors' center, the results of 10 hands operated with the described limited approach currently exceed one year (Fig. 13a-13b). No early recurrence was noted within this time.

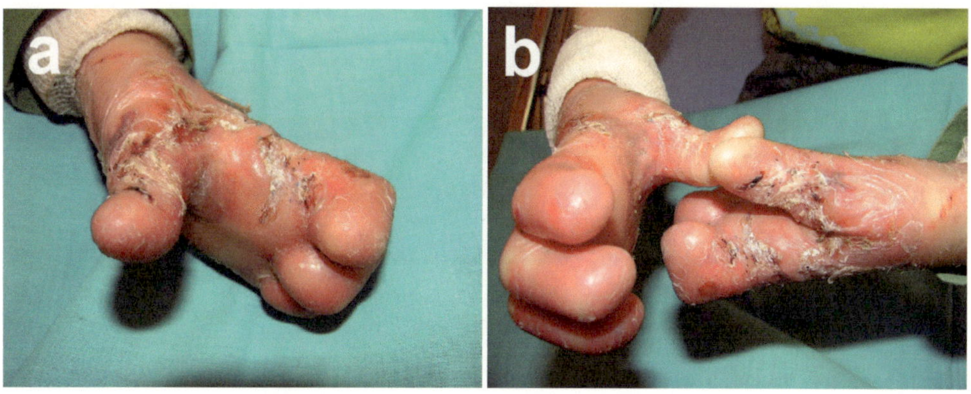

Fig. 13. (a) Left thumb six month after the operation. (b) Right thumb one year after the operation. Patient CC.

The observations indicate that, in comparison with other methods used in parallel, they do not differ significantly. However, this lack of a difference may be associated with the presented indications for surgery, which currently apply to all of the RDEB patients treated in the center. It appears that the treatment of early lesions enhances patient health, irrespective of the selected surgical method. Results of more extensive techniques may be good, even after many years (Fig. 14 a-b). Comparable early results of the limited approach may be similar (Fig.14 c-d). This benefit occurs with both lower financial outlays and decreased psychophysical burden.

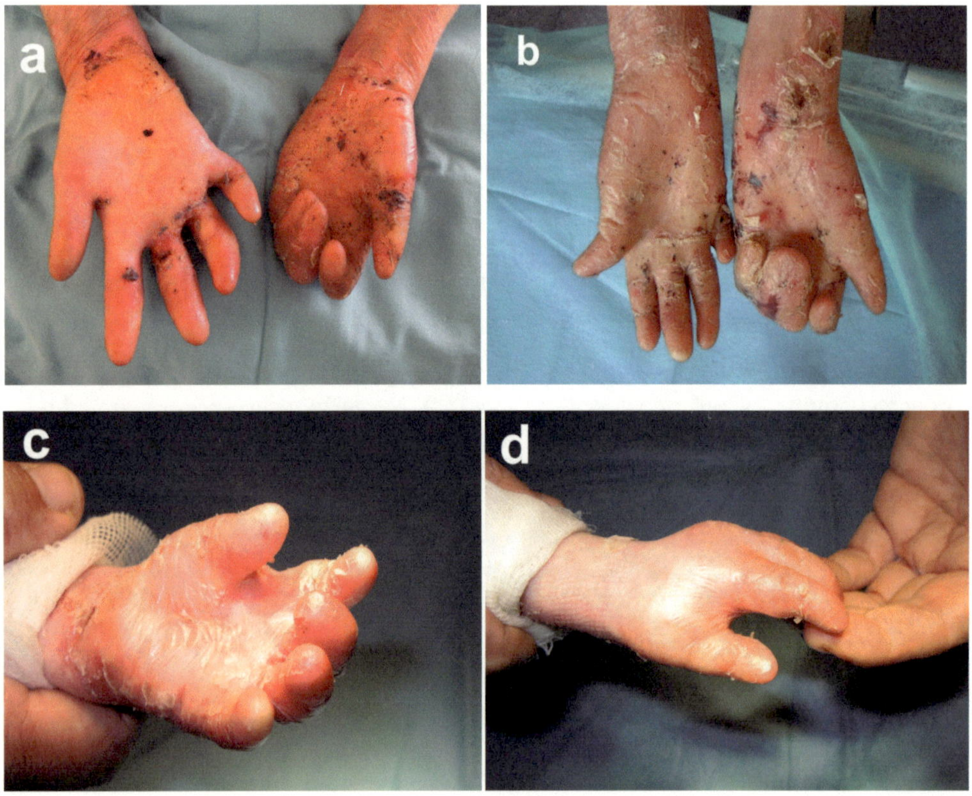

Fig. 14. (a-b) Right hand of the patient eight months and four years after the operation.
(c-d) Patient after the limited surgery (patient AA), at eight months.

3. References

Azizkhan RG, Denyer JE, Mellerio JE, González R, Bacigalupo M, Kantor A, Passalacqua G, Palisson F, Lucky AW. Surgical management of epidermolysis bullosa: Proceedings of the IInd International Symposium on Epidermolysis Bullosa, Santiago, Chile, 2005. Int J Dermatol. 2007;46(8):801-8.

Bernardis C, Box R. Surgery of the hand in recessive dystrophic epidermolysis bullosa. Dermatol Clin. 2010;28(2):335-41, xi.

Brandling-Bennett HA, Morel KD. Common wound colonizers in patients with epidermolysis bullosa. Pediatr Dermatol. 2010;27(1):25-8.

Ciccarelli AO, Rothaus KO, Carter DM, Lin AN. Plastic and reconstructive surgery in epidermolysis bullosa: clinical experience with 110 procedures in 25 patients. Ann Plast Surg. 1995;35(3):254-61.

Cuono C, Finseth F. Epidermolysis bullosa: current concepts and management of the advanced hand deformity. Plast Reconstr Surg. 1978;62(2):280-5.

Devries DT, Johnson LB, Weiner M, Fine JD. Relative extent of skin involvement in inherited epidermolysis bullosa (EB): composite regional anatomic diagrams based on the findings of the National EB Registry, 1986 to 2002. J Am Acad Dermatol. 2004;50(4):572-81.

Eisenberg M, Llewelyn D. Surgical management of hands in children with recessive dystrophic epidermolysis bullosa: use of allogeneic composite cultured skin grafts. Br J Plast Surg. 1998;51(8):608-13.

Fine JD, Johnson LB, Weiner M, Stein A, Cash S, Deleoz J, Devries DT, Suchindran C. Pseudosyndactyly and musculoskeletal contractures in inherited epidermolysis bullosa: experience of the National Epidermolysis Bullosa Registry, 1986-2002. J Hand Surg Br. 2005;30(1):14-22.

Fine JD, Mellerio JE. Extracutaneous manifestations and complications of inherited epidermolysis bullosa: part II. Other organs. J Am Acad Dermatol. 2009;61(3):387-402

Fine JD, Mellerio JE. Extracutaneous manifestations and complications of inherited epidermolysis bullosa: part I. Epithelial associated tissues. J Am Acad Dermatol. 2009;61(3):367-84

Fine JD. Inherited epidermolysis bullosa. Orphanet J Rare Dis. 2010;5:12.

Fivenson DP, Scherschun L, Cohen LV. Apligraf in the treatment of severe mitten deformity associated with recessive dystrophic epidermolysis bullosa. Plast Reconstr Surg. 2003;112(2):584-8.

Goldschneider K, Lucky AW, Mellerio JE, Palisson F, del Carmen Viñuela Miranda M, Azizkhan RG. Perioperative care of patients with epidermolysis bullosa: proceedings of the 5th international symposium on epidermolysis bullosa, Santiago Chile, December 4-6, 2008. Paediatr Anaesth. 2010;20(9):797-804.

Jutkiewicz J, Noszczyk BH, Wrobel M. The use of Biobrane for hand surgery in Epidermolysis bullosa. J Plast Reconstr Aesthet Surg. 2010;63(8):1305-11.

Ladd AL, Kibele A, Gibbons S. Surgical treatment and postoperative splinting of recessive dystrophic epidermolysis bullosa. J Hand Surg Am. 1996;21(5):888-97.

Mellerio JE. Epidermolysis bullosa care in the United Kingdom. Dermatol Clin. 2010 Apr;28(2):395-6, xiv.

Pfendner E, Uitto J, Fine JD. Epidermolysis bullosa carrier frequencies in the US population. J Invest Dermatol. 2001;116(3):483-4.

Pohla-Gubo G, Hintner H. Epidermolysis bullosa care in Austria and the Epidermolysis Bullosa House Austria. Dermatol Clin. 2010;28(2):415-20, xv.

Terrill PJ, Mayou BJ, Pemberton J. Experience in the surgical management of the hand in dystrophic epidermolysis bullosa. Br J Plast Surg. 1992;45(6):435-42.

5

Special Aspects of Forearm Compartment Syndrome in Children

Andreas Martin Fette
University of Pécs, Medical School
Hungary

1. Introduction

Trauma to the wrist and forearm in children resulting in either distal or midshaft fractures are quite common in pediatric surgery practice. The treatment of such fractures is well established and healing in the majority of patients reported as uneventful. However, if there is an extensive muscle hematoma, or extensive swelling due to mangled soft tissue injury, or a heavy bleeding, the situation can suddenly change and run into a disastereous Compartment Syndrome putting muscles, nerves and vessels at risk for destruction. In the following paragraphs our patients collective is presented as an illustrative exemplary and discussed in front of a literature and textbook review.

2. Exemplary patients collective

After suffering an accident with a distal or mid-shaft forearm (Salter Harris I/II, comminute, shaft) fracture, a persistent hemorrhage from the fracture side or a lacerated vessel, eight children (6 male, 2 female) with a Mean age of 12 (range 8 to 15 ½) years developed a forearm Compartment Syndrome (CS) within 1 hour to 1 week requiring fasciotomy. In 3|8 patients an additional mangled upper limb trauma has been notified, in one patient as part of a polytrauma.

All patients displayed clinical signs of elevated compartment pressure in due course. Namely, by elevated compartment pressure measurements in 2|8, immediate impaired neurological function in 1|8, while another 3|8 presented late with signs of Volkmann`s Contracture (VC), Reflex Sympathetic Dystrophy Syndrome (RSDS), or expression of Vanishing Bone (VB) disease.

Primary non-surgical treatment with closed reduction and plaster cast (POP) splinting for fracture treatment respectively splinting alone for sole soft tissue trauma took place in half (4|8) of our patients.

At the time of intervention, open fasciotomy has been performed in each patient according to common incision lines and structures involved. During surgery, the following types of Compartment Syndromes have to be encountered in our exemplary sample:

- 2 | 8 isolated pronator quadratus hematomas
  (deep, distal anterior-flexor compartment)
- 2 | 8 distal/middle anterior-flexor compartments (Fig.1)
- 3 | 8 anterior-flexor and dorsal-extensor compartments
  (exclusively in very late presenters)
- 1 | 8 isolated proximal dorsal-extensor compartment

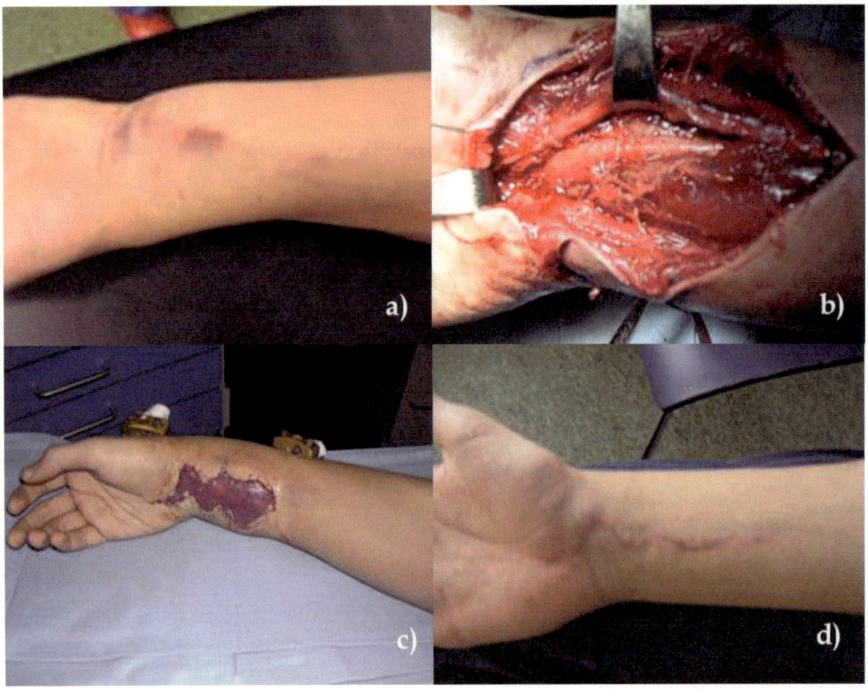

Fig. 1. Classical case; clinical picture: massive swelling, sensivity loss of fingers, in much pain. a) At the time of accident. b) During fasciotomy. c) Temporary closure of the fasciotomy by a foam dressing and a dynamic suture. d) Nicely healing scar after skin closure.

Half of our patients showed a late onset of their CS symptoms after an initial so-called uneventful closed reduction and POP splinting. During fasciotomy, in all fracture patients ORIFs (3 x K-wires, 1 x external fixateur (Fig.2), 1 x ESIN, 2 x combinations) have to be performed to stabilize the bone. The non-fracture patient could be managed by sole splinting entirely.

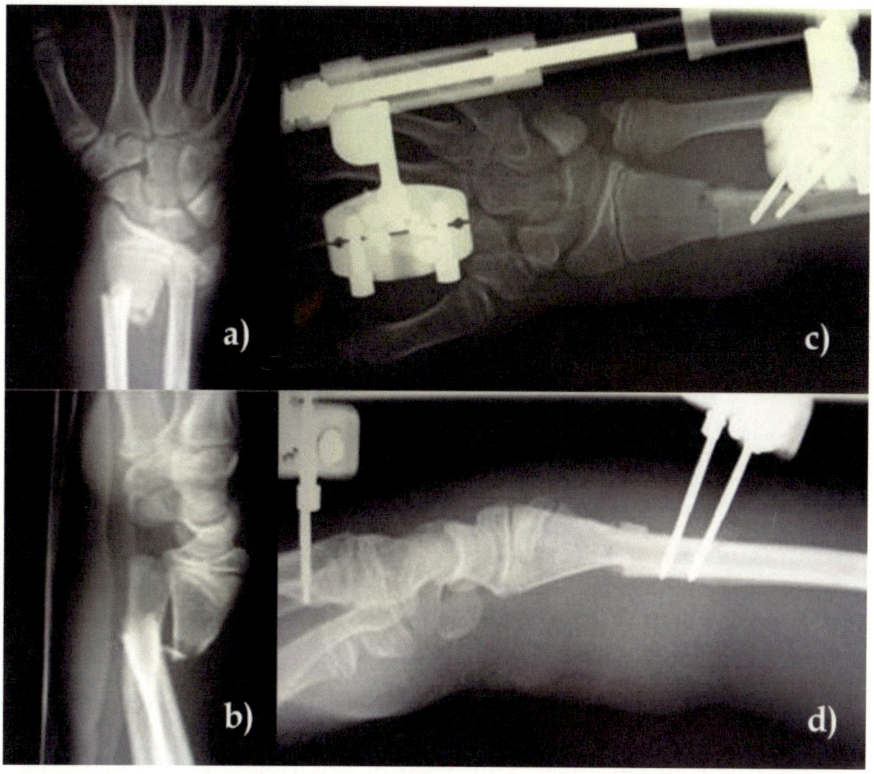

Fig. 2. Classical case; x-rays: a) dislocated distal forearm fracture, plane view. b) dislocated distal forearm fracture, lateral view. c) post reduction and ORIF, plane view. d) post reduction and ORIF, lateral view.

For fasciotomy closure, either a customized foam dressing (polytetrafluorethylene, Epigard®, The Clinipad Corporation) with dynamic sutures (in 5|8) or a topical negative pressure (TNP)/vacuum-assisted closure device (V.A.C.®, KCI Medical, 75-125 mmHg, intermittent mode) (Fig.3) have been used (in 2|8) until final tensionless closure by secondary direct suture.

Three-quarter of our patients showed an uneventful fracture healing with on time removal of implants (ROI) or POP splints; except the polytrauma and Vanishing Bone patients. Direct and tensionless closure of the fasciotomy/skin incision site could be achieved finally in all cases with only minimal scarring at the final follow-up visit. In general, application of the V.A.C.® device resulted in a markedly faster decrease of the soft tissue swelling and edema, which resulted in a much faster closure of the incision site, too (Fig.3).

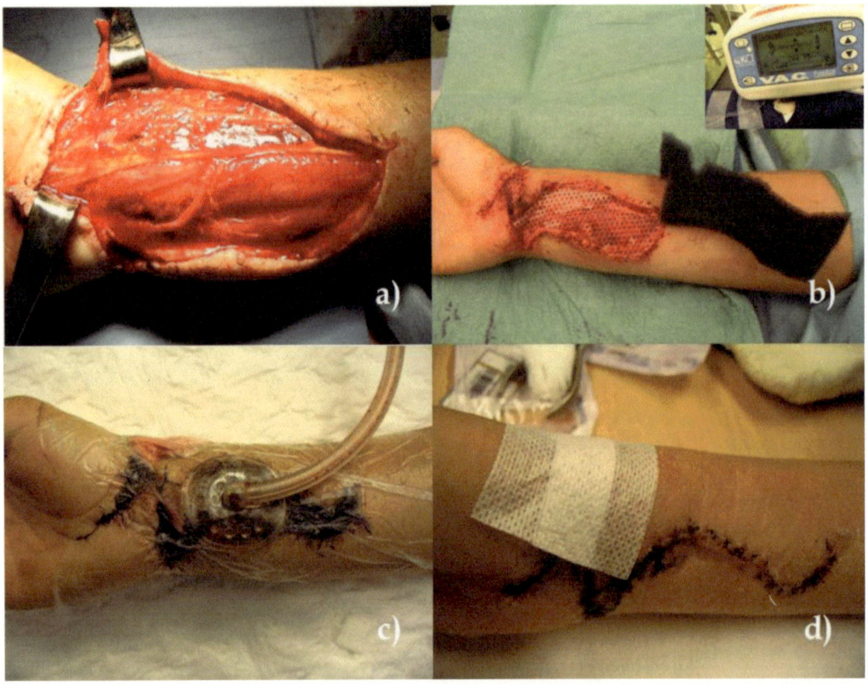

Fig. 3. Special case; clinical picture: massive swelling, increased compartment pressure. a) Immediately after fasciotomy. b) V.A.C.® foam prepared for dynamic suture application. Inlet: V.A.C.® suction unit. c) V.A.C.® dressing in place and in action. d) Nicely healing scar after fast and tensionless skin closure.

In the early presenters (5|8) full ROM, grip and strength could be observed to be back in the majority of patients after 6 to 8 weeks. While in the late presenters (3|8, range 1 to 6 wks after incident) symptoms consistent with RSDS in 1|8, respectively with VC (ie muscle necrosis, contracture) in 2|8 have been expressed. The latter reporting only moderate sequelae after 6 to 9 months of intensive physiotherapy. The latest expressed an additional Vanishing Bone disease and underwent multi-stage secondary reconstruction surgeries to improve his overall forearm function. Our average follow-up comprised 1.5 years.

3. Discussion

The representative findings out of our patient collective, established and progressive management, options and treatment strategies are now discussed in front of a selected literature review.

3.1 Definition of terms: Compartment Syndrome, Volkmann Contracture, Reflex Sympathetic Dystrophy Syndrome and Vanishing Bone disease

A Compartment Syndrome (CS) is defined as the condition in which a raised tissue pressure within the closed skin and soft tissue coat, respectively the tight connective tissue separating muscle groups, leads to a lack of perfusion resulting in neuro-muscular dysfunction and tissue- or organ damage. A Compartment Syndrome has either extrinsic or intrinsic causes, and will be described as acute, subacute, chronic, or recurrent (Bae et al., 2001; Grottkau et al., 2005; Joseph et al., 2006; Krahn, 2005; Mars & Hadley, 1998; Mubarak & Carroll, 1979; Ouellette, 1998; Paletta & Dehghan, 1994; Prasarn & Ouellette, 2009, 2011; Ragland et al., 2005; Ramos et al., 2006; Sawyer, 2010; Wright, 2009).

Volkmann`s contracture (VC) is defined as the end-result of an ischemic injury to the muscles and nerves of the limb. Volkmann`s ischemia is the acute episode of pain aggravated by passive stretching and neurological deficit resulting from ischemia of muscle and nerve. Volkmann`s ischemia, if untreated, leads to Volkmann`s contracture. It is a disorder of the small vessels, then if the pressure in the tissue rises, the capillaries, venules and arterioles get occluded, while the major arteries nearly always remain patent. During the 1970s, numerous investigators established the pathophysiology of Compartment Syndrome as follows: An injury, that would lead to increased intracompartmental pressure. That, if not relieved, would result in Volkmann`s contracture. Although Hamilton first described ischemic contracture in 1850, Richard von Volkmann is credited with describing it in 1881 in his famous article entitled "Ischemic Muscle Paralysis and Contractures". Hildebrand, in 1906, was the first to use the term "Volkmann`s ischemic contracture". The most frequent historical cause of Compartment Syndrome with subsequent Volkmann`s contracture of the upper extremity in children is the supracondylar fracture of the humerus. Recently reported cases on newborns showing contractures and nerve changes at the time of acute presentation describe it as "Neonatal Volkmann`s syndrome" (Bae et al., 2001; Blakemoore et al., 2000; Grottkau et al., 2005; Krahn, 2005; Krenzien et al., 1998; Mubarak & Carroll, 1979; Ouellette, 1998; Paletta & Dehghan, 1994; Preis, 2000; Ragland et al., 2005; Ramos et al., 2006; Wright, 2009).

Reflex Sympathetic Dystrophy Syndrome (RSDS) is a condition that features a group of typical symptoms, including pain (often of "burning" type), tenderness, and swelling of an extremity associated with varying degrees of sweating, warmth and/or coolness, flushing, discoloration, and shiny skin. Other terms it is referred to are "shoulder-hand syndrome", "causalgia" or "Morbus Sudeck". The exact mechanism of development is not well understood. Theories include irritation and abnormal excitation of nerve tissue, leading to abnormal impulses along nerves affecting blood vessels and skin. Triggers, in no particular order and besides others, can be trauma, surgery, nerve irritation by entrapment or shingles, shoulder problems or even any non-associated event in one-third of patients. According to our best knowledge especially in the pediatric age group reports are very sparse. The onset of symptoms can be rapid, gradual incomplete and mono- or bilateral, passing through the stages: acute, dystrophic and atrophic. With the first stage showing early x-ray changes like patchy bone thinning, and the last stage showing significant osteoporosis already (Bae et al., 2001; Cooney et al., 1980; Shield, 2011).

Characterized by spontaneous or posttraumatic progressive resorption of bone, Vanishing Bone (VB) disease is a rare entity. Numerous names have been used in the literature to describe this condition such as phantom bone, massive osteolysis, disappearing or vanishing bone disease, acute spontaneous absorption of bone, hemangiomatosis and lymphangiomatosis, or Gorham and Stout disease. Since it has been first described in 1838, the etiology still remains speculative, the prognosis is unpredictable, and effective therapy still has not been determined. Incidence may be linked to a history of minor trauma, although as many as half of the patients do not have any history of trauma at all. Most cases occur in children or adults < 40 years. Approximately 60 % of all cases with Vanishing Bone disease are reported to occur in men. It has been reported that > 15 % of patients die as a result of their disease and that neurological complications increase the mortality up to 33.3 %. The bones of the upper extremity and the maxillofacial region are the predominant osseous locations of the disease. Multicentric involvement is unusual. Vanishing Bone disease is a rare idiopathic disease leading to extensive loss of bone matrix, which is replaced by proliferating thin-walled vascular channels and fibrous tissue. The process often extends to the soft tissues and adjacent bones, especially at the shoulder girdle. The radiographic appearance becomes diagnostic when unilateral partial or total disappearance of contiguous bones, tapering of bony remnants, and absence of a sclerosing or osteoblastic reaction are present. Radiation and chemotherapy, and antiresorptive medications have all been used with different degrees of success. On the one hand bone grafting techniques yield poor results, indicated by a high incidence of bone graft resorption, however, on the other hand successful reconstructions with bone grafts are reported as well. Recently, the diagnosis was found in the late presenting cases by the residual findings of compartment ischemia and skeletal growth changes in newborns with Compartment Syndrome (Ragland et al., 2005; Rubel et al., 2008; Schnall et al., 1993; Papadakis et al., 2011).

3.2 History and incidence of Compartment Syndrome

First descriptions of "Compartment Syndrome" are found at the beginning of the 19th century by Larrey (1812) and Hamilton (1850), before Richard von Volkmann, a surgeon from Halle in Germany first mentioned "traumatic Compartment Syndrome" in 1881. Later in 1911, Bernhard Bardenheuer first considered fasciotomy as a potential therapy, shortly before JB Murphy in 1914 suggested, that fasciotomy should be used to relieve the pressure in edematous extremities. Finally, PN Jepson established fasciotomy in 1926. Finochietto started research on the Compartment Syndrome of the upper limb in 1920, but the current term "Compartment Syndrome" was not established before 1963 by Reszel et al. from the Mayo Clinic. During the 1940s, numerous reports of "acute anterior compartment syndrome of the leg" due to prolonged marching or other rigorous activities to the extremity appeared. Theories regarding venous obstruction (Brooks 1922) were strongly challenged by Griffiths (1940), who considered that arterial injury with reflex spasm to the collateral vessels has to be considered as the primary cause of Volkmann`s ischemia. Recently, with better definition of the compartment anatomy and the development of pressure measurement devices, it has been realized that such a Volkmann`s ischemic contracture has been caused by an untreated Compartment Syndrome, which could even have been existed before without any major arterial injury. During the 1970s, numerous investigators established the pathophysiology of "Compartment Syndrome" as an injury where increased intracompartmental pressure, if not relieved, might result in a Volkmann`s contracture. Seddon, in 1966, described the four separate compartments of the leg, emphasizing the need for fasciotomy of each compartment being under increased intracompartmental pressure again (Choi et al., 2010; Krahn, 2005; Mubarak & Carroll, 1979; Paletta & Dehghan, 1994).

But still in 1998, less than 50 % of hospitals in ie the United Kingdom had dedicated devices for measuring intracompartmental pressure and it is likely that in less affluent countries even fewer centers would have this opportunity available (Joseph et al., 2006). And this even despite the fact that "Compartment Syndrome" is recognized as a real surgical emergency. With an incidence of 1 to 3 per 1 000 fractures in 2002, if following a supracondylar humerus fracture, which is reported as the most classical incident (Battaglia et al, 2002). Respectively, with a Median annual incidence of 7.3/100.000 in men and 0.3/100.000 in women in Germany in

2005, or an incidence after fractures ranging from 3 % to 17 % (Krahn, 2005). Data of a computerized search of the US National Pediatric Trauma Registry published in the same year reported 85 % of cases as a sequelae of fractures, while 13 % resulted from soft tissue injuries alone. Forearm fractures have been the most common cause in the upper extremity, besides tibia and/or fibula fractures if regarding the lower extremity. Open fractures significantly increased the risk of developing a Compartment Syndrome, either in forearm or leg fractures. Sixty percent of patients went directly from the emergency room to the operating room, suggesting that the other 40 % developed their Compartment Syndrome after admission, or suffered a delayed diagnosis. Boys outnumbered girls by a 1.5 : 1 ratio in the 1 to 4 year old group, with the predominance in adolescent boys increasing to 15 : 1 in the 15 to 19 year old age group. Nearly 94 % of the injuries has been reported as unintentional, nearly 4 % as the result of an assault, and nearly 1 % as self inflicted (Grottkau et al, 2005).

3.3 Compartment Syndrome anatomy and pathophysiology

Anatomic compartments may be best described as those spaces, or potential spaces, who are limited at their binderies by osteo-fascial borders (Berger & Weiss, 2001; Bibbo et al, 2000; Ogden, 2000). Starting distal on the upper extremity, at the level of the hand, there are 10 compartments discernible, each with its own individual fascial layer. Namely, four dorsal interosseous compartments, three palmar interosseous compartments, a thenar compartment, a hypothenar compartment, and an adductor compartment (Shin et al, 1996). At the forearm level, besides the tight fascial membranes subgrouping the muscles into compartments, the tight interosseous membrane between radius and ulna have to be considered, too. Finally resulting in the three major forearm compartments: anterior, posterior and radial. With the anterior and posterior compartment being subdivided in a superficial and deep component each. With each compartment first containing its adjacent muscle groups, and second being traversed by its own nerve-vessel-cable. For example, the median, ulnar, radial, volar-interosseous or posterior one (for details see Fig. 4). The median route contains the median nerve, the ulna route ulnar artery and nerve, while the radial one contains radial artery and the superficial ramus of the radial nerve. The volar-interosseus route accommodates the anterior interosseus nerve and artery, while the posterior one accommodates the posterior interosseus nerve (for details see Fig. 4) (Battaglia et al., 2002, Zhixin et al., 2010; EORIF, 2011).

Trauma is it in most of the cases, that is the incipient factor, resulting in direct tissue damage and tissue hemorrhage. The resultant increase in local venous pressure lowers the arterio-venous pressure gradient, leading to decreased local blood flow and tissue oxygenation. The relative anerobic conditions that follow promote the loss of cellular oxidative processes, which in turn cause the loss of cell membrane ionic gradients, causing cell membrane destruction and cell death. Increased capillary permeability results, causing an increase in tissue edema, and further loss of tissue oxygen tension, which ultimately causes cell death (Bibbo et al., 2000; Krahn, 2005). In an expansile space, any tendency of elevation of tissue pressure can be accommodated by an increase in volume of the space. In a closed compartment, be this osseo-fascial or fascial alone, increasing pressure cannot be accommodated and the resistance to perfusion increases (Mars & Hadley, 1998). But the raise in intracompartmental pressure alone it is not the only thing that matters, because finally it is multifactorial ! Then, each soft tissue trauma releases bradykinin, histamine and other vasoactive substances causing vessel dilatation and increased capillar permeability.

The result is an interstitial edema caused by the penetrating tissue fluids, and at each vessel the wall gets damaged, too. Collagen fibres and thromboactive factors are released leading to disseminated vessel obstruction causing ischemia. The muscle cell react to the trauma among others by damage to the calcium pump. Influx from ions and water into the cell results, and the cell is swelling up. Potassium, creatinine and other substances leave the muscle cell. In extensive muscle damage rhabdomyolysis and myoglobinuria, kidney failure and respiratory insufficiency (= crush syndrome) can be the results. During ischemia the hypoxia is deemed responsible for the excessive dilatation of the vessels. As soon as the cause of the ischemia is solved and a normal perfusion restored, a massive diapedesis of fluid out of the vessel into the interstitium will be the answer. This amount of fluid can not be absorbed by the compartment space. The result will be a progressing increase in pressure. These pathomechanism can account for an increase in intracompartmental volume on up to 60 %. This pressure adds on the compression forces of the triggering agens increasing hypoxia and its sequelae even more (Krahn, 2005).

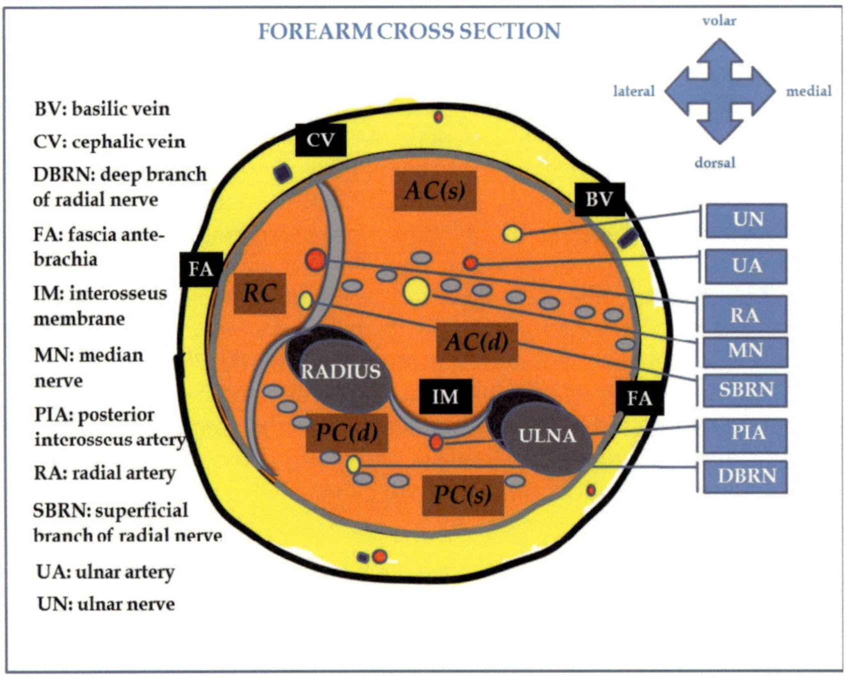

Fig. 4. Cross-section of the forearm. *AC: anterior compartment.* Superfial component accomodating pronator teres muscle, flexor carpi radialis & ulnaris muscle, palmaris longus muscle, flexor digitorum superficalis muscle. Deep component accomodating digitorum profundus muscle, flexor policis longus muscle and pronator quadratus muscle. *PC: posterior compartment.* Superfial component accomodating extensor carpi ulnaris muscle, extensor digitorum muscle, extensor digiti minimi muscle. Deep component accomodating supinator muscle, adductor pollicis longus muscle, extensor pollicis longus & brevis muscle, extensor indicis muscle. *RC: radial compartment* hosting brachioradialis muscle and extensor carpi radialis longus & brevis muscle.

Skeletal muscle can withstand a minimum 4 hours of ischemia; 4 to 8 hours of ischemia have variable outcomes. More than 8 hours of ischemia to skeletal muscle usually produces irreversible damage. However, even after 4 hours of ischemia, complications of muscle ischemia may occur, like ie significant myoglobinuria, that may result in renal failure due to acute tubular necrosis. Peripheral nerve tissue has been shown to maintain normal conduction with up to 1 hour of ischemia. Reversible neuropraxia occurs after 1 to 4 hours and irreversible axonotmesis after 8 hours of ischemia. Progressively higher compartment pressures may result in earlier irreversible changes. Reperfusion injury is also a factor in Compartment Syndromes that develop after tissue perfusion is re-established after an ischemic period. Reperfusion injury involves the production of oxygen free radicals, lipid peroxidation, and calcium influx, resulting in the disruption of the mitochondrial oxidative phosphorylation (Bibbo et al., 2000).

An injury to a major artery (Type I, Holden (1975)) might produce a Compartment Syndrome by one of these two mechanisms as well. First, the Compartment Syndrome may result if there is an inadequate collateral circulation, or if the vessel is only partially occluded, like ie arterial spasm or intima tear. In this situation the decreased perfusion and ischemia of both capillaries and muscles will cause an increase in the permeability of the capillary walls. The resulting edema will cause even more ischemia and the vicious circle will be set up. Second, with complete arterial occlusion, once the circulation is restored a Compartment Syndrome may develop from post-ischemic swelling. With complete arterial occlusion secondary to massive emboli or prolonged use of a tourniquet, in which the circulation is not restored, gangrene and not a Compartment Syndrome will result (Mubarak & Carroll, 1979).

3.4 Typical and atypical causes of forearm Compartment Syndrome

Fractures and fracture hematoma of the upper extremity, in particular those involving the elbow, forearm and wrist, have been reported as the most common causes of Compartment Syndrome in the pediatric population (Bae et al., 2001; Battaglia et al., 2002; Blakemore et al., 2000; Grottkau et al., 2005; Kadiyala & Waters, 1998; Kowtharapu et al., 2008; Krahn, 2005; Mubarak & Carroll, 1979; Paletta & Dehghan, 1994; Preis, 2000; Ramos et al., 2006; Yuan et al., 2004). Considering open vs closed forearm fractures the relative risk for developing a Compartment Syndrome is markedly increased in the open fracture group (Grottkau et al., 2005). Accompanying or fracture-related arterial injury (Choi et al., 2010; Krenzien, 1998; Mars & Hadley, 1998; Mubarak & Carroll, 1979; Ramos et al., 2006), repeated or multiple unsuccessful attempts for reduction, but also simple or undue external compression from bandages, tourniquets, plaster casts, or any position on the operating table during musculo-skeletal surgery, either elective or emergency, can augment to the Compartment Syndrome development risk, too (Bae et al., 2001; Mars & Hadley, 1998; Ramos et al., 2006; Wright, 2009).

As well as other medical procedures or complications thereout like venous access, intravenous fluid infiltration or extravasation, or a subclavian vein thrombosis can do (Bae et al., 2001; Paletta & Dehghan, 1994; Mars & Hadley, 1998). In children, Compartment Syndrome is also a recognized complication of high-energy and crush injuries, small or extensive blunt trauma, or burns (Grottkau et al., 2005; Mars & Hadley, 1998; Prasarn & Ouellette, 2011; Ramos et al., 2006; Shin et al., 1996; Wright, 2009). Not to forget rhabdomyolysis of any origin (Paletta & Dehghan, 1994; Ramos et al., 2006), ischemia-reperfusion events (Bae et al., 2001; Ramos et al., 2006; Shin et al., 1996), all types of infection and septicemia (ie influenza, HIV, enteroviruses) (Bae et al., 2001; Mars & Hadley, 1998), and bleeding disorders (Bae et al., 2001; Paletta & Dehghan, 1994; Ramos et al., 2006). According to more and more frequently arising case reports Compartment Syndrome could also evolve after animal or insect bites (Bae et al., 2001; Mars & Hadley, 1998; Paletta & Dehghan, 1994; Ramos et al., 2006; Sawyer et al., 2010) or suction injures (Shin et al., 1996; Tachi et al., 2001).

However, an untreated Compartment Syndrome might not only be the cause of a Volkmann`s Contracture (VC), Reflexe Sympathetic Dystrophy Syndrome (RSDS) or a Vanishing Bone (VB) disease, vice versa, any of these diseases at any level or stage might trigger the development of a Compartment Syndrome as well, which finally can lead to a complete functional loss of the whole extremity (Cooney et al., 1980; Gousheh, 2010; Landi & Abate, 2010; Papadakis et al., 2011; Raimer et al., 2008; Rubel et al., 2008; Shield, 2011; Schnall et al., 1993; Zhixin et al., 2010). Especially in newborns, there are an increasing number of reports of forearm Compartment Syndromes and associated conditions with disastreous sequelae and outcomes found in current literature reviews (Christiansen, 1983; Landi & Abate, 2010; Ragland et al., 2005; Raimer et al., 2008).

Atypical causes of Compartment Syndrome reported are acute hematogenous osteomyelitis (author`s remark: in the reference case in the lower extremity but in our case in the upper extremity) (Stott, 1997) and myositis ossificans (Melamed & Angel, 2008).

3.5 Clinical signs and symptomes for diagnosis of Compartment Syndrome

Clinical signs and symptomes of a Compartment Syndrome are sometimes masked by polytrauma, a more sinister key trauma, dressings and splintages in place, or by other impressing soft tissue injuries or lesions. However, finding the right diagnosis fast is of key importance to avoid life-long sequelae. This is underscored by recent analyses of closed malpractice claims involving Compartment Syndrome, where the failure of diagnosis is one of the most common cause of litigation against medical professionals in North America. With the average indemnity payment for CS cases of 426 000 US Dollar being considerably higher than the average 136 000 US Dollar indemnity payment for any other orthopedic cases (Choi et al., 2010).

Besides a positive history, the classically described physical findings for Compartment Syndrome are the "7 Ps": *Pain*: progessive, not relieved by narcotics, out of proportion to examination; *Pain with Passive stretch* of the fingers; *Paresthesia*: diminished sense of light touch, pin prick, two-point discrimination; *Pulse*: absent pulses, absent Doppler signals; *Poikilothermia-Pallor*: a cool, pale extremity; *Paralysis*: motor deficits; *Palpation-Pressure*: a tense compartment (Bae et al., 2001; Bibbo et al., 2000; Paletta & Dehghan, 1994; Sawyer et al., 2010). With severe, persistent pain (Johnson & Chalkiadis, 2009; Paletta & Dehghan, 1994) and the tense swelling of the involved extremity (Bibbo et al., 2000; Joseph et al., 2006) being the most common reported physical findings. The individual signs and symptoms are designated as early, middle, or late according to when they become apparent during the clinical progression of the Compartment Syndrome (Sawyer et al., 2010). An adequate sensory neurological examination was not possible in most of the (pediatric) patients due to the poor patient cooperation in this particular age group (Kadiyala & Waters, 1998; Paletta & Dehghan, 1994; Prasarn & Ouellette, 2011). A high index of suspicion for a Compartment Syndrome should always be maintained in all obtunded patients. Obtunded patients are those with a dulled or altered physical or mental status secondary to injury, illness, or anesthesia; those with diminished or absent sensation because of nerve injury or anesthesia, and the mentally ill or disabled. These patients represents the most vulnerable group whose inability to demonstrate the hallmark symptoms and signs of the syndrome put them in jeopardy of a late diagnosis of a Compartment Syndrome and its potentially devastating sequelae. This patient, but not exclusively, should be examined most closely and frequently, and any changes over time must be documented most carefully (Ouellette, 1998; Prasarn & Ouellette, 2011).

According to some authors an increasing analgesic requirement in frequency and dosage might be an early indicator of impending Compartment Syndrome even before classical signs, like "7 Ps" become evident (Bae et al., 2001; Choi et al., 2010; Yang & Cooper, 2010). Since the one of these cardinal symptoms is immense pain, a literature review was undertaken in order to assess the association of epidural analgesia and Compartment Syndrome in children, especially whether epidural analgesia delays the diagnosis, and how to identify patients who might be at risk. Evidence was sought to offer recommendations in the use of epidural analgesia in patients at risk of developing a Compartment Syndrome of the lower (!) limb. Increasing analgesic use, breakthrough pain and pain remote to the surgical site were identified as important early warning signs of minding Compartment Syndrome in the lower limb of a child with a working epidural. The presence of any should trigger immediate examination of the painful site, and active management of the situation (Johnson & Chalkiadis, 2009; Yang & Cooper, 2010).

In the special age group of the newborns, recently, all patients with Compartment Syndrome presented with a sentinel forearm skin lesion. Patterns and involvement ranged from mild skin and subcutaneous lesions to dorsal and volar Compartment Syndrome with or without distal tissue loss, compressive neuropathy, muscle loss, late skeletal changes, and distal bone growth abnormalities (Christiansen et al., 1983; Landi & Abate, 2010; Ragland et al., 2005; Raimer et al., 2008).

In summary, since most of the classic signs and symptoms of Compartment Syndrome are unreliable or unobtainable in the pediatric age group, a high clinical suspicion is needed to make an accurate and timely diagnosis (Bae et al., 2001; Bibbo et al., 2000; Choi et al., 2010; Johnson & Chalkiadis, 2009; Joseph et al., 2006; Kadiyala & Waters, 1998; Paletta & Dehghan, 1994; Prasarn & Ouellette, 2011; Sawyer et al., 2010, Wright, 2009; Yang & Cooper, 2010). Additional tests, such as compartment pressure measurements might be used to establish the diagnosis further (see next paragraph) (Mars & Hadley, 1998; Paletta & Dehghan, 1994).

3.6 Pressure measurements in children with Compartment Syndrome

Confirmation of the diagnosis of Compartment Syndrome currently entails direct recording of the tissue pressure by invasive means and different techniques of invasive recording of intracompartmental pressure have been described in literature so far. As Compartment Syndrome is a progressive phenomenon, a single recording of normal compartment pressure at one point of time does not imply that all is well. Tissue pressure can build up gradually and rise to unacceptable limits. Consequently, it may be necessary to monitor intracompartmental pressure sequentially. This can be done by repeated measurements involving skin punctures on each occasion or by leaving an indwelling catheter till the clinical situation warrants it. Both of these options have obvious disadvantages, particularly in children (Battaglia et al., 2002; Bibbo et al, 2000; Choi et al., 2010; Joseph et al., 2006; Kowtharapu et al., 2008; Krahn, 2005; Mars & Hadley,1998; Ouellette, 1998; Paletta &

Dehghan, 1994). Therefore, in allday practice in children continous monitoring is used less and in the majority of cases, compartment pressure is measured in the operating room after induction of general anesthesia to confirm the diagnosis and document the compartment pressure before fasciotomy is performed (Paletta & Dehghan, 1994).

Besides a lot of commercially available compartment pressure measurement devices, there are other handmade devices in use like a handheld saline infusion manometer (Fig.5) or arterial line and pressure transducer devices (Bibbo et al, 2000; Choi et al., 2010; Krahn, 2005; Paletta & Dehghan, 1994). A standard 18-gauge hypodermic needle connected to an arterial line and pressure transducer is also an acceptable method for measuring compartment pressure (Bibbo et al, 2000; Paletta & Dehghan, 1994). This technique has the advantage of being readily available in most emergency departments, and it has been demonstrated to correlate well with compartment pressure readings taken otherwise from commercial compartment pressure measuring devices (Bibbo et al, 2000).

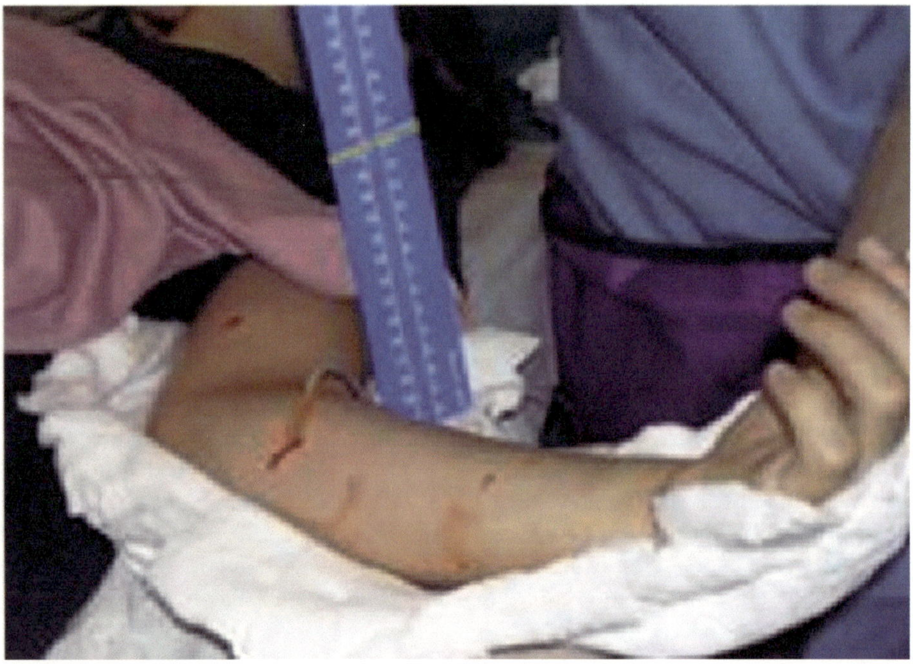

Fig. 5. Compartment pressure measurement device in place.

In order to assess the feasibility of using measurement of tissue hardness as a method of diagnosing Compartment Syndrome non-invasively in children, a simple handheld device to measure tissue hardness was fabricated. The relationship between hardness and compartmental pressure was studied in an experimental model and in three fresh amputated lower limbs. Experimental data from this study suggest that there is a nonlinear relationship between intracompartmental pressure and tissue hardness. The study also showed that tissue hardness can be measured reproducibly in the forearm of children with this device. However, further refinement of the measuring device and well designed clinical trials are needed to establish whether CS can finally be diagnosed reliably by measuring tissue hardness non-invasively alone (Joseph et al., 2006).

At the tissue level an increase in compartment pressure leads to compression of the venous and lymphatic outflow. When this obstruction to outflow is greater than the mean arterial pressure, decreased tissue perfusion and ischemia occur. But adequate cell nutrition, and hence viliability, is dependent upon this adequate tissue perfusion with adequate diffusion of nutritients, including oxygen, within the tissue. While the ultimate driving pressure is the mean arterial blood pressure, it is the pressure in the microcirculation, opposed by tissue and venous pressures, which determines the adequacy of nutrient bloodflow in the capillaries. Cell viability can therefore be threatened by any mechanism, which elevates venous and tissue pressures or which reduces mean arterial pressure, and it is the relationship between these two competiting forces which determines the outcome. In an expansile space, any tendency of tissue pressure elevation can be balanced by an increase in volume of the space. In a closed compartment, either osseo-fascial or fascial alone, the increasing pressure cannot be balanced and resistance to perfusion increases (Mars & Hadley, 1998; Sawyer et al., 2010).

Some investigators believe, that this occurs at a compartment pressure of 40 mmHg or more, while others believe it occurs when the pressure gradient between arterial inflow and venous outflow approaches 30 to 40 mmHg of mean arterial pressure (Krahn, 2005; Mars & Hadley, 1998; Sawyer et al., 2010). Other trauma protocols consider compartment pressure to be significantly elevated when the pressure reading falls within 30 points of the diastolic blood (mmHg) pressure; with the utility of comparing this compartment pressure reading to the patient`s diastolic blood pressure to be proven in experimental Compartment Syndrome models to be predicitive of the threshold for neuromuscular ischemic damage (Bae et al., 2001; Bibbo et al, 2000; Krahn, 2005). The normal pressure in a muscle compartment is reported to be less than 10 to 12 mmHg and the blood flow in the capillary circulation is reported to cease when compartment pressure exceed 35 mmHg (Ramos et al., 2006). But intracompartmental pressure are reported to vary within the lowest pressure measured at 25 mmHg and the highest at 86 mmHg (Krahn, 2005; Paletta & Dehghan, 1994, Sawyer, 2010). And authors are cited, that peak compartment pressures do not influence the patient`s outcome at all (Battaglia et al., 2002; Krahn, 2005), respectively that they even vary considerably periprocedural (ie pre- and post reduction) and according to the site of location, as well as amongst individuals themselves (Battaglia et al., 2002). While some authors recommend decompression at an absolute compartment pressure, others believe that there is no absolute pressure defining Compartment Syndrome at all. However, the overall experience suggest that in children, directly measured compartment pressures are useful data, but should not deter fasciotomy in patients with obvious deteriorating physical findings or displaying the classical signs and symptoms already mentioned (Bibbo et al., 2000; Krahn, 2005; Kowtharapu et al., 2008; Ouellette, 1998; Ramos et al., 2006).

Briefly summarized: Besides the typical clinical findings, initial and repeated compartment pressure measurements are a recommended diagnostic tool, but it is an invasive and scarring procedure, time consuming and the value of the readings is often limited or at least questionable. And peak intracompartmental pressure do not necessarily match with the severity of the condition of the patient in due course.

3.7 Management and treatment of Compartment Syndrome

Surgery remains the mainstay in treatment for acute Compartment Syndrome and definitive treatment must consist of emergent fasciotomy of ALL involved compartments. With early diagnosis and expeditious treatment being of key importance (Bae et al., 2001; Battaglia et al., 2002; Berger & Weiss, 2001; Bibbo et al., 2000; Blakemore et al., 2000; Choi et al., 2010; Christiansen et al., 1983; Cooney et al., 1980; Gousheh, 2010; Grottkau et al., 2005; Kadiyala & Waters, 1998; Kowtharapu et al., 2008; Krahn, 2005; Krenzien et al., 1998; Landi & Abate, 2010; Mars & Hadley,1998; Mubarak & Carroll, 1979; Ogden, 2000; Ouellette, 1998; Paletta & Dehghan, 1994; Prasarn et al., 2009; Prasarn & Ouellette, 2011; Preis 2000; Ragland et al., 2005; Ramos et al., 2006; Sawyer et al., 2010; Shin et al., 1996; Stott et al., 1997; Tachi et al., 2001; Yuan et al., 2004; Zhixin et al., 2010).

Fasciotomy should always be performed according to the individual compartments and structures most likely involved, and according to the common incision lines regularly used in hand surgery practice. Ensuring a full and complete fasciotomy is also essential, since an incomplete fasciotomy poses a considerable risk for damaging the forearm structures even further. Getting proper access to the region of interest is essential, but any additional (surgical) trauma to the tissue must be reduced to a minimum. Any bleeder must be stopped meticiously. Incision lines should never cross skin folds perpendicular and never leave badly perfused flaps or skin margins behind (Berger & Weiss, 2001; Krenzien et al., 1998; Ogden, 2000). Splinting, elevation, and delayed wound closure usually follows the simple compartment fasciotomy (Bae et al., 2010; Battaglia et al., 2002; Blakemore et al., 2000; Choi et al., 2010; Cooney et al., 1980; Christiansen et al., 1983; Kowtharapu et al., 2008; Krahn, 2005; Landi & Abate, 2010; Mars & Hadley, 1998; Mubarak & Carroll, 1979; Ogden, 2000; Ouellette, 1998; Prasarn et al., 2009; Prasarn & Ouellette, 2011; Ragland et al., 2005; Ramos et al., 2006; Sawyer wt al, 2010; Shin et al., 1996; Stott et al., 1997; Zhixin et al., 2010).

Concomitant fractures will be fixed according to actual guidelines and textbooks, using either cast splintage or ORIF techniques. The latter becoming more and more prefered (Dietz et al., 1997; Fette et al., 2009; Grottkau et al., 2005; Kadiyala & Waters, 1998; Ogden, 2000; Preis, 2000; Yuan et al., 2004), since in those limbs being at risk for Compartment Syndrome, bony fixation like ie percutaneous pinning or intramedullary fixation prevents problems usually noticed with the standard cast treatment (Fette, 2010, Grottkau et al., 2005; Kadiyala & Waters, 1998; Ogden, 2000; Preis, 2000). However, there is also an increased incidence of Compartment Syndrome reported for patients treated with intramedullary fixation (ESIN), especially for the ones with long surgery times and long use of intraoperative fluoroscopy, when compared to patients treated with closed reduction and casting alone (Yuan et al., 2004). Any bone reconstruction must be stable enough right from the beginning for an early (self-) mobilization by the child or a guided pediatric physio- or occupational therapy. Removal of implants usually can be scheduled according to common standards and protocols (Dietz et al., 1997; Fette et al., 2009; Fette, 2010; Grottkau et al., 2005; Kadiyala & Waters, 1998; Ogden, 2000; Preis, 2000; Yuan et al., 2004).

Concomitant nerve-, vessel- or tendon injuries upgrade the simple Compartment Syndrome into a complex one. In principle, surgical therapy comprises freeing of the delicate structures and their meticulous (micro-) surgical repair to restore function as much as possible, quite often as a multi-staged and interdisciplinary procedure (Berger & Weiss, 2001; Cooney et al., 1980; Fette, 2010; Gousheh, 2010; Krenzien et al., 1998; Landi & Abate, 2010; Ogden, 2000; Ragland et al., 2005; Raimer et al., 2008, Zhixin et al., 2010).

The same applies for potential trigger or potential in due course morbidities like Volkmann`s Contracture, Reflex Sympathetic Dystrophy Syndrome or Vanishing Bone disease. Here usually the whole armentarium of non-surgical and reconstructive-surgical treatment modalities are required. These include invigorating activities and extensive physio- and occupational therapy, if indicated as well (Fette et al., 2002; Papadakis et al., 2011; Schnall et al., 1993; Shield, 2011).

Classical management of the fasciotomy is delayed primary (= secondary) closure. The splitted fascia and skin are usually covered by impregnated gauze and cotton wool or by a foam dressing. The margins in most cases are approximated by a dynamic suture, until the swelling has settled down completely, and the skin can be finally closed by direct suture. Respectively, by a skin graft or even more rarely by a flap (Fette et al., 2002; Paletta & Dehghan, 1994; Tachi et al., 2001). Modern treatment takes advantage of the topical negative pressure therapy (ie V. A. C.®, KCI Medical, Wiesbaden/Germany). The wound surface is protected by a silicone sheet, the wound margins by a hydrocolloid, just before the foam is applied, and fixed to the wound margins by stitches or staples. This altogether is sealed by foil, the TRAC™ pad is installed and the negative pressure in continuous mode (authors remark: 75 mmHg) set up by the V. A. C.® machine. As soon as the swelling went down (24 to 72 hours), the machine is switched to intermittend mode and the negative pressure can be increased in the majority of cases. Immediately putting some "massage-like" and stretching effect on the tissue and skin margins and therefore acting like a "tissue expander"-device. Making fasciotomy closure finally fast, easy and complete tension-free (Fette & Epp 2007; Fette, 2008; Fette & Doede, 2009; Willy, 2005).

3.8 Outcome after fasciotomy for forearm Compartment Syndrome

Early recognition and expeditious treatment are essential to obtain a good clinical outcome and prevent permanent disability (Bae et al., 2001; Prasarn & Ouellette, 2011; Shin et al., 1996; Ramos et al., 2006; Wright, 2009). Thus, the large majority of the patients will achieve full restoration of function (Bae et al., 2001; Gousheh, 2010; Prasarn & Ouellette, 2011; Shin et al., 1996; Ramos et al., 2006; Tachi et al., 2001). However, a well and uneventful healed fasciotomy after a Compartment Syndrome regularly gets a 10 % occupational disability credit in the German medical appraisal system (Krahn, 2005). Improved approaches to assessment and better management, together with early recognition, helped to reduce the bad outcomes (Krahn, 2005; Shin et al., 1996; Wright, 2009). But there is still a considerable risk for developing Volkmann`s Contracture with significant morbidity (Cooney et al., Gousheh, 2010; Krahn, 2005; Kretzien et al., 1998; Landi & Abate, 2010; Mubarak & Carroll, 1979; Ragland et al., 2005; Raimer et al. 2008; Paletta & Dehghan, 1994), Reflex Sympathetic Dystrophy Syndrome (Shield, 2011; Cooney et al., 1980), or Vanishing Bone disease (Papadakis et al., 2011; Rubel et al., 2008; Schnall et al., 1993) anyway. Recent reports on this entire entity focusing especially on newborns showed even more complex and disastrous outcomes requiring even more complex and demanding reconstructive procedures than ever seen previously in the past (Christiansen et al., 1993; Landi & Abate 2010; Ragland et al., 2005; Raimer et al., 2008).

According to a historical report, the volar and occasionally the volar and dorsal compartment together are mainly involved in older patients with supracondylar humerus and forearm fractures (Mubarak & Carroll, 1979).

Average time to surgical intervention from the time of increasing signs and symptoms are reported to be around 18-25 (range 1-96) hours (Bae et al., 2001), but there are others reporting >> 24 hours delay in the initial diagnostic process as well (Mubarak & Carroll, 1979). Full functional recovery is anticipated within 6 months in most patients (Bae et al., 2001), and average follow-up reported is 22 months (Prasarn et al., 2009).

Since there is no specific predictor or indicator, nor a clinical sign or symptom or any technical or lab investigation to diagnose a Compartment Syndrome fast and safely, the most powerful indicator is the suspicion of the attending (pediatric) surgeon. Compartment pressure measurements might be helpful and indicative, but especially in the pediatric age group it has to be considered, that they are painful, invasive and need specified technical equipment, that is not commonly available. Surely, this high tech equipment can be replaced by components easily available in any pediatric surgery department or ER, but their set-up is time consuming and measurements taken still less reliable. Overall experience in diagnosing (pediatric) Compartment Syndrome among ER or pediatric surgery staff is usually limited, as well as it is with putting a pressure probe device in action. And so far there are still no table of normal values available and compartment pressure can vary considerably in due course and even within the individual. Conditions like polytrauma, splintage, Volkmann Contracture, Reflex Sympathetic Dystrophy Syndrome or Vanishing Bone disease might mask or even trigger the underlying Compartment Syndrome. Waiting for the so-called historical signs, impalpable pulse and neurological deficit, is too dangerous, then when realising them it is much too late.

4. Conclusion

The potential risk of an even late onset Compartment Syndrome should always be considered in all children presenting with a remarkable forearm injury. Clinical signs and symptoms are various, inconstant and unreliable. The only consistent finding is the suspicion of the attending surgeon. Immediate surgical release of the Compartment Syndrome, stable fixation of the concomitant fracture and meticulous repair of all important anatomic structures involved is mandatory to prevent these children from disastreous sequelae and outcomes. By reducing the swelling and in parallel stretching the skin, the V.A.C.® device, throughout the intermittend mode, facilitates and fastens the tensionless direct closure of the fasciotomy site.

5. References

Bae, DS, Kadiyala, RK & Waters, PM. (2001). Acute Compartment Syndrome in Children: Contemporary Diagnosis, Treatment, and Outcome. *Journal of Pediatric Orthopaedics*, Vol.21, No.5, pp. 680-688

Battaglia, TC, Armstrong, DG & Schwend, RM. (2002). Factors affecting forearm compartment pressures in children with supracondylar fractures of the humerus. *Journal of Pediatric Orthopedics*, Vol.22, pp. 431-439

Berger, RA & Weiss, APC (Eds). (2001). *Hand Surgery*. Lippincott Williams & Wilkins, Wolters-Kluwer Company, Philadelphia-Baltimore-New York-London-Buenos Aires-Hongkong-Sydney-Tokio

Bibbo, Ch, Lin, SS & Cunningham, FJ. (2000). Acute traumatic compartment syndrome of the foot in children. *Pediatric Emergency Care*, Vol.16, No.4. pp 244-248

Blakemore, LC, Cooperman, DR, Thompson, GH, Wathey, C & Ballock, RT. (2000). Compartment Syndrome in Ipsilateral Humerus and Forearm Fractures in Children. *Clinical Orthopaedics And Related Research*, No. 376, pp. 32-38

Choi, PD, Melikian, R & Skaggs, DL. (2010). Risk factors for vascular repair and compartment syndrome in the pulseless supracondylar humerus fracture in children. *Journal of Pediatric Orthopedics*, Vol.30, No.1 (Jan-Feb 2010), pp. 50-56

Christiansen, SD, Desai, NS, Pulito, AR & Slack, MR. (1983). Ischemic extremities due to compartment syndrome in a septic neonate. *Journal Of Pediatric Surgery*, Vol.18, No.5 (October 1983), pp. 641-643

Cooney, WP III, Dobyns, JH & Linscheid, RL. (1980). Complications of Colles` Fractures. *Journal of Bone and Joint Surgery A*, Vol.62, No.4 (June 1980), pp. 613-619

Dietz, HG, Schmittenbecher, PP & Illing, P. (1997). *Intramedulläre Osteosynthese im Wachstumsalter*. Urban & Schwarzenberg, München, Wien, Baltimore

eorif. CompartmentSyndrome, In: *eorif.com*, accessed 07/08/2011, Available from: http:// eorif.com/General/CompartmentSyndrome.html

Fette, A, Mayr, J & Pierer, G. (2002). Forearm reconstruction in a scholargirl suffering polytrauma and mangled upper limb injury, In: *Proceedings of 8 th Congress of FESSH, A Collection Of Free Papers*, Hovius S, pp. 115-118, Monduzzi Editore, International Proceedings Division, ISBN 88-323-2522-5

Fette, A & Epp, B. (2007). VAC-KCI. Vielseitig Anwendbares Concept für KinderChirurgische Indikationen. *Direct-fmch*, Supplement zum 3-Länder- Kongress in Luzern/Schweiz, März 2007

Fette, A. (2008). Wundbehandlung mit der Wundvakuumversiegelung/VAC® - Therapie in der Kinderchirurgie. Fallbeispiele von „Nutzniessern, Opfern, Befürwortern und Gegnern". *European Surgery (Acta Chirurgica Austriaca)*, Vol.40, Suppl 222/08, pp. 58-62

Fette, A & Doede, Th. (2009). Update Vakuumversiegelung in der plastischen Chirurgie im Kindesalter, *Kongressband Festsymposium 50 Jahre Kinderchirurgie in Rostock*, Stuhldreier, G, Shaker Verlag, ISBN 978-3-8322-8769-6, Aachen

Fette, A, Feichter, S, Zettl, A, Haecker, FM & Mayr J. (2009). Elastisch-stabile Markraumschienung (ESMS) von Unterarmschaftfrakturen im Kindesalter. *Obere Extremität Schulter Ellenbogen Hand*, Vol.4, pp. 55-62, DOI 10.1007/s11678-008-008-2

Fette, A. (2010). Challenges on the injured pediatric elbow joint, In: *Hand Surgery 2010 IFSSH*, Chung, MS & BAEK, GH, pp. 347-349, HS Gong Konnja Publishing, ISBN 978-89-6278-331-5, Seoul, Korea

Gousheh, J. (2010). Surgical Treatment of Old Volkmann Syndrome, In: *Hand Surgery 2010 IFSSH*, Chung, MS & BAEK, GH, pp. 308-309, HS Gong Konnja Publishing, ISBN 978-89-6278-331-5, Seoul, Korea

Grottkau, BE, Epps, HR & Di Scala, C. (2005). Compartment syndrome in children and adolescents. *Journal of Pediatric Surgery*, Vol.40, pp. 678-682

Johnson, DJG & Chalkiadis, GA.(2009). Review article. Does epidural analgesia delay the diagnosis of lower limb compartment syndrome in children. *Pediatric Anesthesia*, Vol.19, pp. 83-91, DOI: 10.1111/j.1460-9592.2008.02894.x

Joseph, B, Varghese, RA, Mulpuri, K, Paravatty, S, Kamath, S & Nagaraja N. (2006). Measurement of tissue hardness: can this be a method of diagnosing compartment syndrome noninvasively in children ? *Journal of Pediatric Orthopaedics*, Vol.15, No.6, pp. 443-448

Kadiyala, RK & Waters, PM. (1998). Upper extremity pediatric compartment syndrome. *Hand Clinics*, Vol.14, No.3 (August 1998), pp. 467-475

Kowtharapu, DN, Thabet, AM, Holmes, L jr & Kruse, R. (2008). Osteochondral flap avulsion fracture in a child with forearm compartment syndrome. *Orthopedics*, Vol.31, No.8 (Aug 2008), pp. 805

Krahn, NE. (2005). Das akute Kompartmentsyndrom. Funktionelle Resultate und Lebensqualität nach operative Behandlung. Inaugural - Dissertation, Bochum (accessed: 23/07/2011)

Krenzien, J, Richter, H, Gussmann, A & Schildknecht, A. (1998). Das Compartmentsyndrom und die Volkmann Kontraktur - sind sie bei der supracondylären Humerusfraktur vermeidbar ?? *Chirurg*, Vol. 69, pp. 1252-1256

Landi, A & Abate M. (2010). The Perinatal Compartment Syndrome, In: *Hand Surgery 2010 IFSSH*, Chung, MS & BAEK, GH, pp. 303-305, HS Gong Konnja Publishing, ISBN 978-89-6278-331-5, Seoul, Korea

Mars, M & Hadley, GP. (1998). Raised compartment pressure in children: a basis of management. *Injury*, Vol.29, No.3, pp. 183-185, PH: S0020-1383(97)00172-1

Melamed, E & Angel, D. (2008). Myositis ossificans mimicking compartment syndrome of the forearm. *Orthopedics*, Vol.31, No.12 (Dec 2008), case report

Mubarak, SJ & Carroll, NC. (1979). Volkmann`s Contracture in children: aetiology and prevention. *The Journal of Bone and Joint Surgery B*, Vol.61, No.3 (August 1979), pp. 285-293

Ogden, JA. (Ed). (2000). *Skeletal Injury Of The Child. Third edition.* Chapter 10, pp. 316-320, Springer Verlag, Berlin Heidelberg New York. ISBN 0 - 387-985107

Ouellette, EA. (1998). Compartment syndromes in obtunded patients. *Hand Clinics*, Vol.14, No.3 (August 1998), pp. 431 - 50

Paletta, CE & Dehghan, K. (1994). Compartment syndrome in children. *Ann Plast Surg*, Vol.32, No.2 (February 1994), pp. 141-144

Papadakis, SA, Khaldi, L, Babourda, EC, Papadakis, S, Mitsitsikas, Th & Sapkas, G Vanishing Bone Disease: Review and Case Reports, In: *Ortho Supersite*, accessed 23/07/2011, Available from: http://www.orthosupersite.com/print.aspx?rid=26 425

Prasarn, ML, Ouellette EA, Livingstone A & Guiffrida AY. (2009). Acute pediatric upper extremity compartment syndrome in the absence of fracture. *Journal of Pediatric Orthopedics*, Vol.29, No.3 (Apr-May 2009), pp. 263-268

Prasarn ML & Ouellette EA. (2011). Acute compartment syndrome of the upper extremity. *Journal of the American Academy of Orthopaedic Surgeons*, Vol.19, No.1 (Jan 2011), pp. 49-58

Preis, J. (2000). Volkmann`s contracture and supracondylar fractures of the humerus in children. *Rozhledy V Chirurgii*, Vol.79, No.8 (August 2000), pp. 357-363

Ragland, R III, Moukoko, D, Ezaki, M, Carter, PR & Mills, J. (2005). Forearm Compartment Syndrome In The Newborn: Report of 24 cases. *The Journal of Hand Surgery A*, Vol.30, No.5 (September 2005), pp. 997-1003

Raimer, L, McCarthy, RA, Raimer, D & Colome-Grimmer, M. (2008). Congenital Volkmann ischemic contracture: a case report. *Pediatric Dermatology*, Vol.25, No.3 (May-June 2008), pp. 352-354

Ramos, C, Whyte, CM & Harris, BH. (2006). Nontraumatic compartment syndrome of the extremities in children. *Journal of Pediatric Surgery*, Vol.41, pp. E5-E7, DOI:10.1016/j.jpedsurg.2006.08.042

Rubel, IF, Carrer, A, Gilles, JJ, Howard, R & Cohen G. (2008). Progressive Gorham disease of the forearm. *Orthopedics*, Vol.31, No.3 (March 2008), 284.

Sawyer, JR, Kellum, EL, Creek, AT & Wood, GW III. (2010). Acute compartment syndrome of the hand after a wasp sting: a case report. *Journal of Pediatric Orthpaedics B*, Vol.19, No.1, pp. 82-85, DOI: 10.1097/BPB.0b013e32832d83f7

Schnall, SB, Vowels, J, Schwinn, CP & Wong, D. (1993). Disappearing bone disease of the upper extremity. *Orthop Rev*, Vol.22, No.3 (May 1993), pp. 617-620

Shield, WC jr. Reflex Sympathetic Dystrophy Syndrome, In: *Medicinenet*, accessed 23/07/2011, Available from: http://www.medinet.com/reflex_sympathetic_ dystrophy_ syndrome/article.htm

Shin, AY, Chambers, H, Wilkins, KE & Buckwell A. (1996). Suction injuries in children leading to acute compartment syndrome of the interossesous muscles of the hand: case reports. *J Hand Surgery A*, Vol.21, pp. 675-678

Stott, NS, Zionts, LE, Holtom, PD & Patzakis, MJ. (1997). Acute Hematogenous Osteomyelitis. An Unusual Cause of Compartment Syndrome in a Child. *Clinical* Orthopaedics *And Related Research*, No.317, pp. 219-222

Tachi, M, Hirabayashi, S & Kuroda, E. (2001). Unusual development of acute compartment syndrome caused by a suction injury: a case report. *Scandinavian Journal of Plastic & Reconstructive Surgery & Hand Surgery*, Vol.35, No.3 (Sept 2001), pp. 329-330

Willy, Ch. (Ed.). (2005). *Die Vakuumtherapie: Grundlagen, Indikationen, Fallbeispiele, praktische Tipps*. Kösel Verlag

Wright, E. (2009). Neurovascular impairment and compartment syndrome. Paediatric Nursing, Vol. 21, No.3 April 2009), pp. 26-29

Yang, J & Cooper, MG. (2010). Compartment syndrome and patient controlled analgesia in children - analgesic complication or early warning system. *Anaesthesia & Intensive Care*, Vol.38, No.2 (March 2010), pp. 359-363

Yuan, PS, Pring, ME, Gaynor, TP, Mubarak SJ & Newton PO. (2004). Compartment syndrome following intramedullary fixation of pediatric forearm fractures. *Journal of Pediatric Orthopedics*, Vol.24, No.4 (Jul-Aug 2004), pp. 370-375

Zhixin, Z, Yuehai, P, Laijin, L & Lei, Ch. (2010). Diagnosis and Treatment of the Deeper Compartment Syndrome of Forearm After Bone Fracture, In: *Hand Surgery 2010 IFSSH*, Chung, MS & BAEK, GH, pp. 306-307, HS Gong Konnja Publishing, ISBN 978-89-6278-331-5, Seoul, Korea

Part 3

Hip

6

The Genotoxic Potential of Novel Materials Used in Modern Hip Replacements for Young Patients

Aikaterini Tsaousi
University of Bristol
United Kingdom

1. Introduction

Total hip replacement (THR), one of the most successful and cost effective surgical interventions introduced in the last 50 or so years in medicine and the second most common elective operation in the UK (Sheldon et al., 1996, Garellick et al., 1998), owes most of its success to the introduction of hard-on-soft arthroplasty by Charnley. Arthroplasty (from the Greek 'arthrosis' = 'joint' and '-plasty' = 'the making of') describes the surgical reconstruction or replacement of a malformed, degenerated or traumatised joint. THR is the treatment of choice for conditions that affect both the articular surfaces (i.e. acetabulum and femur) of the hip joint. Worldwide, approximately one million artificial hips are implanted annually (Smith & Learmonth, 1996). Problems with polyethylene (PE) wear debris from soft-on-hard articulations (causing an infiltration of macrophages, eventually leading to destruction of bone and soft tissue and initiating loosening of the implant) led to the development of hard-on-hard bearing combinations for artificial hips as the latter produce minimal wear and therefore implant failure is delayed.

Until recently, THRs have been reserved primarily for the elderly and with relatively short post-operative life expectancies there was no need for studies investigating the long term effects, since on average, prosthetic joints are relatively trouble-free for 10-15 years (Havelin et al., 2000). However, due to their success, a greater number of THRs are nowadays performed on increasingly younger, more active patients. In England a substantial proportion of THR patients (>12%, i.e. >10.000 individuals yearly) are below 60 (NHS, 2006). Bearing in mind that the use of artificial hips is more rigorous in younger patients and that life expectancy continues to increase, it is time that the question of possible adverse long term effects following implantation needs to be addressed. Most importantly, concerns for potential carcinogenicity of THRs is reasonable to be raised, since both soluble and particulate wear debris originating from the prostheses are biopersistant and are found systemically in the human body following the operation. In this chapter I discuss the proposed links between hip replacements and carcinogenesis to date by summarizing the relevant literature while presenting important background information regarding THRs, the generation of wear debris from hip prostheses, its biopersistence and the extent of its dissemination in the human body. This review is mainly focused on materials currently being used as bearing surfaces in artificial hips for younger patients.

2. Basic anatomy of the hip joint and indications for THR therapy

The hip joint is a multiaxial ball and socket synovial joint formed between the spherical head of the femur and the hollow cup-shaped acetabulum of the pelvis, which in turn forms at the union of 3 pelvic bones (the ileum, ischium and pubis). The depth of the acetabulum is increased by a fibro-cartilaginous rim (labrum) which grips the head of the femur and secures it in the joint. The head of the femur is attached to the femur by a thin neck region. Both joint surfaces are covered with a strong layer of articular hyaline cartilage, except for a small area in the head of the femur, the fovea or pit, from which an intracapsular ligament attaches directly to the acetabulum. A strong fibrous capsule is attached to the rim of the articular cartilage, enclosing the joint cavity. Thickened strands of this capsule form ligaments which support the joint. The whole joint cavity is lined by a membrane, the synovium, the cells of which secrete an oily fluid that lubricates the articulating surfaces and allows smooth movement of the ball within the socket. A network of blood vessels, lymph vessels and nerves is also present (Standring, 2004). The hip joint(s) form the primary connection between the lower limb(s) and the axial skeleton of the trunk and pelvis. Its primary function is to support the weight of the body in both static (e.g. standing) and dynamic (e.g. walking or running) postures. Its strong but loose fibrous capsule permits a large range of movement (second only to the shoulder).

Joint injuries are caused either by trauma or by gradual wear and tear due to aging and/or congenital predisposing factors. The hip joint frequently succumbs to degenerative and inflammatory diseases causing severe pain and stiffness, e.g. osteoarthritis and rheumatoid arthritis. Osteoarthritis, the most common form of chronic joint disease, results primarily from destruction and/or degeneration of the cartilage at the articular surfaces with age. In younger people, it may be the result of congenital dysplasia and/or dislocation, damage caused by fracture, previous inflammation etc. In fact, any situation which puts an unusual stress on the joint(s) can predispose to osteoarthritis (Flugsrud et al., 2002). Rheumatoid arthritis is an inflammatory disease of the connective tissue. It is more common in women and presents mainly between the ages of 25 and 55. Affected joints become swollen and tender due to inflammation of the synovium and escape of synovial fluid into the joint cavity. Although the disease often burns itself out in time, damaged joints continue to disintegrate, causing severe pain and stiffness. Hip joint fractures can occur at any age although they are more frequent in the elderly as they are closely associated with osteoporosis (i.e. a reduction in bone density due to decreased bone formation and/or increased bone resorption resulting in brittle bones). Osteoporosis' incidence increases with age and is most commonly seen in post-menopausal women but it can also begin very early in life. THR therapy aims to relieve pain and increases the patient's quality of life by comprehensively restoring the structure and function of the hip joint via complete replacement of the head of the femur and the lining of the joint socket on the pelvis with artificial materials (Smith & Learmonth, 1996, Garellick et al., 1998).

3. A brief history of THR and the modern artificial hips – Design & materials

The first recorded THR was performed in 1938 by Philip Wiles, using a total hip made entirely of stainless steel. The acetabular cup was fixed with two screws while the femoral component was secured by a bolt that passed through the neck of the femur (Amstutz &

Grigoris, 1996). The next major development was in 1951; the McKee-Farrar total hip was again made entirely of stainless steel however the stem was fixed using acrylic cement. In the late 1950s McKee and Farrar started operating more frequently with a Cobalt-based alloy (CoCrMo) as the principle bearing material. Various types of prostheses, including the McKee-Farrar, Ring, Stanmore and Muller designs, employed this bearing surface during the 1950s-1960s and it was not until the 1970s that metal-on-metal (MOM) articulation lost favour, mainly due to the successful design of the Charnley artificial hip which completely replaced all the other designs (Charnley, 1972). Accelerated corrosion because of improper selection of materials or faulty fabrication techniques (Jacobs et al., 1998a), and concerns about possible carcinogenesis (Heath et al., 1971), metal sensitivity and high infection rates eventually led to the abandonment of MOM articulation as soon as a better option was available (Amstutz & Grigoris, 1996).

While studying animal joint lubrication, Charnley realized that a cartilage substitute was necessary in order to allow artificial joints to function at the extreme low-friction level, as seen in nature. His innovative design consisted of a metal (hard) femoral component, a plastic (soft) acetabular component and bone cement. In 1958, he replaced an eroded arthritic socket with a thick walled Teflon cup, within which a small femoral head articulated, attached to an acrylic-fixed stem. The small (22.25mm) femoral head chosen was aiming for a decreased wear rate, however it had relatively poor stability (the larger the head of a replacement, the less likely it is to dislocate, but the more wear debris will be produced due to the increased articulating surface area) and failed quickly due to massive inflammation following PE wear production. In 1961, Charnley substituted Teflon with high molecular weight polyethylene (HMWPE) which is 500-1000 times more resistant to wear. In the 1970s, Boutin was the first to introduce alumina ceramic as a bearing surface in orthopaedics (Boutin, 1971). Ceramic-on-ceramic (COC) articulations produced minimal wear however early results were discouraging as these prostheses were very prone to fractures (Boutin et al., 1988). Thus, for over two decades, the Charnley Low Friction Arthroplasty design was the preferred system worldwide, far surpassing the other available options. Thousands of people were successfully relieved from their hip pain and the long-term results became more predictable. John Charnley was knighted for his efforts (Cornell & Ranawat, 1986a, b) and many similar designs (pioneered by Charnley) followed.

The current/modern artificial hips have three parts: (a) a rod or stem, which fits into the femur to provide stability and is usually made from metal (Ti- or CoCr-based alloys) while cement (poly-methyl-methacrylate) is sometimes used to fix it firmly in place; (b) a head or ball, which replaces the spherical head of the femur and is made of either hard, smooth metal (usually CoCr alloy) or ceramic (usually Al_2O_3) and (c) a shell or cup which replaces the faulty hip socket and allows bone to grow onto. Sometimes, a liner is used that locks into the shell and this in turn articulates with the ball. The cup can therefore be made of one or more materials, but the actual articulating surface that touches the ball is commonly made of CoCr-alloy, alumina or ultra high-molecular weight-polyethylene (UHMWPE). Each part is manufactured in various sizes in order to accommodate various body sizes and types. In some designs the stem and ball are one piece whilst other designs are modular, allowing additional customization for a better fit. In the U.S., all implant devices must be approved by the Food & Drugs Authority (FDA) and similar purpose governing bodies exist worldwide. In the U.K. approval must be given by the Medicines & Healthcare products

Regulatory Agency (MHRA) prior to clinical use of any THR implants. It is worth mentioning that an implant device may be approved in one country but not in another; e.g. COC total hips were widely used in Europe before they were made available in the U.S. (see www.mhra.gov.uk and www.fda.gov/Medical Devices).

In summary, finally, surface choices in modern THRs can be divided into hard-on-soft metal-on-polyethylene (MOP) or ceramic-on-polyethylene (COP) and hard-on-hard metal-on-metal (MOM) and ceramic-on-ceramic (COC) bearings.

4. Why do implanted artificial hips fail after all?

The ideal implant should stay in situ and function trouble-free indefinitely or at least for the whole of a patient's life. However, this is not an ideal world and revision operations following THRs are often needed after 10-15 years if not sooner (Jacobs et al., 1998b). So why do hip prostheses fail? Initial acute complications following THRs include improper placement, cement extrusion and dislocation. Although dislocation can also occur as a late complication, it is most common in the immediate postoperative period (Manaster, 1996). Late complications include failure of any of the components of the prosthesis, mechanical (aseptic) loosening, bone fracture, heterotopic ossification (bone formation), loosening following infection and osteolysis (also termed aggressive granulomatosis or debris synovitis) (Tigges et al., 1994). In approximately 20% of patients, the artificial hip becomes loose within 20 years after implantation (Doorn et al., 1996a, Doorn et al., 1996b) while aseptic loosening in THR accounts for approximately 75% of revision procedures (Amstutz et al., 1992). In an early study, Dobbs et al evaluated the survival of THR prostheses by measuring whether they were still in situ; MOM articulations were found to have lower survival rates than MOP ones (53% and 88% respectively); nonetheless, the predominant reason for failure/revision in both cases appeared to be loosening of the prostheses' components and authors blamed wear production for triggering osteolysis (Dobbs, 1980).

Initially termed 'cement disease' (Jones & Hungerford, 1987), osteolysis is now understood to be a biological response to particulate wear debris and may originate at several locations around a THR. Willert was among the first to hypothesize that aseptic loosening of THRs was caused by the local macrophage response to wear debris (Willert, 1977). Goldring et al subsequently described the synovial-like nature of the bone-implant interface in patients with loose THRs and showed that cells within the periprosthetic membrane had the capacity to produce large amounts of several 'bone resorbing factors' (Goldring et al., 1983). Although these initial reports were in cemented implants, similar processes have been identified recently in cementless implants (Ingham & Fisher, 2005). Interestingly, Havelin et al reported a significant increase in the annual number of revision operations in Norway mainly due to an increase of wear debris production and osteolysis without loosening. This finding presents a different situation to what was observed in earlier years, where most prostheses failed after aseptic loosening of their components (Havelin et al., 2000).

Osteolysis remains the main problem of THRs leading to revision surgery and a plethora of research studies have identified the generation of particulate wear debris from the articulating surfaces as a key factor. The amount of wear particles that are generated, their chemical composition, size and shape influence the induction of osteolysis (Meneghini et al., 2005). Micron and submicron wear particles (particularly of PE) have been identified as the main cause of loosening of artificial hips, following osteolysis (Ingham & Fisher, 2000). The current hypothesis is that particulate wear debris released from the prostheses can invoke a biological response in the surrounding tissue. Adjacent to THRs, one can find synovial tissue, fibrous tissue, lymphocytes (occasionally) and foreign-body inflammatory cells (macrophages and giant cells) that are present roughly in proportion to the number of particles surrounding the prosthesis (Schmalzried & Callaghan, 1999). The macrophages appear to be the most relevant and important cells with respect to this biological reaction. As wear particles are released, macrophages ingest them in an attempt to clear them, become stimulated and release cytokines. The inflammatory response is marked by the accumulation of more macrophages at the implant site attracted via released cytokines (Ingham & Fisher, 2005). A chain of cytochemical events leads to the production of foreign body giant cells that release chemical mediators able to activate osteoclasts (Wang et al., 1997). During osteolysis, the activated osteoclasts resorb bone, with subsequent loss of integrity of the implant-bone interface, resulting in loosening of the implant and/or cyst formation and finally implant failure (Archibeck et al., 2000, Horowitz et al., 1993, Schmalzried et al., 1992, Wang et al., 1997). The number and the size of the wear particles appear to be the most important factors in determining the potential to elicit a biological response (Ingham & Fisher, 2000, 2005). Importantly, aseptic loosening and/or osteolysis requiring revision have also been reported for hard-on-hard, minimally wearing THRs using MOM and COC bearings (Harris, 1994, Yoon et al., 1998).

5. Modes of wear and the generation of different types of wear debris from hip prostheses

Wear is the removal of material that occurs as a result of the motion between two opposing surfaces, under load (Schmalzried & Callaghan, 1999). In THRs, these can be either the primary bearing surfaces of an articulating couple or secondary surfaces. The conditions under which the prosthesis was functioning when the wear occurred have been termed the wear modes. Mode 1 wear results from the motion of two primary bearing surfaces against each other, as intended; this is unavoidable. Mode 2 wear results from a primary bearing surface moving against a secondary surface that it was not intended to come in contact with (e.g. when a femoral head penetrates a modular PE liner and articulates with its metal backing). Mode 3 wear results from primary surfaces sliding against each other but with third body particles interposed (thus the contaminant particles directly abrade one or both of the primary surfaces which are in turn transiently or permanently roughened, leading to a higher mode 1 wear rate). Mode 4 wear results from rubbing together two secondary surfaces (e.g. a liner with a backing) and particulate debris generated this way can migrate to the primary bearing surfaces leading to third body wear.

There are four fundamental mechanisms through which wear debris can be generated: adhesion, abrasion, corrosion and fatigue. Adhesion involves the bonding of opposing surfaces when they are pressed together under load. Adhesive wear occurs when fragments usually from the weaker of two relatively smooth bearing surfaces break off and adhere to the opposing surface. A so-called transfer film may be formed, whose disruption and reformation may lead to extreme fluctuations in wear rate (McKellop et al., 1981). Abrasion is the mechanical process of surface grinding that takes place as a result of friction. Abrasive wear occurs when asperities found on a relatively hard articulating surface cut and plough through a softer/smoother surface during the sliding motion, forming a series of grooves in the smoother surface. This results in the removal of material. The same process can also take place when other wear particles (e.g. cement), generated elsewhere, are caught between two bearing surfaces and exacerbate the wear process by scratching and scoring them; wear produced this way is called 'third body' (Sedel, 1992, Hamadouche et al., 2002). Corrosion is the deterioration of essential properties in a material due to reactions with its surroundings. There are several types of corrosive processes and corrosive wear can occur in the presence of a 'hostile' environment such as the human body. Regarding bearing surfaces, corrosion products can form a passivation layer which is continuously worn away by the sliding action of the articulating surfaces; thus corrosion can progress further generating both soluble and particulate wear debris. Fatigue arises when local stresses exceed the fatigue strength of a material, leading to its failure after a certain number of loading cycles and the release of wear debris from its surface and/or its fracture. In articulating surfaces, fatigue wear occurs during repeated sliding or rolling over the same area, in the presence of local surface features or bearing pair incongruities (i.e. unmatches). This produces accumulations of concentrated local cyclic stresses which exceed the fatigue limit of either material in the wear couple. Such concentrated cyclic surface loading leads to the formation of surface and subsurface cracks which can lead to surface break-up and the release of large fragments (Schmalzried & Callaghan, 1999).

Notably, deformation of any of the bearing surfaces is expected to result in increased (Mode 1) wear. Acetabular (component) deformation can be observed as a consequence of the press-fit technique, which is employed to fix equatorial over-sized implant cups in place without cement (Squire et al., 2006). As completely spherical cups have a considerable risk of being pushed out of the acetabulum due to the so called 'rebound effect' (combination of strong forces all around the cup), over-sizing cups around their equator allows a more reliable fixation by compression forces only. Nonetheless, cup deformation could adversely affect the bearing clearance (Springer et al., 2011) and thus the fluid film lubrication of MOM bearings, possibly leading to increased adhesive and/or abrasive wear. Deformation has also been implicated during difficult intra operative assembly of COC bearings (Langdown et al., 2007).

In general, one can discriminate between particulate and soluble wear debris. Evidently, particulate wear debris can be produced by any of the above described wear mechanisms while soluble wear can occur only by the corrosive wear mechanism and basically consist of soluble ionic forms of metals, either from the implant surface itself or from the surface of released wear particles. Particulate corrosion debris is also generated by an electrochemical process in which metal ions released from an implant surface subsequently form metal salt precipitates. Such corrosion products may be generated from any metal surface but most commonly originate from MOM modular interfaces (Urban et al., 2004). Importantly, the generation of wear debris in a prosthetic hip from different mechanisms (described above) can occur either simultaneously or at different times over the lifetime of the prosthesis.

6. Wear rates and the choice of modern bearings for young patients

In vivo measurements from tissue retrieval studies often report on the amount of the prostheses debris produced (either particle mass or particle number) per gram of dried tissue. Such investigations have shown that the number of wear particles surrounding THRs can range from 8.5×10^{8} to 5.7×10^{11} per gram of dry tissue (Hirakawa et al., 1996). However, given that the concentration of wear debris decreases with increasing distance from the bearing surfaces and that a great amount of wear particles may not stay adjacent to the prostheses but rather be carried to very distant sites (see section 7), the adequacy of such measurements for the calculation of wear rates in vivo is questionable. Wear rates in vivo can be perhaps more adequately calculated using measurements of linear or volumetric wear from retrieved implants. Linear wear is reported in length units and values represent the depth of several ridges found on randomly chosen sample areas from the surface of retrieved components. Volumetric wear can be calculated from numerous linear wear measurements, using certain equations/formulas and assuming that the femoral ball (or acetabular lining) is originally a perfect sphere with a radius to best fit non-worn regions of each component (McKellop et al., 1996).

In vitro hip simulator studies report wear rates per million cycles (Mc), since 1 Mc is thought to correspond to an implant's moderate use for a year. In fact, such studies could be considered more accurate, since wear debris can in fact be collected. Wear can also be presented as weight loss and then converted to volumetric wear using the alloy's density. However, questions have arisen as to the correspondence between the wear particles generated in vitro and those observed clinically in vivo (Savio et al., 1994). Nevertheless, hip simulator studies have proven particularly useful in identifying the wear pattern/profile of total hip systems; thus such studies have shown that unlike MOP systems which show linear ratios of wear over time, modern MOM prostheses have an early high wear ratio phase (run-in) followed by a lower wear ratio phase (steady-state) (Anissian et al., 2001). The same biphasic profile is observed also with modern COC articulations (Hatton et al., 2002) and it is speculated that the initial wear phase is due to a polishing effect resulting from the motion of the head against the cup (Mode 1 wear) while the following phase is mostly due to third body wear. Hard-on-soft Charnley type couples like MOP have a single, constant rate of wear production since there is no 'polishing effect' i.e. it is the soft lining of the cup that always wears out.

PE wear rates from MOP articulations reported both in vivo and in vitro range in general from 30-100mm^3 per year. In the U.S., COP is the most common alternative bearing combination used in THR patients as it has been shown to reduce wear rates when compared with conventional MOP by 10% to 50% for periods exceeding 10 years (Jazrawi et al., 1998). However, other studies have not reported significant differences between MOP and COP wear rates (Schmalzried et al., 1998). Anissian et al calculated the run-in and steady-state wear rates of modern MOM articulations to be 2.22mm^3/Mc and 1.0mm^3/Mc, respectively. However, higher wear rates have been estimated from in vivo studies. McKellop et al concluded that the long term maximum wear rates of any design could be approximately 6μm per year - corresponding to a maximum mean volumetric wear of 6mm^3 metal particles per year (McKellop et al., 1996). One reason for the differences observed between in vivo and in vitro reported wear rates could be the nature of the lubricant used in simulators. The tribologic performance of a joint largely depends on the existence of a fluid (lubricant) film and the amount of coverage it confers to its surfaces and lubrication has a major influence on the amount of abrasive and especially adhesive wear (Walker, 1971). Another confounding variable appears to be the presence of surface coatings, which have been reported on both ceramic and metallic implants (Streicher et al., 1996, Lu & McKellop,

1997). It may be that the bearing surfaces in a hip simulator are actually articulating on such (smoother) coatings instead of the implant surfaces. Using low protein serum as a synovial fluid substitute, adding EDTA to reduce protein precipitates and running simulator tests at speeds that prevent heat generation are some of the modifications thought to result in decreased coating phenomena (Medley et al., 1996). Chan et al concluded that low surface roughness and small clearance between the head and cup are necessary for adequate fluid film lubrication and therefore for less wear production to occur; they suggested that if these parameters are optimal, all other engineering and manufacturing factors do not have a significant effect on the production of wear debris. Their simulator tests also showed that the volumetric wear of MOM articulation is 2000 times smaller than that of MOP articulation (Chan et al., 1999).

In more recent hip simulator studies a technique called microseparation is employed, where the ball and socket separate slightly during the swing phase of gait, to produce (higher) wear rates that are more relevant clinically (i.e. are similar to the ones reported in vivo). It has been proposed that microseparation could occur in any hip prosthesis and it may be involved in the initiation of 'stripe' wear, a small band of wear observed to occur around the rim of acetabular cups in retrieved COC hip prostheses (Mittelmeier & Heisel, 1992). Neck and socket impingement is another way of generating stripe wear (Nizard et al., 1992). Nevelos et al, by introducing microseparation of the COC prostheses, reproduced for the first time clinically relevant wear rates (typically 1-5mm^3 per annum), wear patterns and mechanisms (Nevelos et al., 1999). Other microseparation studies reported wear rates of 1-2mm^3/Mc (1.24mm^3/Mc for modern prostheses and 1.74m m^3/Mc for the first generation ones). The wear stripe often seen clinically on the femoral head was reproduced on both prosthesis types. The degree of rim contact depended on clearance and the authors postulated that clinically, microseparation may depend on factors like components' alignment, position, soft tissue tension and muscle forces. Interestingly, two size-ranges of particles were found under in vitro microseparation testing: small (nanometre scale) and large (micrometre scale) particles (Tipper et al., 2002). Nanometre sized ceramic wear particles were first described in periprosthetic tissues in a study that also revealed a bimodal size distribution of alumina ceramic particles in vivo (Hatton et al., 2002).

According to the above, it is evident that hard-on-soft Charnley type bearings demonstrate more wear for the same time period than hard-on-hard bearings (MOM and COC) as predicted, but are less susceptible to catastrophic failure. Modern hard-on-hard surfaces are mainly only sensitive to failure due to surgical technique (e.g. fixation, component positioning). Artificial hips that produce little wear are thought to be more durable and have a lesser risk for osteolysis, loosening and revision; hence, given a correct surgical implantation technique, modern hard-on-hard bearings are the preferred choice for younger, more active patients who have good quality bone tissue (Figure 1). Judging by wear debris production rate alone, ceramics provide the most desirable bearing surfaces (Savio et al., 1994) with alumina COC THRs having the lowest wear rates of any bearing surface combinations (Boutin et al., 1988). It has been calculated that the debris produced from an alumina-alumina THR where the femoral head is not too small, no stress risers occur from implantation, the acetabular cup is aligned properly, and an adequate clearance is maintained between the ceramic components may be as little as 1/4000 that of an equivalent MOP design (Sedel, 1992, Hamadouche & Sedel, 2000, Hamadouche et al., 2002).

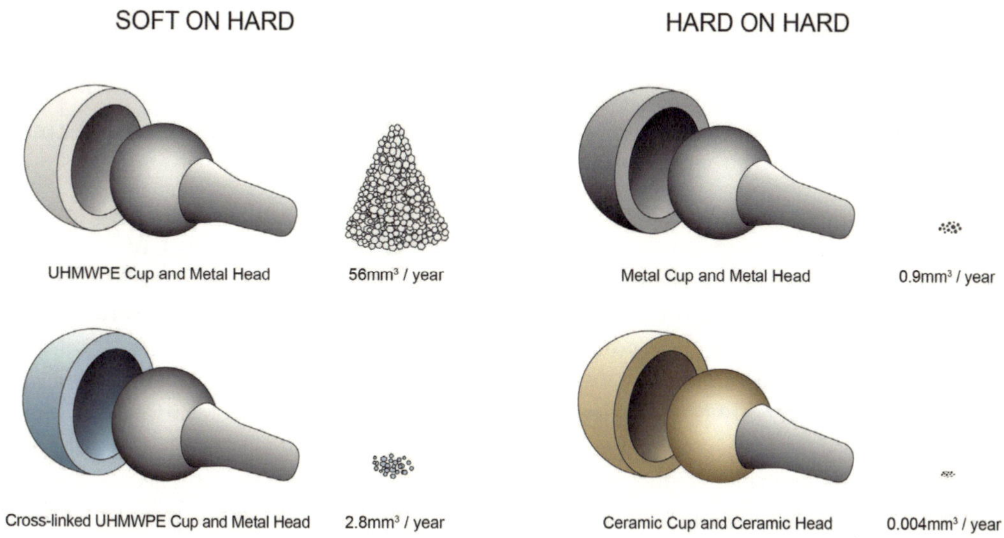

Fig. 1. Volumetric wear rates (estimates) of modern THR cup and head combinations. Data taken from Heisel et al., 2004.

Savio et al reviewed and compared descriptions of wear debris from many in vivo (revisions, autopsies) and in vitro (hip simulators) sources. The authors concluded that the type (composition) of THR materials plays a critical role in regards to the size, shape, volume and number of particles that are produced both in vivo and in vitro. More specifically, they hypothesised that the size of wear particles (minimum wear diameter) should be inversely proportional to a material's modulus of elasticity (i.e. its hardness) and they have consequently predicted that ceramic wear particles should be the smallest, polymeric ones the largest and metallic ones of an intermediate size (Savio et al., 1994). Simulator tests (Chan et al., 1999) support the above hypothesis and so do analyses of particles that are produced in vivo (Doorn et al., 1998). Nonetheless, hard-on-hard bearings, although producing far smaller volumes of wear than conventional Charnley type couples, may produce a similar active total surface area of debris. The very small (nanometre) size of metallic debris released by MOM bearings (Archibeck et al., 2000), combined with the fact that the bioavailability of metal is thought to be a function of the total surface area of the released debris rather than on its volume or weight (Shanbhag et al., 1997), casts doubt on the supposition that the net adverse biologic response will be reduced by modern MOM designs even though the volumetric wear is reduced. COC articulations are also reported to release nanometre sized particles (Hatton et al., 2002).

In addition to abrasive, adhesive and surface fatigue wear, metal alloys may suffer from corrosion. Corrosion can affect the whole surface of the implant or just a specific region (e.g. could be confined to an area of wear from mechanical stress). It is estimated that 30μg of metal ions (i.e. soluble wear) may be released from a prosthetic hip each day (Hennig et al., 1992, Merritt & Brown, 1996). Ions are shown to react with other molecules forming several types of particulate corrosion wear. Jacobs et al analysed particulate corrosion products from retrieved implants and surrounding tissues. Particles of metal oxides, metal chlorides, and chromium phosphate corrosion products were identified on implants of 10 designs from 6 manufacturers. The most abundant solid corrosion product was an amorphous chromium orthophosphate hydrate-rich material (Jacobs et al., 1995).

7. Dissemination and biopersistance of wear debris from implanted artificial hips

As mentioned, wear debris can be both soluble (ions) and particulate. Ions may only be formed from metal components of artificial hips as they are the result of corrosion. Importantly, even in COC articulations, the stem is usually made of metal (Co-based or Ti-based alloy) and therefore, the existence of corrosion wear (both soluble and particulate) is applicable to all modern prostheses. Ions may stay bound to local tissue or bind to protein moieties that are transported via the bloodstream and lymphatics to remote organs. In an early post-mortem study, an increase in the concentrations of Co and Cr in remote tissues (liver and spleen) of a patient with bilateral Co-based alloy total hip components was reported; interestingly, Cr was found in a higher level than Co (Dobbs & Minski, 1980). Michel et al also reported on two post-mortem specimens with CoCr alloy components: in both cases high levels of Co and Cr were detected in adjacent tissues while a wide systemic effect was observed with increased concentrations of Co found in the heart, liver, spleen and lymphatic tissue and of Cr in the aorta, heart, liver, pancreas and spleen (Michel et al., 1991).

Elevated levels of Co and Cr ions in the serum, blood and/or urine of patients have been reported numerous times following both MOP and MOM THRs. In an early cohort study Black et al showed that Cr levels increased significantly (peaked) immediately after primary THRs; this peak was reduced six months post-operatively but it did not fall below control levels (Black et al., 1983). After a similar study, Sunderman et al suggested that a substantial increase of serum and urine Co levels seen in two patients was associated with loosening of their prosthesis (Sunderman et al., 1989). In a later retrospective study whole blood and serum were analysed from CoCr alloy MOP THR patients who had their artificial hips in place for up to 18 years. None of the devices were loose and no increase in the serum levels of Cr was documented, however, in 4 patients massive Co enrichments were seen as a consequence of implant corrosion while the levels of Co in the serum were significantly higher than controls up to more than 10 years postoperatively; moreover, significant Co and Cr enrichment was seen in several tissues and organs (Michel et al., 1991). Not surprisingly, joint failure can result in large increases in the amount of soluble metal ions detected in urine and/or blood (Jacobs et al., 1998a). According to Schaffer et al the levels of both Co and Cr in blood and urine increase continuously; at 2-3 years post-operatively more than a quarter of the patients retrospectively studied exceeded German occupational exposure limits (Schaffer et al., 1999). A more recent study showed a steady increase in both metal elements for up to 2-3 years postoperatively, depending on the type/brand of metal alloy, while subsequently metal levels declined although still remaining markedly above control levels (i.e. immediately after the operation). Thus, it has been proposed that the rises and declines of metal levels over time are the result of biomechanical influences on the implant's tribology (Lhotka et al., 2003). Simulation experiments support this view, since the pattern of metal levels observed in the blood and urine of MOM patients correlate with the (biphasic) wear pattern of the prosthesis per se (Anissian et al., 2001).

Importantly, Jacobs et al reported that younger patients had significantly higher levels of systemic metal release than older patients and postulated a more active lifestyle as the underlying factor (Jacobs et al., 1998a). A recent study by Dunstan et al in young (mean age 45 years) patients supports this view; moreover, it shows that MOM articulations released significantly higher levels of Co and Cr when compared to MOP ones while further elevation of metal levels was observed in patients with loose MOM THRs (Dunstan et al., 2005). Several in vivo and simulator studies have presented evidence that higher patient activity has as a result higher wear rates. Hence, it has been proposed that wear is a function of use, not time (Schmalzried et al., 2000). The case of a long distance runner with a MOM artificial hip supports this view: Metal (Co) levels in his blood were increased following completion of a marathon run and returned back to baseline levels 4 weeks later (Brodner et al., 2003). A contradictory study, after monitoring 7 recipients of well functioning MOM hips during a 2 week long physical activity challenge, suggested that serum metal levels are not affected by patient activity; therefore periodic measurements of serum ion levels could be used to monitor the tribologic (lubrication, friction, and wear) performance of MOM bearings without adjusting for patient activity (Heisel et al., 2005). However, the low number of participants, the use of only one external control and the fact that patients were not monitored past this period of physical exercise coupled with the existence of other contradictory reports (e.g. the case of the marathon runner) show that a correlation between MOM patient activity and systemic metal release can neither be proven nor excluded. When Jacobs et al explored the prospects for using blood, serum and/or urine metal levels to monitor the performance of MOM THRs, they concluded that it would be premature to recommend metal concentration analysis on a routine clinical basis since interpretation of values requires an extensive database with correlative clinical information (Jacobs et al., 2004). In summary, leaching of soluble wear (metal ions) following primary THR is not an occurrence of merely local significance, but one that affects the trace element status of the entire organism and over extended periods of time.

Particulate wear from artificial hip joints is also shown to be biopersistant and capable of systemic dissemination. Particulate corrosion debris (metal precipitates) from modular MOM junctions have been found locally and in sites remote from the hip (Urban et al., 1994). Cr phosphate particles have been found in the liver, spleen and para-aortic lymph nodes of patients with corroded but otherwise successful THRs (Jacobs et al., 1995). In a post-mortem study, Case et al reported an accumulation of wear particles in periprosthetic tissues and a systemic dissemination of huge numbers of sub-microscopic metal particles within the bone marrow, the local and distal lymph nodes, the liver and the spleen; in one case even in the frontal cortex of the brain. Interestingly, PE debris was not detected in these remote sites, despite its usual abundance in periprosthetic tissues, while the levels of metal were higher in the subjects that had a loose, worn implant (Case et al., 1994). A major parameter affecting the dissemination of particles in various tissues is their size; while bigger particles stay close to the periprosthetic tissues, smaller particles can travel further (Savio et al., 1994). Dissemination of THR metallic wear particles to the liver, spleen and abdominal lymph nodes was identified in other later studies (Shea et al., 1997, Urban et al., 2000). A recent post-mortem analysis showed that metallic particles were present in the liver and spleen of 73% of patients with a prior failure and revision of their THR. Particles generated by previous component failures were present in the liver or spleen a decade or more later and suggesting that particle deposition in the organs is cumulative (Urban et al., 2004).

The dissemination properties and systemic effects of ceramic wear debris remain unknown. Because ceramics are insoluble in biological media (i.e. there is no production of ions/corrosion products at physiological pH), biocompatibility concerns do not relate to soluble wear debris. Although there are no reports of systemic dissemination of ceramic particles, ceramic particles have been observed in periprosthetic tissues (Savio et al., 1994). Similarities of their pale colour to the normal colour of tissues may mean that dissemination of particles to distant sites is harder to identify in the case of ceramics. The low wear rates and the very recent clinical use of COC articulations might also explain the absence of such reports. Based on reports on their observed size and shape however, there is no reason to believe that ceramic particles could not systemically disseminate and accumulate with time in various parts of our bodies, just as metal particles do.

8. Proposed links between total hip replacements and cancer

Given that wear debris from THR implants can disseminate (locally and systemically) and are biopersistant (mainly particulates), their carcinogenic potential is a real concern; especially as their use in younger patients, who may have a post-operative life expectancy of more than 30 years, is constantly increasing. Hard-on-hard bearings (i.e. MOM and COC) are usually the preferable option for such patients because they have been shown to generate less wear debris compared to conventional Charnley-type prostheses and are therefore thought to have less of a risk for early implant failure. But even for successful, durable THRs with minimal wear rates, the production and accumulation of wear debris over time cannot be avoided; and notably the use of a THR implant will inevitably be more rigorous and last longer in younger patients. The International Agency for Research on Cancer (IARC), a body within the World Health Organization (WHO) responsible for evaluating carcinogenic risks to humans, in a recent evaluation of surgical implants and other foreign bodies implanted (WHO, 1999) categorized all foreign bodies of Co-based, Cr-based and Ti-based alloys in Group 3, i.e. 'not classifiable as to their carcinogenicity to humans'. Ceramic implants were also under the same group.

8.1 Case reports, human cohort and epidemiology studies

There are relatively few reports of malignant tumours associated with total joint replacement (TJR) in humans, but the number of cases is increasing. Early published reports included cases of malignant soft tissue tumours such as chondrosarcoma, malignant fibrous histiocytoma, rhabdomyosarcoma, osteosarcoma and haemangio-endothelioma associated with joint replacement surgery (Swann, 1984, Jacobs et al., 1992). These have led to calls for the establishment of a central registry for implant related tumours (Apley, 1989). In 1992, the editor of a well established orthopaedic journal wrote 'the 24 tumours thus far made public show no pattern in their histological type or in the timing of their appearance'. Nonetheless, he mentioned the importance of concerted efforts under way to accumulate cases of malignant neoplasms associated with TJRs, so as to better define the risks prospectively (Goodfellow, 1992).

During the past 30 years there have been sporadic case reports documenting the development of malignant neoplasms adjacent/proximate to artificial hips. Jacobs et al listed 18 reported cases in which malignancy was associated with MOM THRs. In most cases, malignant fibrous histiocytomas were reported at or near the femoral bone. The rest of the cases included osteosarcomas, fibrosarcomas or epitheloid sarcomas (Jacobs et al., 1992). Five years later, Cole et al listed 23 hip implant related tumours; malignant fibrous histiocytoma in ten patients and osteosarcomas in four while malignant epithelioid hemangio-endothelioma, chondrosarcoma, fibrosarcoma, synovial sarcoma, spindle-cell sarcoma, epithelioid sarcoma and an adenocarcinoma had each been reported once. Interestingly, only in two of these cases the acetabulum was the primary tumour site (Cole et al., 1997). A relatively large number of case reports have described neoplasms originating from bone or soft connective tissue in the region of metal implants. However, a recent analytical study did not report an increased risk of soft-tissue sarcoma after metal implants (Adams et al., 2003). Notably, the study compared the incidence of soft-tissue sarcoma after metal implantation to the general population's incidence of soft-tissue sarcomas, regardless of their presentation site. The results could possibly be much different if the comparison was made to the general population's incidence of soft-tissue sarcomas solely at the hip region. There are few well documented cases of malignant lymphoma following THR surgery. Radhi et al reported the only case of soft tissue lymphoma in the quadriceps muscle overlying an implanted hip 4 years postoperatively (Radhi et al., 1998). Ito and Shimizu reported a case of non-Hodgkin's lymphoma expanding from the ischium to involve the acetabular floor of an implanted THR (Ito & Shimizu, 1999). Ganapathi et al reported a B-cell lymphoma at the site of a chronic discharging sinus overlying a femoral periprosthetic fracture; the sinus formed at the time of the primary THR and continued to discharge for 12 years, until the patient died (Ganapathi et al., 2001). Other cases reported have developed after chronic osteomyelitis (Dodion et al., 1982). Lymphomas and other cancers developing at a site of a metallic implant may theoretically result from the carcinogenicity of the metallic alloy, in particular from prostheses made of CoCr. However, there is growing evidence that some soft tissue malignant lymphomas occur after long standing antigenic stimulation in patients with a defective immune system (Radhi et al., 1998). Startlingly, regarding ceramics and carcinogenesis, there has been only one case report on an aggressive soft tissue sarcoma 15 months after implantation of a ceramic Ti-stem COP THR (Schuh et al., 2004). However, this could be due to the fact that COC articulations have only recently been re-introduced for clinical use, therefore there is a limited experience with ceramics in comparison to metals.

It has been suggested that given the small number of reported cases of tumours around THR implants over the vast number of THRs performed, an association between joint replacement and local malignancy may be coincidental (Goodfellow, 1992). However, if one considers that wear debris from hip prostheses do not stay bound to periprosthetic tissues but disseminate throughout the body and accumulate in tissues/organs far from the hip, it is evident that looking for tumours only adjacent to the prostheses to draw conclusions as to the carcinogenicity of THR implants is not enough. To establish whether a link exists between such implants and malignancy, one must look at large scale epidemiology studies. In 1988, Gillespie et al studied more than 1000 patients and acknowledged the incidence of cancer 10 years after total hip replacement. There was a 3-fold increase in the prevalence of leukaemia and lymphomata in patients with Co-alloy THRs along with a puzzling decrease in the incidences of breast and colon cancer. The authors hypothesised that chronic stimulation of the immune system from soluble and particulate wear of metal-on-metal THRs could encourage the emergence of lymphoreticular malignancies but increased immune surveillance could also inhibit the development of certain epithelial cancers (Gillespie et al., 1988). In a follow-up study, Visuri et al reported similar findings (Visuri & Koskenvuo, 1991). A later cohort study (Mathiesen et al., 1995) failed to confirm an increased prevalence of haematological malignancies following THR however, the number of patients followed was small and the post-operative follow up period of the patients was rather short. Nyren et al included a greater number of patients but still failed to link haematological malignancies with MOM implants. Instead, the authors reported a small but significant increase in kidney and prostate cancers in patients with THR (Nyren et al., 1995). A more recent study with over 400 patients, compared the incidence of cancer (9.5 years post-operatively) in patients with MOM or MOP articulations with that of the general population. Supporting Gillespie's puzzling findings, the authors reported that the total cancer incidence in both groups of patients was less than expected in the general population. Nonetheless, a significant increase in the incidence of leukaemia and lymphomas was shown for patients with MOM prosthesis only (Visuri et al., 1996).

In 1996, Gillespie et al presented an overview of the 4 relevant epidemiological studies published before mid 1995 with conflicting results. The results of the two earlier studies (Gillespie et al., 1988, Visuri & Koskenvuo, 1991) suggested a sustained increase in the risk of lymphoma and leukaemia after THR while the results of the two more recent studies (Mathiesen et al., 1995, Nyren et al., 1995) did not confirm this; although in one of them an increased risk was observed in the first year after implantation. The authors mention that 'the heterogeneity may be statistical in origin, but could also have a biologic explanation in the greater proportion of metal on metal prostheses used before 1973 (Gillespie et al., 1996). Gillespie et al had also performed 2 matched cohort studies and a case control study. In conclusion, neither the results of the matched studies of patients (operated on after 1973) nor the results of the latter 2 published epidemiological studies indicated a significantly increased risk of lymphoma or leukaemia following THR. Nonetheless, Gillespie et al tactfully advised that 'if metal on metal articulations were to be reintroduced, careful surveillance would be essential'. As joint replacement surgery is becoming one of the most common surgical procedures, the widespread epidemiological debate on the frequency of haematological malignancies in these patients remains to date.

The IARC has recently reviewed the epidemiological data for the risk of malignancy after THR (McGregor et al., 2000). It was noted that epidemiology studies compared patients with orthopaedic implants with the general population, thus failing to take into consideration several possible confounding factors/variables (e.g. immunosuppressive therapy, prevalence of rheumatoid arthritis). Moreover, the follow up period of most studies was considered to be too short after exposure to investigate the development of cancer, as carcinogens usually have a long latency period (i.e. the time from exposure to a carcinogen until the clinical presentation of a tumour/malignancy). Asbestos particles for example are known to produce cancer between 22 and 37 years after exposure (Barrett, 1994). It was also noted that the mutagenicity and carcinogenicity of biomaterials are influenced by their exact composition, their surface properties, the composition and rate of release of leachable materials, the physical environment and degradation (which may lead to formation of compounds with different mutagenic properties). Therefore, since most epidemiology studies of orthopaedic implants have not taken into account the type of metal alloy used in each case, most of this information was considered inadequate. Unfortunately, no epidemiological data relevant to the carcinogenicity of ceramic implants is available to date. Therefore, orthopaedic implants according to IARC remain non-classifiable (WHO, 1999).

In molecular epidemiology, the occurrence of DNA damage has been explored for its links to the development of cancer. The frequency of cells with structural chromosomal aberrations in peripheral blood lymphocytes is the first genotoxicity biomarker that has shown a clear association with cancer risk. In two separate large (>1500 subjects) cohort studies, the level of chromosomal aberrations in peripheral blood lymphocytes was measured in healthy individuals at the start of the study, and the development of cancer was monitored over several decades. High levels of chromosomal aberrations were clearly associated with increased total cancer incidence in one cohort and increased total cancer mortality in the other cohort, suggesting that DNA lesions responsible for chromosomal aberrations are clearly associated with cancer risk (Hagmar et al., 2004). An important preliminary cohort study by Case et al used blood and bone marrow samples from 71 patients at revision arthroplasty and 30 controls (prior to primary arthroplasty) to test for chromosomal aberrations. Cells adjacent to the prosthesis had a higher chromosomal aberration rate compared to that seen in iliac crest bone marrow cells from the same patients at revision surgery. Both samples taken at revision surgery had higher chromosomal aberration rates than those seen preoperatively in femoral bone marrow cells in controls. The authors also noted the occurrence of clonal expansion of lymphocytes in 2 out of 21 patients studied at revision arthroplasty, which was performed more than 10 years after primary THR (Case et al., 1996). In a follow-up study, Doherty et al used peripheral blood lymphocytes from 31 MOM THR patients presenting at revision and over 30 controls (prior to having a THR) for cytogenetic analysis. They showed that at revision arthroplasty there was a 3-fold increase in aneuploidy and a 2-fold increase in random chromosomal translocations which could not be explained by confounding variables (smoking, gender, age and diagnostic radiographs). Most interestingly, metal alloy specific differences were seen: In the lymphocytes of Ti-alloy prostheses recipients there was a 5-fold increase in aneuploidy but no increase in chromosomal translocations; by contrast, in the lympocytes of CoCr-alloy recipients there was a 2.5 fold increase in aneuploidy and a 3.5 increase in chromosomal translocations. In lymphocytes from patients with stainless steel prostheses there was no increase in either aneuploidy or chromosomal translocations. Therefore, the authors suggested that although chromosomal translocations and aneuploidy can be seen in normal (non-THR) patients and are known to accumulate with time, genetic changes in THR patients may depend on the type of prosthesis (Doherty et al., 2001). Finally, in a more recent prospective study, Ladon et al investigated changes in metal levels and chromosome aberrations in patients within 2 years of receiving MOM THRs. A statistically significant increase of both chromosome translocations and aneuploidy was seen in peripheral blood lymphocytes at 6, 12 and 24 months post-operatively. The changes were generally progressive with time but the change in aneuploidy was much greater than in chromosome translocations. Although there was a significant increase of both Co and Cr ion concentrations, no significant correlations were found between chromosome translocation indices and Co or Cr concentration in whole blood while the clinical consequences of these observed changes remain unknown (Ladon et al., 2004).

8.2 Animal studies

In vivo investigations into the carcinogenicity of orthopaedic implant related materials were undertaken as early as the 1950s, prompted by the clinical observation that workers in nickel and chromate refining/smelting plants had increased risks of nasal and lung tumours. Oppenheimer et al were the first to clearly establish the potential carcinogenicity of implants: they placed various metal foils subcutaneously in rats and observed malignant tumours develop (Oppenheimer et al., 1956). One year later, Heath et al observed rhabdomyosarcomas following intramuscular injection of Co powder in more than half of the rats studied (Heath, 1957). Heath et al also demonstrated the development of sarcomata in rats bearing CoCrMo wear particles from total joint prostheses (Heath et al., 1971). However, tumourigenesis due to CoCrMo could not be confirmed in later studies by Meachim (Meachim et al., 1982).

Swanson et al were the first to test wear debris collected directly from orthopaedic implants. They used simulators to produce Vitallium (CoCrMo) powder, resuspended it in horse serum and injected it into rats; local sarcomas developed in 15 of 41 animals within 4-18 months (Swanson et al., 1973). In 1977, Gaechter et al used intramuscular implantation of solid alloy implants but, after evaluating seven alloys (260 animals in total) for 2 years, failed to demonstrate a carcinogenic hazard. Notably, they recorded 19 malignant sarcomas, all remote from the implantation site (Gaechter et al., 1977). In a follow up study, Memoli et al implanted rats with a variety of alloys in solid rod, powdered and sintered aggregate form and observed the animals (until they died or) for 30 months. A slight increase in sarcomata was noted in rats bearing metal alloy implants with high contents of Co, Cr or Ni and the development of lymphomas with osseous involvement was also more common in these animals. Interestingly, tumours were more commonly seen in rats that received (metal) powders compared to those that received rods or sintered implants (Memoli et al., 1986). Howie et al published a contradictory study on the effects of intra-articular CoCr-alloy wear particles in rats, where they noted no tumours after observing the animals for more than 1 year (Howie & Vernon-Roberts, 1988). Although carcinogenicity of various (mostly metal) implant materials has been documented in several animal studies, a more recent study investigating the carcinogenic effects of intra-articular powder administration of CoCrMo and TiAlV alloys in rats disputed these early findings, suggesting that such particles if carcinogenic are only weakly so (Lewis et al., 1995). The authors used particulate wear debris created in a simulator and observed the animals for 2 years (or until there was evidence of tumours). The negative carcinogenesis results of this study should be interpreted with caution, since the number of animals used per experimental group was low (8-12 rats), and the observation period was rather short. Bouchard et al assessed the carcinogenicity of CoCrMo versus TiAlV implants in a long-term study in rats. Importantly, the existence of implant associated tumours correlated with loose implants; none with well fixed in situ implants. Histologically the tumours were categorized as dermatofibrosarcoma, fibrosarcoma, malignant histiocytoma, lymphoma and osteosarcoma, seen both adjacent to the implantation site and in remote sites - most prevalent in the pituitary and mammary glands. The authors suggested a foreign-body (immunological) reaction as the primary mechanism of carcinogenesis, as a significantly increased accumulation of chronic inflammatory tissues was seen around loose rather than fixed implants (Bouchard et al., 1996). Animal studies using alumina ceramics as implant materials are virtually absent from the literature, however, in one study in rats subcutaneous implantation of discs of aluminium oxide ceramic produced local sarcomas (Kirkpatrick et al., 2000).

There are many limitations as to what extent the carcinogenicity of human THR implants can be evaluated in animal studies. First of all, there are differences in the composition of the materials tested, although this is not surprising given the developments in the production of implants over the years. There are also some differences in the methods of preparation of materials for administration but mainly there is great variation in the proposed routes of administration and the site(s) of implantation. A priori, the intra-articular route of administration seems to be the most appropriate for arthroplasty carcinogenesis models and as early as 1988 intraarticular injections had been proposed as the route of choice for such studies (Howie & Vernon-Roberts, 1988). Furthermore, there is observed variation as to the physical form (foils, solids, particles) of the materials used and an increasing trend to use small particulates rather than solid implants; possibly since the important role of wear particles for implant failure in THR was recognized. Finally, the differences in the periods of time that the animals were observed following implantation and in the number of animals that were used in each case make critical evaluation of such studies difficult. The relevance of animal models for evaluation of THR cancer risk in humans is still questionable, especially as it is well documented that different animals and even strains/species of the same animal have different susceptibility to tumour formation (Gibb, 1992). Several calls and recommendations for the 'standardization' of animal carcinogenicity studies have been made (Courtland & William, 1996). Importantly, the IARC recently states 'despite the large number of animal studies, none have proven truly conclusive as to the carcinogenicity of implant materials, resulting only in indefinite statements at best regarding excessive tumour formation in animals exposed to wear debris from orthopaedic implants' (WHO, 1999).

8.3 In vitro studies

A cancerous substance is termed capable of inducing a cancerous phenotype; for in vivo evaluations this means the induction of solid tumours and/or haematological malignancies while in cell culture models scientists look for cancer biomarkers and/or neoplastic transformation. The latter is an attainment of certain heritable characteristics from a cell, such as loss of contact inhibition and continuous growth/division, which can lead to clonal expansion. Neoplastic transformation is often the result of one or more heritable genetic alterations and in fact all recognized carcinogens are also genotoxic. Thus, in vitro testing of potential carcinogens has initially largely relied on the use of several genotoxicity tests (e.g. the Ames test, which measures the ability of a chemical to induce mutations in bacteria). On the other hand, not all acquired genetic alterations lead to neoplastic transformation (i.e. cancerous phenotypes) hence not all mutagens/genotoxins are carcinogens. Concerns for the potential carcinogenicity of THR implants relate mostly to the systemic existence of both soluble and particulate wear debris for long periods of time following implantation. Even for successful THRs the generation of mode 1 wear from the intended ball-on-socket articulation (see section 5) is inevitable and so is its dissemination throughout the body. Currently, due to their low wear rates, the preferred articulating couples for implantation in young patients are MOM (mainly CoCr alloy) and COC (mainly alumina). Unlike ceramics, there is a long clinical experience with metals. However, the genotoxicity of orthopaedic metal alloys has been investigated in-vitro mainly by testing their soluble ions, since until recently it has always being assumed that the effects of metal particles could be attributed solely to their ionic form(s). Lison et al have shown this to be a misjudgement when they showed that Co metal particles induced DNA damage via free radicals by a mechanism which was independent of the existence of soluble Co (II) ions; in fact they proved that Co atoms from the surface of the particle were able to reduce oxygen, thus forming reactive oxygen species (ROS) (Lison et al., 2001). Notably, there are only a few in-vitro studies relevant to the potential carcinogenicity of orthopaedic metals which employed metal particulates rather than their ions.

Particulate corrosion debris from metal bearings includes insoluble metal salts. Patierno et al actually indicated that the water-insoluble (particulate) Cr VI salts are more potent carcinogens than the water soluble ones, since only the particulate Cr (VI) compounds induced neoplastic transformation of mouse embryo cells (Patierno et al., 1988). In later studies, Wise et al used chromosome damage as a measurable genotoxic endpoint to study the genotoxicity of both particulate and soluble Cr (VI) in primary human bronchial fibroblasts at concentrations of low, medium and high toxicity. The scientists used lead chromate ($PbCrO_4$) and sodium chromate (Na_2CrO_4) as prototypical particulate and soluble Cr VI salts, respectively, to show that the amount of chromosomal damage increased with increasing concentrations after 24h to both compounds (and so did the cytotoxicity levels) (Wise et al., 2002). Other studies have showed that metallic Co particles were able to induce DNA breaks and micronuclei in human peripheral lymphocytes in a dose dependent manner (Anard et al., 1997, Van Goethem et al., 1997). De Boeck et al showed that despite a relatively large interexperimental and interdonor variability, the DNA-damaging potential of the Co-tungsten carbide mixture was higher than that of Co metal and Co chloride which had comparable responses (De Boeck et al., 2003). Metallic Co and its compounds without tungsten carbide are classified by the IARC as being 'possibly carcinogenic to humans' (WHO, 1991) while Co metal containing tungsten carbide was recently classified as 'probably carcinogenic to humans' (WHO, 2006).

Perhaps the most relevant study to the potential carcinogenicity of CoCr-alloy wear debris was performed by Davies et al; using primary human fibroblasts as a cell culture model the authors reported on metal-specific differences in the level/types of DNA damage induced by synovial fluid retrieved at revision surgery from 24 patients. Synovial fluid taken during revision surgery from all 6 samples from CoCr MOM prostheses and 4 of 6 samples from CoCr MOP prostheses, but none of 6 samples from stainless steel MOP prostheses caused significant DNA damage. Particulate-free samples of phosphate buffered saline where CoCr alloy was left to corrode also caused DNA damage and the authors suggested that this depended mainly on a synergistic effect between the Co and Cr ions produced by corrosion (Davies et al., 2005). Notably, the retrieved synovial fluid is thought to contain both soluble and particulate CoCr-alloy wear debris. Studies from our group have shown that CoCr alloy particles cause genotoxic damage in primary human fibroblasts while factors such as particle size and cell age may influence the genotoxic outcomes (Papageorgiou et al., 2007a, Papageorgiou et al., 2007b). There is a lack of in vitro carcinogenicity and/or genotoxicity studies for particulate alumina. Alumina's biocompatibility has been evaluated by Takami et al using the Ames test in bacteria; no mutagenic activity was observed in 5 tester strains of Salmonella typhimurium. In addition, no cytotoxicity was observed in mouse fibroblast cells following incubation with Al_2O_3 disks in cultures for up to 48 hours (Takami et al., 1997).

However, a more relevant study by Dopp et al reported that alumina ceramic fibres were genotoxic to human amniotic fluid cells causing both numerical and structural chromosomal aberrations (Dopp et al., 1997). More recently, our group has shown that alumina particles can be genotoxic to human cells in vitro (Tsaousi et al., 2010).

The cellular mechanisms of carcinogenesis have been the subject of a vast amount of in vitro studies in the field of cancer research. Such studies have elucidated the cause-effect links for most of the recognized human carcinogens. Interestingly, out of all listed carcinogens to date (according to the IARC), asbestos is the only substance of a 'particulate' nature. Studies investigating the effects of particulate matter in relation to lung cancer have shown that the carcinogenicity of particles and/or fibres follows different rules to chemical carcinogenesis. Particles and fibres form a rather specific group among all toxicants, and their physicochemical behaviour in genotoxicity tests is usually very different from that of soluble chemicals, especially the nature of their interaction with DNA. During/after exposure, chemicals may interact directly with DNA and/or indirectly (e.g. following metabolic activation and/or cell signalling events). On the other hand, particulate matter is thought to interact with DNA only following internalization (i.e. phagocytosis), while indirect action on DNA is possible without the need for metabolic activation (e.g. via formation of ROS related to surface properties and/or interaction with mitotic spindle apparatus). Another major difference is seen in the kinetics of exposure. Chemicals show a classical pharmacokinetic behaviour: distribution, biotransformation, elimination. Particulate kinetics on the other hand depends on deposition, clearance, durability, overload, etc. Furthermore, particulates are believed to have a 'carrier' function in vivo (Donaldson & Stone, 2003, Speit, 2002, Oberdorster, 2002).

Both CoCr alloy and ceramic THR systems are 'not yet classifiable as to their carcinogenicity to humans', although Cr (VI) is accepted around the world as a human lung carcinogen (WHO, 1990) and soluble Co (II) salts have recently been classified as possibly carcinogenic to humans (WHO, 2006). This may be in part due to the lack of enough convincing evidence that CoCr particulate wear debris can be genotoxic. However, for ceramic THR systems, the main reason is probably that they have only recently been introduced to the market. In vitro studies from our group have shown that both CoCr alloy and Al_2O_3 particles are genotoxic to human cells (Papageorgiou et al., 2007a, Tsaousi et al., 2010). Importantly, it has recently been shown that cobalt-chromium nanoparticles can damage human cells across an intact cellular barrier without having to cross the barrier, by intercellular signaling possibly through cell-cell junctions (Case et al, 2009).

9. Conclusion

THR is generally considered as a treatment option when pain is so severe that it impedes normal function despite the use of anti-inflammatory medication. As an elective procedure, it is a decision reached after careful consideration of its comparative benefits over its potential risks. When the editor of JBJS invited surgeons to submit reports of any tumour associated with replaced joints he wrote 'although the benefits of joint replacement might outweigh any risks a thousand-fold, that is no excuse for suppressing the facts'. As modern non-corroded MOM and COC THRs commonly used for young patients will still inevitably generate particulate wear over time, it is our belief that research should focus more on its long-term genotoxicity and therefore carcinogenic potential. The genotoxicity of different materials should also be taken into account for the design and development of all prosthetic implants. Finally, THR surgeons should consider lifestyle factors further than the levels of physical activity such as the likelihood of having children.

10. Acknowledgements

I would like to thank Mr James O'Shaughnessy for the artwork and Miss Stamatia Goni for her valuable comments and suggestions. Also thanks to Miss Veerle Verheyden and the School of Clinical Science, University of Bristol, for generously supporting this publication.

11. References

Adams, J.E.et al. 2003. Prosthetic Implant Associated Sacromas: A Case Report Emphasing Surface Evaluation and Spectroscopic Trace Metal Analysis. *Annals of Diagnostic Pathology,* 7, 35-46.

Amstutz, H.C.et al. 1992. Mechanism and clinical significance of wear debris-induced osteolysis. *Clin Orthop Relat Res,* 7-18.

Amstutz, H.C. & Grigoris, P. 1996. Metal on metal bearings in hip arthroplasty. *Clin Orthop Relat Res,* S11-34.

Anard, D.et al. 1997. In vitro genotoxic effects of hard metal particles assessed by alkaline single cell gel and elution assays. *Carcinogenesis,* 18, 177-84.

Anissian, H.L.et al. 2001. The wear pattern in metal-on-metal hip prostheses. *J Biomed Mater Res,* 58, 673-8.

Apley, A.G. 1989. Malignacy and Joint Replacement: the Tip of an Iceberg? *The Journal of Bone and Joint Surgery,* 71-B, 1.

Archibeck, M.J.et al. 2000. Alternate bearing surfaces in total joint arthroplasty: biologic considerations. *Clin Orthop Relat Res,* 12-21.

Barrett, J.C. 1994. Cellular and molecular mechanisms of asbestos carcinogenicity: implications for biopersistence. *Environ Health Perspect,* 102 Suppl 5, 19-23.

Black, J.et al. 1983. Serum concentrations of chromium, cobalt and nickel after total hip replacement: a six month study. *Biomaterials,* 4, 160-4.

Bouchard, P.R.et al. 1996. Carcinogenicity of CoCrMo (F-75) implants in the rat. *J Biomed Mater Res,* 32, 37-44.

Boutin, P. 1971. [Alumina and its use in surgery of the hip. (Experimental study)]. *Presse Med,* 79, 639-40.

Boutin, P.et al. 1988. The use of dense alumina-alumina ceramic combination in total hip replacement. *J Biomed Mater Res,* 22, 1203-32.

Brodner, W.et al. 2003. Serum cobalt levels after metal-on-metal total hip arthroplasty. *J Bone Joint Surg Am,* 85-A, 2168-73.

Case, C.P.et al. 1996. Preliminary observations on possible premalignant changes in bone marrow adjacent to worn total hip arthroplasty implants. *Clin Orthop Relat Res,* S269-79.

Case, C.P.et al. 1994. Widespread dissemination of metal debris from implants. *J Bone Joint Surg Br,* 76, 701-12.

Chan, F.W.et al. 1999. The Otto Aufranc Award. Wear and lubrication of metal-on-metal hip implants. *Clin Orthop Relat Res,* 10-24.

Charnley, J. 1972. The long-term results of low-friction arthroplasty of the hip performed as a primary intervention. *J Bone Joint Surg Br,* 54, 61-76.

Cole, B.J.et al. 1997. Malignant fibrous histiocytoma at the site of a total hip replacement: review of the literature and case report. *Skeletal Radiol,* 26, 559-63.

Cornell, C.N. & Ranawat, C.S. 1986a. The impact of modern cement techniques on acetabular fixation in cemented total hip replacement. *J Arthroplasty,* 1, 197-202.

Cornell, C.N. & Ranawat, C.S. 1986b. Survivorship analysis of total hip replacements. Results in a series of active patients who were less than fifty-five years old. *J Bone Joint Surg Am,* 68, 1430-4.

Courtland, L.G. & William, S.J. 1996. Metal Carcinogenesis in Total Joint Arthroplasty: Animal Models. *Clinical Orthopedics and Related Research,* 329S, S264-68.

Davies, A.P.et al. 2005. Metal-specific differences in levels of DNA damage caused by synovial fluid recovered at revision arthroplasty. *J Bone Joint Surg Br,* 87, 1439-44.

De Boeck, M.et al. 2003. In vitro genotoxic effects of different combinations of cobalt and metallic carbide particles. *Mutagenesis,* 18, 177-86.

Dobbs, H.S. 1980. Survivorship of total hip replacements. *J Bone Joint Surg Br,* 62-B, 168-73.

Dobbs, H.S. & Minski, M.J. 1980. Metal ion release after total hip replacement. *Biomaterials,* 1, 193-8.

Dodion, P.et al. 1982. Immunoblastic lymphoma at the site of an infected vitallium bone plate. *Histopathology,* 6, 807-13.

Doherty, A.T.et al. 2001. Increased chromosome translocations and aneuploidy in peripheral blood lymphocytes of patients having revision arthroplasty of the hip. *J Bone Joint Surg Br,* 83, 1075-81.

Donaldson, K. & Stone, V. 2003. Current hypotheses on the mechanisms of toxicity of ultrafine particles. *Ann Ist Super Sanita,* 39, 405-10.

Doorn, P.F.et al. 1996a. Metal versus polyethylene wear particles in total hip replacements. A review. *Clin Orthop Relat Res,* S206-16.

Doorn, P.F.et al. 1998. Metal wear particle characterization from metal on metal total hip replacements: transmission electron microscopy study of periprosthetic tissues and isolated particles. *J Biomed Mater Res,* 42, 103-11.

Doorn, P.F.et al. 1996b. Tissue reaction to metal on metal total hip prostheses. *Clin Orthop Relat Res,* S187-205.

Dopp, E.et al. 1997. Induction of micronuclei, hyperdiploidy and chromosomal breakage affecting the centric/pericentric regions of chromosomes 1 and 9 in human amniotic fluid cells after treatment with asbestos and ceramic fibers. *Mutat Res,* 377, 77-87.

Dunstan, E.et al. 2005. Metal ion levels after metal-on-metal proximal femoral replacements: a 30-year follow-up. *J Bone Joint Surg Br,* 87, 628-31.

Flugsrud, G.B.et al. 2002. Risk factors for total hip replacement due to primary osteoarthritis: a cohort study in 50,034 persons. *Arthritis Rheum,* 46, 675-82.

Gaechter, A.et al. 1977. Metal carcinogenesis: a study of the carcinogenic activity of solid metal alloys in rats. *J Bone Joint Surg Am,* 59, 622-4.

Ganapathi, M.et al. 2001. Periprosthetic high-grade B-cell lymphoma complicating an infected revision total hip arthroplasty. *J Arthroplasty,* 16, 229-32.

Garellick, G.et al. 1998. Life expectancy and cost utility after total hip replacement. *Clin Orthop Relat Res,* 141-51.

Gibb, F. 1992. Differences in animal and human responses in carcinogenic metals. *Progress in Clinical and Biological Research,* 374, 369-79.

Gillespie, W.J.et al. 1988. The incidence of cancer following total hip replacement. *J Bone Joint Surg Br,* 70, 539-42.

Gillespie, W.J.et al. 1996. Development of hematopoietic cancers after implantation of total joint replacement. *Clin Orthop Relat Res*, S290-6.

Goldring, S.R.et al. 1983. The synovial-like membrane at the bone-cement interface in loose total hip replacements and its proposed role in bone lysis. *J Bone Joint Surg Am,* 65, 575-84.

Goodfellow, J. 1992. MAlignacy and Joint Replacement. *The Journal of Bone and Joint Surgery,* 74-B, 645.

Hagmar, L.et al. 2004. Impact of types of lymphocyte chromosomal aberrations on human cancer risk: results from Nordic and Italian cohorts. *Cancer Res,* 64, 2258-63.

Hamadouche, M.et al. 2002. Alumina-on-alumina total hip arthroplasty: a minimum 18.5-year follow-up study. *J Bone Joint Surg Am,* 84-A, 69-77.

Hamadouche, M. & SEDEL, L. 2000. Ceramics in orthopaedics. *J Bone Joint Surg Br,* 82, 1095-9.

Harris, W.H. 1994. Osteolysis and particle disease in hip replacement. A review. *Acta Orthop Scand,* 65, 113-23.

Hatton, A.et al. 2002. Alumina-alumina artificial hip joints. Part I: a histological analysis and characterisation of wear debris by laser capture microdissection of tissues retrieved at revision. *Biomaterials,* 23, 3429-40.

Havelin, L.I.et al. 2000. The Norwegian Arthroplasty Register: 11 years and 73,000 arthroplasties. *Acta Orthop Scand,* 71, 337-53.

Heath, J.C. 1957. The production of malignant tumours by cobalt in the rat. *British Journal of Cancer,* 10, 668-73.

Heath, J.C.et al. 1971. Carcinogenic properties of wear particles from prostheses made in cobalt-chromium alloy. *Lancet,* 1, 564-6.

Heisel, C.et al. 2004. Bearing surface options for total hip replacement in young patients. *Instr Course Lect,* 53, 49-65.

Heisel, C.et al. 2005. The relationship between activity and ions in patients with metal-on-metal bearing hip prostheses. *J Bone Joint Surg Am,* 87, 781-7.

Hennig, F.F.et al. 1992. Nickel-, chrom- and cobalt-concentrations in human tissue and body fluids of hip prosthesis patients. *J Trace Elem Electrolytes Health Dis,* 6, 239-43.

Hirakawa, K.et al. 1996. Characterization and comparison of wear debris from failed total hip implants of different types. *J Bone Joint Surg Am,* 78, 1235-43.

Horowitz, S.M.et al. 1993. Studies of the mechanism by which the mechanical failure of polymethylmethacrylate leads to bone resorption. *J Bone Joint Surg Am,* 75, 802-13.

Howie, D.W. & Vernon-Roberts, B. 1988. The synovial response to intraarticular cobalt-chrome wear particles. *Clin Orthop Relat Res*, 244-54.

Ingham, E. & Fisher, J. 2000. Biological reactions to wear debris in total joint replacement. *Proc Inst Mech Eng [H],* 214, 21-37.

Ingham, E. & Fisher, J. 2005. The role of macrophages in osteolysis of total joint replacement. *Biomaterials,* 26, 1271-86.

Ito, H. & Shimizu, A. 1999. Malignant lymphoma at the site of a total hip replacement. *Orthopedics,* 22, 82-4.

Jacobs, J.J.et al. 1998a. Corrosion of metal orthopaedic implants. *J Bone Joint Surg Am,* 80, 268-82.

Jacobs, J.J.et al. 1992. Early sarcomatous degeneration near a cementless hip replacement. A case report and review. *J Bone Joint Surg Br,* 74, 740-4.

Jacobs, J.J.et al. 2004. Can metal levels be used to monitor metal-on-metal hip arthroplasties? *J Arthroplasty,* 19, 59-65.

Jacobs, J.J.et al. 1998b. Metal release in patients who have had a primary total hip arthroplasty. A prospective, controlled, longitudinal study. *J Bone Joint Surg Am,* 80, 1447-58.

Jacobs, J.J.et al. 1995. Local and distant products from modularity. *Clin Orthop Relat Res,* 94-105.

Jazrawi, L.M.et al. 1998. Alternative bearing surfaces for total joint arthroplasty. *J Am Acad Orthop Surg,* 6, 198-203.

Jones, L.C. & Hungerford, D.S. 1987. Cement disease. *Clin Orthop Relat Res,* 192-206.

Kirkpatrick, C.J.et al. 2000. Biomaterial-induced sarcoma: A novel model to study preneoplastic change. *Am J Pathol,* 156, 1455-67.

Ladon, D.et al. 2004. Changes in metal levels and chromosome aberrations in the peripheral blood of patients after metal-on-metal hip arthroplasty. *J Arthroplasty,* 19, 78-83.

Langdown, A.J.et al. 2007. Incomplete seating of the liner with the Trident acetabular system: a cause for concern? *J Bone Joint Surg Br,* 89, 291-5.

Lewis, C.G.et al. 1995. Intraarticular carcinogenesis bioassays of CoCrMo and TiAlV alloys in rats. *J Arthroplasty,* 10, 75-82.

Lhotka, C.et al. 2003. Four-year study of cobalt and chromium blood levels in patients managed with two different metal-on-metal total hip replacements. *J Orthop Res,* 21, 189-95.

Lison, D.et al. 2001. Update on the genotoxicity and carcinogenicity of cobalt compounds. *Occup Environ Med,* 58, 619-25.

Lu, Z. & Mckellop, H. 1997. Frictional heating of bearing materials tested in a hip joint wear simulator. *Proc Inst Mech Eng [H],* 211, 101-8.

Manaster, B.J. 1996. From the RSNA refresher courses. Total hip arthroplasty: radiographic evaluation. *Radiographics,* 16, 645-60.

Mathiesen, E.B.et al. 1995. Total hip replacement and cancer. A cohort study. *J Bone Joint Surg Br,* 77, 345-50.

Mcgregor, D.B.et al. 2000. Evaluation of the carcinogenic risks to humans associated with surgical implants and other foreign bodies - a report of an IARC Monographs Programme Meeting. International Agency for Research on Cancer. *Eur J Cancer,* 36, 307-13.

Mckellop, H.et al. 1981. Friction and wear properties of polymer, metal, and ceramic prosthetic joint materials evaluated on a multichannel screening device. *J Biomed Mater Res,* 15, 619-53.

Mckellop, H.et al. 1996. In vivo wear of three types of metal on metal hip prostheses during two decades of use. *Clin Orthop Relat Res,* S128-40.

Meachim, G.et al. 1982. A study of sarcogenicity associated with Co-Cr-Mo particles implanted in animal muscle. *J Biomed Mater Res,* 16, 407-16.

Medley, J.B.et al. 1996. Comparison of alloys and designs in a hip simulator study of metal on metal implants. *Clin Orthop Relat Res,* S148-59.

Memoli, V.A.et al. 1986. Malignant neoplasms associated with orthopedic implant materials in rats. *J Orthop Res,* 4, 346-55.

Meneghini, R.M.et al. 2005. The biology of alternative bearing surfaces in total joint arthroplasty. *Instr Course Lect,* 54, 481-93.

Merritt, K. & Brown, S.A. 1996. Distribution of cobalt chromium wear and corrosion products and biologic reactions. *Clin Orthop Relat Res,* S233-43.

Michel, R.et al. 1991. Systemic effects of implanted prostheses made of cobalt-chromium alloys. *Arch Orthop Trauma Surg,* 110, 61-74.

Mittelmeier, H. & Heisel, J. 1992. Sixteen-years' experience with ceramic hip prostheses. *Clin Orthop Relat Res,* 64-72.

Nevelos, J.E.et al. 1999. Analysis of retrieved alumina ceramic components from Mittelmeier total hip prostheses. *Biomaterials,* 20, 1833-40.

Nhs. 2006. *Main Operations: Summary 2005-2006* [Online]. The Information Center (England). Available: http://www.hesonline.nhs.uk/Ease/servlet/ContentServer?siteID=1937&categoryID=204 [Accessed 05/10/07].

Nizard, R.S.et al. 1992. Ten-year survivorship of cemented ceramic-ceramic total hip prosthesis. *Clin Orthop Relat Res,* 53-63.

Nyren, O.et al. 1995. Cancer risk after hip replacement with metal implants: a population-based cohort study in Sweden. *J Natl Cancer Inst,* 87, 28-33.

Oberdorster, G. 2002. Toxicokinetics and effects of fibrous and nonfibrous particles. *Inhal Toxicol,* 14, 29-56.

Oppenheimer, B.S.et al. 1956. Carcinogenic effect of metals in rodents. *Cancer Res,* 16, 439-41.

Papageorgiou, I.et al. 2007a. The effect of nano- and micron-sized particles of cobalt-chromium alloy on human fibroblasts in vitro. *Biomaterials,* 28, 2946-58.

Papageorgiou, I.et al. 2007b. Genotoxic effects of particles of surgical cobalt chrome alloy on human cells of different age in vitro. *Mutat Res,* 619, 45-58.

Patierno, S.R.et al. 1988. Transformation of C3H/10T1/2 mouse embryo cells to focus formation and anchorage independence by insoluble lead chromate but not soluble calcium chromate: relationship to mutagenesis and internalization of lead chromate particles. *Cancer Res,* 48, 5280-8.

Radhi, J.M.et al. 1998. Soft tissue malignant lymphoma at sites of previous surgery. *J Clin Pathol,* 51, 629-32.

Savio, J.A., 3RDet al. 1994. Size and shape of biomaterial wear debris. *Clin Mater,* 15, 101-47.

Schaffer, A.W.et al. 1999. Increased blood cobalt and chromium after total hip replacement. *J Toxicol Clin Toxicol,* 37, 839-44.

Schmalzried, T.P. & Callaghan, J.J. 1999. Wear in total hip and knee replacements. *J Bone Joint Surg Am,* 81, 115-36.

Schmalzried, T.P.et al. 1998. The multifactorial nature of polyethylene wear in vivo. *J Bone Joint Surg Am,* 80, 1234-42; discussion 42-3.

Schmalzried, T.P.et al. 1992. Periprosthetic bone loss in total hip arthroplasty. Polyethylene wear debris and the concept of the effective joint space. *J Bone Joint Surg Am,* 74, 849-63.

Schmalzried, T.P.et al. 2000. The John Charnley Award. Wear is a function of use, not time. *Clin Orthop Relat Res,* 36-46.

Schuh, A.et al. 2004. Malignant fibrous histiocytoma at the site of a total hip arthroplasty. *Clin Orthop Relat Res*, 218-22.

Sedel, L. 1992. Ceramic hips. *J Bone Joint Surg Br*, 74, 331-2.

Shanbhag, A.S.et al. 1997. Effects of particles on fibroblast proliferation and bone resorption in vitro. *Clin Orthop Relat Res*, 205-17.

Shea, K.G.et al. 1997. Lymphoreticular dissemination of metal particles after primary joint replacements. *Clin Orthop Relat Res*, 219-26.

Sheldon, T.et al. 1996. On the evidence. Provision revision. *Health Serv J*, 106, 34-5.

Smith, J. & Learmonth, I.D. 1996. *Your Operation: Hip Replacement*, Hodder & Stoughton, Headway.

Speit, G. 2002. Appropriate in vitro test conditions for genotoxicity testing of fibers. *Inhal Toxicol*, 14, 79-90.

Springer, B.D.et al. 2011. Deformation of 1-Piece Metal Acetabular Components. *J Arthroplasty*.

Squire, M.et al. 2006. Acetabular component deformation with press-fit fixation. *J Arthroplasty*, 21, 72-7.

Standring, S. 2004. *Gray's Anatomy: The Anatomical Basis of Clinical Practice*, Churchill Livingstone.

Streicher, R.M.et al. 1996. Metal-on-metal articulation for artificial hip joints: laboratory study and clinical results. *Proc Inst Mech Eng [H]*, 210, 223-32.

Sunderman, F.W., JR.et al. 1989. Cobalt, chromium, and nickel concentrations in body fluids of patients with porous-coated knee or hip prostheses. *J Orthop Res*, 7, 307-15.

Swann, M. 1984. Malignant soft-tissue tumour at the site of a total hip replacement. *The Journal of Bone and Joint Surgery*, 66-B, 629-31.

Swanson, S.A.et al. 1973. Laboratory tests on total joint replacement prostheses. *J Bone Joint Surg Br*, 55, 759-73.

Takami, Y.et al. 1997. Biocompatibility of alumina ceramic and polyethylene as materials for pivot bearings of a centrifugal blood pump. *J Biomed Mater Res*, 36, 381-6.

Tigges, S.et al. 1994. Complications of hip arthroplasty causing periprosthetic radiolucency on plain radiographs. *AJR Am J Roentgenol*, 162, 1387-91.

Tipper, J.L.et al. 2002. Alumina-alumina artificial hip joints. Part II: characterisation of the wear debris from in vitro hip joint simulations. *Biomaterials*, 23, 3441-8.

Tsaousi, A.et al. 2010. The in vitro genotoxicity of orthopaedic ceramic (Al(2)O(3)) and metal (CoCr alloy) particles. *Mutation Research-Genetic Toxicology and Environmental Mutagenesis*, 697, 1-9.

Urban, R.M.et al. 1994. Migration of corrosion products from modular hip prostheses. Particle microanalysis and histopathological findings. *J Bone Joint Surg Am*, 76, 1345-59.

Urban, R.M.et al. 2000. Dissemination of wear particles to the liver, spleen, and abdominal lymph nodes of patients with hip or knee replacement. *J Bone Joint Surg Am*, 82, 457-76.

Urban, R.M.et al. 2004. Accumulation in liver and spleen of metal particles generated at nonbearing surfaces in hip arthroplasty. *J Arthroplasty*, 19, 94-101.

Van Goethem, F.et al. 1997. Comparative evaluation of the in vitro micronucleus test and the alkaline single cell gel electrophoresis assay for the detection of DNA damaging agents: genotoxic effects of cobalt powder, tungsten carbide and cobalt-tungsten carbide. *Mutat Res,* 392, 31-43.

Visuri, T. & Koskenvuo, M. 1991. Cancer risk after Mckee-Farrar total hip replacement. *Orthopedics,* 14, 137-42.

Visuri, T.et al. 1996. Cancer risk after metal on metal and polyethylene on metal total hip arthroplasty. *Clin Orthop Relat Res,* S280-9.

Walker, P.S.A.G., B.L 1971. The Triboloby (friction, lubrication and wear) of all metal artificial hip joints. *Wear,* 17, 285-99.

Wang, J.Y.et al. 1997. Prosthetic metals interfere with the functions of human osteoblast cells in vitro. *Clin Orthop Relat Res,* 216-26.

Who 1990. Volume 49: Chromium, Nickel and Welding. *IARC: Monographs on the Evaluation of Carcinogenic Risks to Humans.*

Who 1991. Volume 52: Cobalt and Cobalt Compounds. *IARC Monographs on the Evaluation of Carcinogenic Risks to Humans.*

Who 1999. Volume 74: Surgical Implants and Other Foreign Bodies. *IARC Monographs on the Evaluation of Carcinogennic Risks to Humans.*

Who 2006. Cobalt in Hard Metals and Cobalt Sulfate, Gallium Arsenide, Indium Phosphide and Vanadium Pentoxide. . *IARC Monographs on the Evaluation of Carcinogenic Risks to Humans.*

Willert, H.G. 1977. Reactions of the articular capsule to wear products of artificial joint prostheses. *J Biomed Mater Res,* 11, 157-64.

Wise, J.P., SR.et al. 2002. The cytotoxicity and genotoxicity of particulate and soluble hexavalent chromium in human lung cells. *Mutat Res,* 517, 221-9.

Yoon, T.R.et al. 1998. Osteolysis in association with a total hip arthroplasty with ceramic bearing surfaces. *J Bone Joint Surg Am,* 80, 1459-68.

7

Total Hip Arthroplasty After Previous Acetabulum Fracture Surgery

Babak Siavashi
Tehran University of Medical Sciences, Sina Hospital
Iran

1. Introduction

In recent years because of more car accidents and high energy traumas, acetabulum and pelvic fractures are happened more.

Because acetabulum is a part of hip joint, its fracture is important. At first, it is a weight bearing joint and it is involved in approximately all movements of body. In daily living, it must tolerate about 5-7 times body weight. For example, in the position of one leg stance about 3.5 times body weight is transmitted to hip joint. Even in sitting position and also in supine position and straight leg rising, hip joint is under pressure. Because it is a weight bearing joint, it should be smooth without step in articular surface to be harmonic and congruent with the head of femur. Hip joint is a ball and socket joint with wide range of motion. Lower limb is attached by it to body and because of long lever arm of femur and tibia, transmitted force to joint is extremely high.

In the past, acetabulum surgery and fixation of it was not as common as today. Many patients were treated with long time skeletal traction (for about 3 months). This type of treatment has some complications. The joint is not reduced anatomically and articular surface is not smooth and a step remains in joint surface which lead to destructive joint disease (DJD) and arthrosis after union of fracture. It means that it is united in malreduced position ,therefore malunion occurs. In some instances ,joint particles do not come near each other even with heavy skeletal traction so there may be nonunion in some regions of acetabulum and a defect may remain in a wall or column of acetabulum. If in the future this patient need total joint replacement, there may be wide range of acetabular deficiencies from cavitary and segmental deficiencies to the most sever one named pelvic discontinuity which should be repaired before implantation of acetabular cup. This is a complicated and difficult surgery to reconstruct acetabulum and prepare it for total hip arhtroplasty. Long term skeletal traction has some other complications. Bed rest for a long period of time may lead to bed sore on buttocks and sacrum and discomfort. Muscle atrophy and weakness around hip and knee joint appears after complete bed rest for a long time. Kidney stones and gastrointestinal malfunction are other complications of long term skeletal traction.

Because of social deprivation, psychological problems may be seen in an active patient who should rest for about 3 months in bed for skeletal traction. But, with open reduction and internal fixation of acetabulum fracture, patient can be out of bed with crutches and be present in community .Also ,he or she can move his or her joints and prevent muscle atrophy.

For these reasons, open reduction and internal fixation of acetabulum fracture is advised in recent years. The philosophy of this procedure is not only restoration of smooth articular surface and cartilage of hip joint, but also it brings different parts of acetabulum near each other for union with each other. If in future because of joint destruction and arthrosis total joint replacement is necessary, there will be a good and stable bone stock for implantation of acetabular cup and there will be no missed segment or pelvic discontinuity.

But unfortunately, acetabulum surgery and internal fixation of columns and walls of it is not free of complications. Infection, sciatic nerve injury, avascular necrosis (AVN) of head of femur and late destructive joint disease (DJD) of hip and leg length discrepancy (LLD) are some examples. Some of these complications have no definitive treatment (like sciatic nerve injury) but other complications as DJD and AVN of head of femur can be managed in the best way with total joint replacement.

But hip joint replacement after previous operation for internal fixation of fractured acetabulum is not a simple and straight forward operation and needs special attentions. The aim of this chapter is to discuss about indications of total hip arthroplasty after acetabulum fracture surgery, pre operative planning, approaches and needed equipments and post operative rehabilitation after this kind of total joint replacement.

2. Indications of total hip arthroplasy after actabulum fracture fixation

In post operative period, acutely or chroncally, there may be some complications which may be solved by total hip replacement. One of them is avascular necrosis of head of femur. Some acetabular fractures are truly fracture dislocations and even after reduction and rigid fixation, because of injury to vascular supply of head of femur, necrosis and collapse of head of femur develop in early period or as a late complication. Specially with posterior approach to hip joint (Kocher langen beck approach), there may be injury to main vascular supply of head of femur (medial femoral circumflex artery). With disruption of blood input to the head of femur, signs and symptoms of necrosis will be appeared. Because of rapid progression of collapse and joint destruction in these cases, minor surgeries like core decompression and osteotomies are ineffective and finally total joint replacement is inevitable.

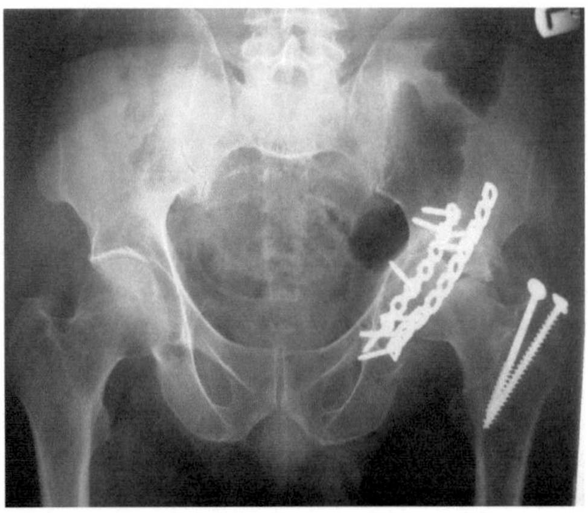

Fig. 1. Avascular necrosis of head of femur.

One of the most common complications of acetabular fractures are destructive joint disease. Because even with surgery and open reduction of acetabulum, anatomic reduction may not be possible(after some days because of contracture of soft tissues, joint particles may not come near each other and perfect reduction may not be achieved) and remaining steps in joint surface may lead to destructive joint disease after union of fracture and weight bearing on lower extremity.

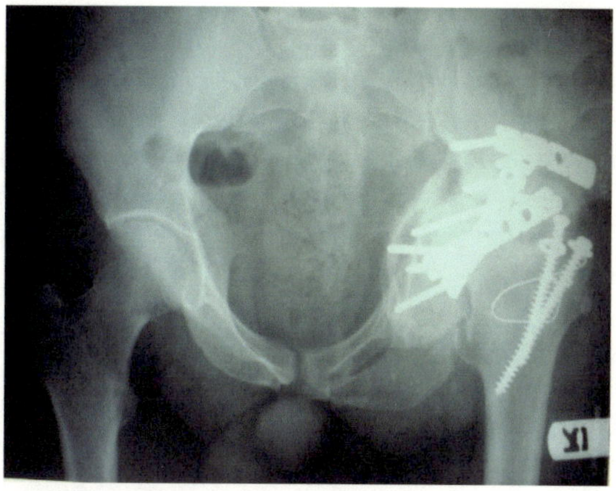

Fig. 2. Destructive joint disease after acetabulum fracture.

Painful joint after acetabulum fracture may be due to chondrolysis of articular cartilage and may be sever enough to be treated with total joint replacement.

These are main indications for total hip replacement after fixation of acetabulum fracture but there are some other indications for total hip replacement .

Infection and resorption of head of femur after acetabulum surgery can be treated with debridement and irrigation and intravenous antibiotic therapy. After complete eradication of infection, total hip replacement can be done.

In some situations, internal fixation may be failed. It may be treated with refixation of fracture but sometimes with fixation failure there may be injury to the head of femur or acetabular walls and reconstruction of them may be impossible and joint replacement may be the be the best treatment .

Leg length discrepancy may appear after collapse of femoral head after avascular necrosis. So, leg length discrepancy itself is not the indication of joint replacement .But in parallel with treatment of avascular necrosis of femoral head, length of lower extremity can be increased and leg length discrepancy can be corrected.

3. Preoperative planning

Total hip arthroplasty after surgical fixation of acetabular fracture is a technical demanding operation. So, it should be done after complete assessment of both patient and bony pelvis.

At first, infection as a cause of hip destruction and resorption of head of femur should be ruled out. Complete blood cell count (CBC), Erythrocyte sedimentation rate (ESR) and C reactive protein (CRP) should be checked. Whole body bone scan (triphasic) can be helpful in this manner. If there is high probability of infection as a cause of joint destruction then aspiration of hip joint will be helpful.

High quality radiography can show the bone stock of pelvis for implantation of acetabular cup and femoral stem of prosthesis. One of the purposes of fixation of acetabulum fracture is to reconstruct bony frame of pelvis for future total hip replacement.

Iliac and Obturator views of pelvis and acetabulum can show more details of columns and walls (anterior and posterior) and bony union of acetabulum. Computerized Tomography scan (CT scan), specially axial cuts, can show the quality and quantity of posterior wall and column and union of them. Also, exact position of hardwares(plates and screws) can be showed. It can be estimated if plates and screws may interfere with joint arthroplasty specially insertion of acetabular cup. Medial wall of acetabulum and its integrity can be shown with axial CT scan.

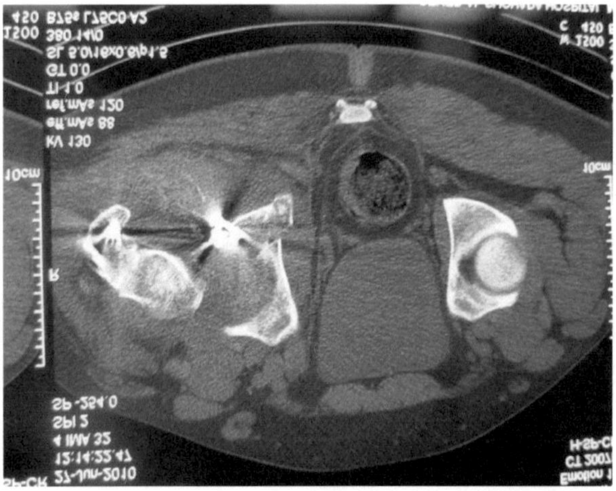

Fig. 3. axial CT scan.

If posterior or anterior walls or columns are deficient, before insertion of acetabular cup, they should be reconstructed with allografts (distal femur allograft is a good source of both cortical and cancellous bone) or autografts (remaining parts of head and neck of femur or iliac bone) and the surgeon should prepare himself for these procedures. In the case of medial wall defect metallic meshes are used for reconstruction of it.

Templating of hip joint is very useful so the surgeon can estimate the exact bone defects of acetabulum and the needed size of cup.

Preoperative scanogram can show true leg length discrepancy and the surgeon can estimate the best cut for femoral neck and the size of head of prosthesis.

Abductor function is important for successful total hip arthroplasty. Abductor function and its strength can be evaluated with physical examination and with Electromyography and nerve conduction velocity (EMG/NCV) with special attention to gluteous medius muscle.

4. Approaches

Factors that guide the surgeon to choose the best approach for total hip arthroplasty after acetabulum surgery are : 1- previous approach to hip joint for acetabulum fixation 2- deficiencies in anterior or posterior wall or column of acetabulum and need to reconstruct them 3- surgeon experience 4- condition of soft tissue and skin

Because of previous surgery, there is fibrosis in the tract of incision and around hip joint. This fibrotic tissue in one hand, limits soft tissue mobility and make the operation more difficult and on the other hand, increases bleeding in the field of operation. Because of tightness in the soft tissue and limited exposure, sometimes it is better to do osteotomy of greater trochanter .This osteotomy not only makes exposure better and wider, but also helps the surgeon to save abductors. Also, sometimes for better exposure of the acetabulum for preparation of it for implantation of acetabular cup, there may need to forcefully retract the muscles. This violence to muscles can damage them and predispose infection. Forceful exposure may transmit the energy to shaft or proximal femur and break them.

In my opinion, exploration of sciatic nerve is not always necessary. Because of fibrotic tissue around sciatic nerve from previous operation and exploration of it, dissection of sciatic nerve is very difficult and dangerous, it may itself damage the fibers of nerve. For this reason, after exposure of hip joint and identification of remaining capsule, by staying close to bone and retraction of sciatic nerve with the fibrotic tissue around it, acetabulum can be identified and can be prepared for implantation of acetabular cup.

If it is not necessary for preparation of acetabulum for implantation of cup, it is not wise to search for all of hardwares (plate and screws) for fixation of acetabulum fracture and their removal. Because this not only damage more soft tissue and weaken posterior support of hip joint and predisposes the prosthesis to dislocation, but also, it may destroy bony support and bone stock of acetabulum and make implantation of cup weaker than usual.

Because of difference in the composition of metal back of acetabular cup and the plate and screws for fixation of acetabulum fracture, there may be galvanic wear of implants and cup of acetabulum. This is a cause of sooner than normal loosening of prosthesis.

Some times, before reaming acetabulum, no hardware or screws are visible behind cartilage of hip joint. After first or second ream, screws come in the field and appear and make more reaming impossible. In this manner, screw or plate removal is necessary.

After exposure of hip joint and acetabulum, union and competency of posterior column and wall should be checked with a probe so the surgeon should be sure about the stability of peripheral ring of acetabulum and its boundries before implantation of acetabular cup. If the fixation is imperfect, so re fixation and plating and bone grafting may be necessary.

5. Equipments

If it is possible, because of lower age of patients in this category, it is better to use cementless cup and cementless stem for total hip arthroplasty. But in some situations, it may be better to use cemented cup. For example, in deficient posterior wall or column and reconstructions of them with structural bone (allograft or outograft), if it is large and bone contact between host bone and cup is minimal (less than 30%), it may compromise osteointegration and also the cup can not be inserted with press fit technique, so cemented cup is preferred. It is accepted that if more than 1/3 of cup is in contact with graft, it is better to use cemented prosthesis. About femoral stem,because of younger age of these patients, nearly always it is better to use cementless stems.

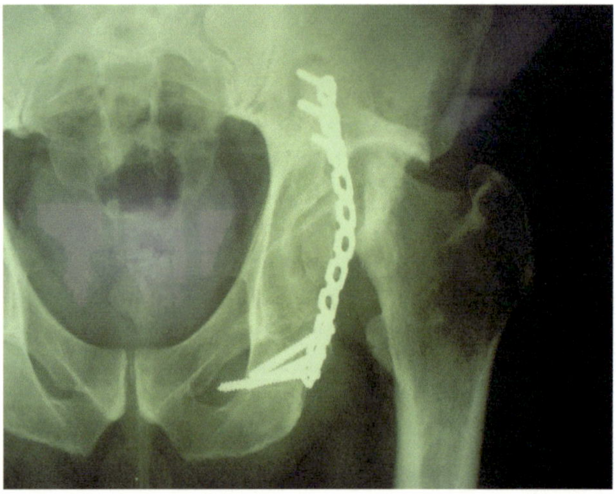

Fig. 4. bone defect of acetabulum.

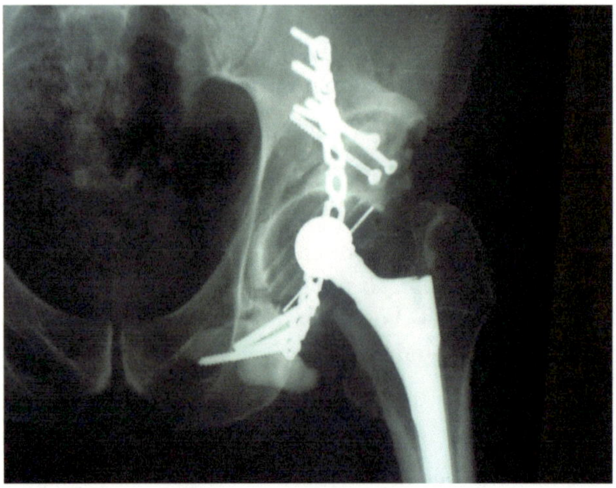

Fig. 5. reconstruction of defect with bone graft and cemented cup.

If trochanteric osteotomy has been done for previous acetabulum surgery, screw removal is not necessary always for insertion of femoral stem. Surgeon can start preparation of femur for insertion of femoral stem, if the screws are found in the way of broaches, then removal of screws should be done.

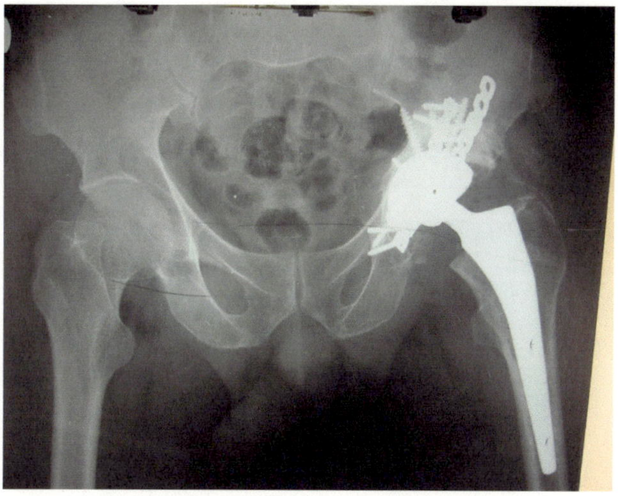

Fig. 6. Cement less cup and cementless stem.

Because removing screws which are inserted for fixation of greater trochanter may damage some fibers of abductor muscles, so, it is better to leave screws in place unless they are located in the tract of insertion of femoral stem.

In rare situations, if even largest cup cannot cover the whole periphery of acetabulum, it may be necessary to use reinforcement acetabular rings or cages. If it should be done, after implantation of cages and fixation of it to iliac bone, behind it, particles of bone grafts (mostly allograft), should be inserted and then cemented cup should be used inside the ring.

If medial wall is deficient, it should be covered with mesh and over it particulated chips bone (allograft or autograft) should be inserted and then acetabular cup or reinforcement ring should be used.

In some cases, hip arthroplasty may be necessary because of absorption of head of femur after avascular necrosis of head. In these cases, even acetabular cartilage seems normal, it is better to do total hip replacement instead of bipolar prosthesis. Because of younger age of these patients and higher demand of them, wear of acetabulum progresses rapidly and another surgery to change bipolar to total hip arthroplasy may be necessary soon.

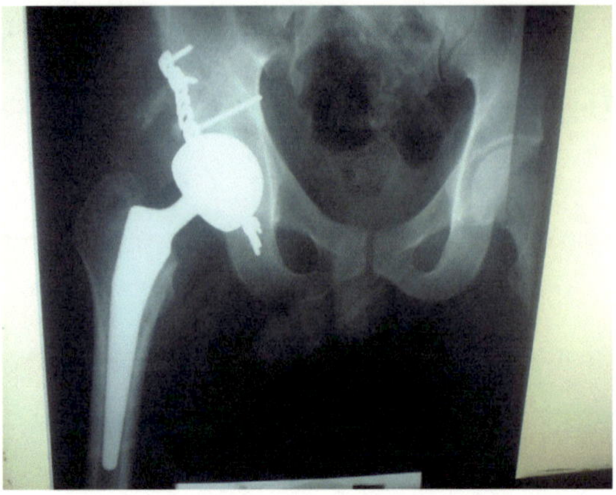

Fig. 7. Bipolar prosthesis for avascular necrosis of head of femur after acetabulum fracture fixation.

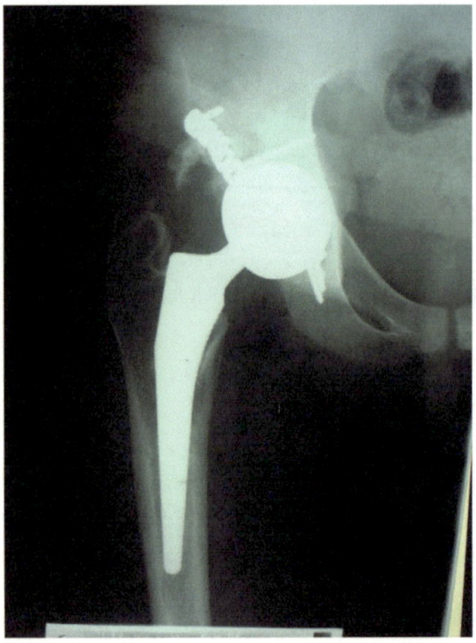

Fig. 8. Rapid wear of acetabulum with bipolar prosthesis (after 5 months).

6. A kind of revision surgery

As it shows, total hip arthroplasty after previous acetabulum surgery is a kind of revision surgery. Because there is a large amount of fibrotic tissues remaining from previous surgery and previous approaches, exposure is limited. Also, there are various defects of walls or columns of acetabulum. Some of these defects are created from resorption of bone and some are created during new exposure and device removal.

Rate of dislocation of prosthesis is higher than primary arthroplasties in these cases as in revision total hip arthroplasties. Also, there is higher risk of infection and sciatic nerve palsy.

These similarities should alert both the surgeon and the patient to be realistic about this operation and preoperative discussion is mandatory for reaching the best results.

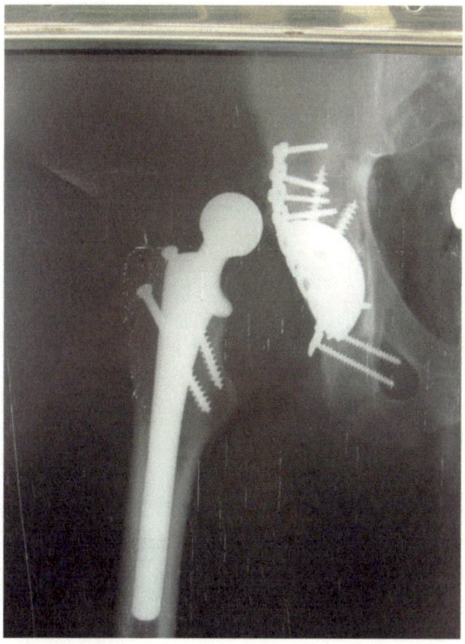

Fig. 9. Dislocation of total hip prosthesis.

7. Post operation period

As other total hip arthroplasties, after operation and before full clearance of anesthesia and sedation, it is wise to use abduction pillows between two legs. If trochanteric osteotomy has been done or if there is weakness of abductor muscles, then for a period of time (approximately 3 months) abduction brace is useful. It not only prevents adduction of lower extremities, but also can limit flexion. With limitation of adduction and flexion, the position of dislocation can be prevented. Because there is no capsule of hip joint and there is deficient and damaged posterior soft tissues after several approaches and operations, hip may be unstable in some degrees of flextion so limitation of flextion while posterior soft tissues are repaired and strong fibrosis develop in the field, is useful.

Because of using cementless prosthesis or using bone grafts for reconstruction of acetabulum, nearly always it is not possible to permit patient to have full weight bearing on his leg. Therefore, we advise touch weight bearing postoperatively.

8. Attention

Risk factors of acetabulum fracture which after fixation may end to total hip replacement seems to be the following items:

1. Posterosuperior wall fracture
2. Posterior wall and column fracture
3. Trochanteric osteotomy
4. Nonanatomic reduction
5. Sever primary displacement of fragments
6. Delayed surgical fixation of acetabulum fracture
7. Comminuted fractures with several particles
8. Intaarticular placement of screws

Fractures of posterosuperior wall of acetabulum may lead to total hip replacement more than fracture of direct posterior wall fracture.

The underlying reasons for this are :

a. Posterosuperior fragment is involved more than posterior wall with weight bearing, so the quality of its reduction is more critical for future destructive joint disease than pure posterior wall segment
b. Reduction and fixation of posterosuperior segment needs more dissection of soft tissue and release of surrounding tissuesand may compromise blood supply to the head of femur (may incidentally damage articular supply of head of femur)
c. For better exposure of posteriosuperior wall of acetabulum, trochanteric osteotomy is more needed. This osteotomy potentially may injure vascular supply of femoral head from arteries around and beneath short external rotators and finally lead to avascular necrosis of head of femur.
d. Fractures of posterosuperior segment are more high energy traumas and the initial impact to the acetabulum is more sever than pure posterior wall fractures. This high energy mechanism of fracture may itself be the cause of cartilage damage and destructive joint disease in the future.

In acetabular fractures which in early phase (usually around 3 months) avascular necrosis of femoral head appears, direct vascular injury to the head of femur is the main cause of head necrosis. But in late necrosis, other factors influence too.

Delayed open reduction and fixation of acetabular fracture is a cause of hip destructive joint disease. Because after 2-3 weeks soft tissue contracture develop and reduction and fixation of segments of joint needs more soft tissue dissection ,with this soft tissue dissection, vascular injury to the head of femur is highly possible. Also, after 2-3 weeks, joint particles can not be anatomically reduced and even small steps and gaps in articular surface of acetabulum may remain. In this way, sever displacement of acetabular segments also lead to poor reduction.

Some times, non intentional placement of screws in joint are the cause of joint damage. So, if there is doubt about position of screws, intraoperative x ray imagings (C-arm or radiography) or postoperative CT scan (specially axial and coronal cuts) are very helpful. If there is a screw in the joint, do not hesitate to remove it and insert another one in correct direction. The best position of screws are toward ischial tuberosity (inferior screws) and toward ilium and iliac bone (superior screws). The most dangerous screws are those that are inserted in the field of acetabular cavity. Even intraoperative C-arm, cannot guaranty safe positioning of screws so special attention to direction of hand during screw insertion is more important.

In few cases, necrosis may develop in acetabular fragments not in the head of femur. So, dissection of all soft tissues from the acetabular segments specially detachment of capsule of hip joint and the periosteum from the wall fragments is forbidden because it can damage the remaining nutrients to the segment.

9. References

[1] Márcio KatzI; Marcos Antônio Akira OkumaI; Alexandre Leme Godoy dos SantosII; Cesar Luiz Betoni GuglielmettiIII; Marcos Hideyo SakakiIV; Arnaldo Valdir Zumiotti. Epidemiology of high-energy trauma injuries among the elderly. *Acta ortop. bras.* vol.16 no.5 São Paulo 2008

[2] Souza RB, Powers CM. Differences in hip kinematics, muscle strength, and muscle activation between subjects with and without patellofemoral pain. *J Orthop Sports Phys Ther.* 2009 Jan;39(1):12-9.
[3] B Noehren1, J Scholz2, I Davis The effect of real-time gait retraining on hip kinematics, pain and function in subjects with patellofemoral pain syndrome *Br J Sports Med* doi:10.1136/bjsm.2009.069112
[4] Thomas Trumble, *Christopher H. Allan, *John Miyano, *John M. Clark, Susan Ott,D. E. Casey Jones, ‡Patrick Fernacola, *Marteinn Magnusson, and *Allan Tencer A Preliminary Study of Joint Surface Changes After an Intraarticular Fracture: A Sheep Model of a Tibia Fracture With Weight Bearing After Internal Fixation. *Journal of Orthopaedic Trauma* Vol. 15, No. 5, pp. 326–332 © 2001 Lippincott Williams & Wilkins, Inc., Philadelphia
[5] Letournel E. Diagnosis and treatment of nonunions and malunions of acetabular fractures. *Orthop Clin North Am.* 1990 Oct;21(4):769-88.
[6] Joel M. Matta, MD; Tania A. Ferguson, MD. Total Hip Replacement After Acetabular Fracture *Orthopedics* September 2005;28(9):959.
[7] Mears DC, Velyvis JH.Primary total hip arthroplasty after acetabular fracture. *Instr Course Lect.* 2001;50:335-54.
[8] D Murphy,M Kaliszer,J Rice.Outcomes after acetabulum fracture::prognostic factors and their inter relationships *Injury*, Volume 34, Issue 7, Pages 512-517 (July 2003)
[9] al-Qahtani S., O'Connor G.: Acetabular fractures before and after the introduction of seatbelt legislation. *Can J Surg* 1996; 39:317-320.
[10] Alexander R.D., Grimm L., Vrahas M.S.: The effect of knee immobilization on degree of hip flexion: A clinical correlation with posterior wall acetabular fractures. *Am J Orthop* 1997; 26:345-347.
[11] Allen T.L., Carter J.L., Morris B.J., et al: Retrievable vena cava filters in trauma patients for high-risk prophylaxis and prevention of pulmonary embolism. *Am J Surg* 2005; 189:656-661.
[12] Alonso J.E., Davila R., Bradley E.: Extended iliofemoral versus triradiate approaches in management of associated acetabular fractures. *Clin Orthop Relat Res* 1994; 305:81-87.
[13] Alonso J.E., Volgas D.A., Giordano V., et al: A review of the treatment of hip dislocations associated with acetabular fractures. *Clin Orthop Relat Res* 2000; 377:32-43.
[14] Anglen J.O., Bagby C., George R.: A randomized comparison of sequential-gradient calf compression with intermittent plantar compression for prevention of venous thrombosis in orthopedic trauma patients: Preliminary results. *Am J Orthop* 1998; 27:53-58.
[15] Anglen J.O., Burd T.A., Hendricks K.J., et al: The "Gull Sign": A harbinger of failure for internal fixation of geriatric acetabular fractures. *J Orthop Trauma* 2003; 17:625-634.
[16] Anglen J.O., Hughes M.: Trochanteric osteotomy for incarcerated hip dislocation due to interposed posterior wall fragments. *Orthopedics* 2004; 27:213-216.
[17] Anglen J.O., Moore K.D.: Prevention of heterotopic bone formation after acetabular fracture fixation by single-dose radiation therapy: A preliminary report. *J Orthop Trauma* 1996; 10:258-263.
[18] Arrington E.D., Hochschild D.P., Steinagle T.J., et al: Monitoring of somatosensory and motor evoked potentials during open reduction and internal fixation of pelvis and acetabular fractures. *Orthopedics* 2000; 23:1081-1083.

[19] Attias N., Lindsey R.W., Starr A.J., et al: The use of a virtual three-dimensional model to evaluate the intraosseous space available for percutaneous screw fixation of acetabular fractures. *J Bone Joint Surg* [Br] 2005; 87:1520-1523.
[20] Bacarese-Hamilton I.A., Bhamra M.: Small bowel entrapment following acetabular fracture. *Injury* 1991; 22:242-244.
[21] Bartlett C.S., DiFelice G.S., Buly R.L., et al: Cardiac arrest as a result of intraabdominal extravasation of fluid during arthroscopic removal of a loose body from the hip joint of a patient with an acetabular fracture. J Orthop Trauma 1998; 12:294-299.
[22] Baumgaertner M.R.: Fractures of the posterior wall of the acetabulum. *J Am Acad Orthop Surg* 1999; 7:54-65.
[23] Beaule P.E., Dorey F.J., Matta J.M.: Letournel classification for acetabular fractures. Assessment of interobserver and intraobserver reliability. *J Bone Joint Surg* [Am] 2003; 85:1704-1709.
[24] Beaule P.E., Griffin D.B., Matta J.M.: The Levine anterior approach for total hip replacement as the treatment for an acute acetabular fracture. *J Orthop Trauma* 2004; 18:623-629.
[25] Berg E.E.: Charcot arthropathy after acetabular fracture. *J Bone Joint Surg [Br]* 1997; 79:742-745.
[26] Berton C., Bachour F., Migaud H., et al: [A new type of acetabular fracture: "True" posterosuperior fracture, a case report]. *Rev Chir Orthop Reparatrice Appar Mot* 2007; 93:93-97.
[27] Bhandari M., Matta J., Ferguson T., et al: Predictors of clinical and radiological outcome in patients with fractures of the acetabulum and concomitant posterior dislocation of the hip. *J Bone Joint Surg [Br]* 2006; 88:1618-1624.
[28] Borer D.S., Starr A.J., Reinert C.M., et al: The effect of screening for deep vein thrombosis on the prevalence of pulmonary embolism in patients with fractures of the pelvis or acetabulum: A review of 973 patients. *J Orthop Trauma* 2005; 19:92-95.
[29] Borrelli Jr. J., Goldfarb C., Catalano L., et al: Assessment of articular fragment displacement in acetabular fractures: A comparison of computerized tomography and plain radiographs. *J Orthop Trauma* 2002; 16:449-456.discussion 456–457
[30] Borrelli Jr. J., Goldfarb C., Ricci W., et al: Functional outcome after isolated acetabular fractures. *J Orthop Trauma* 2002; 16:73-81.
[31] Borrelli Jr. J., Ricci W.M., Anglen J.O., et al: Muscle strength recovery and its effects on outcome after open reduction and internal fixation of acetabular fractures. *J Orthop Trauma* 2006; 20:388-395.
[32] Bosse M.J.: Posterior acetabular wall fractures: A technique for screw placement. *J Orthop Trauma* 1991; 5:167-172.
[33] Bosse M.J., Poka A., Reinert C.M., et al: Preoperative angiographic assessment of the superior gluteal artery in acetabular fractures requiring extensile surgical exposures. *J Orthop Trauma* 1988; 2:303-307.
[34] Bosse M.J., Poka A., Reinert C.M., et al: Heterotopic ossification as a complication of acetabular fracture. Prophylaxis with low-dose irradiation. *J Bone Joint Surg [Am]* 1988; 70:1231-1237.
[35] Bray T.J., Esser M., Fulkerson L.: Osteotomy of the trochanter in open reduction and internal fixation of acetabular fractures. *J Bone Joint Surg [Am]* 1987; 69:711-717.

Part 4

Basic Science

8

Bisphosphonates and Bone

Sirmahan Cakarer, Firat Selvi and Cengizhan Keskin
Istanbul University, Dentistry Faculty,
Department of Oral and Maxillofacial Surgery
Turkey

1. Introduction

Bisphosphonates are pyrophosphate analogues which were used for over a century in industry (mainly in the textile and oil industries) as antiscaling and anticorrosive agents because of their property of inhibition of calcium carbonate precipitation. After the discovery of biological effects of bisphosphonates more than 30 years ago, they have now become indispensable in medicine for the treatment of skeletal complications of malignancy, Paget's disease, osteoporosis, multiple myeloma, hypercalcemia and fibrous dysplasia.

Bisphosphonates can be classified into two groups regarding their administration routes as orally or intravenously. The biological action mechanism of bisphosphonates on bone is maintained by their inhibitory effects on osteoclasts.

The general side effects and complications associated with bisphosphonates are esophageal or gastric irritation, atypical bone fractures, osteonecrosis of the jaws and ocular inflammation. Among these complications, Bisphosphonate-related Osteonecrosis of the Jaws (BRONJ) attracts clinical attention because of it's difficult management and its pathogenesis still being unclear.

The present chapter reviews history, classification, pharmacokinetics, clinical relevance and the mechanism of action of bisphosphonates. This chapter also focuses on the common side effects associated with these drugs, including mainly the Bisphosphonate-related Osteonecrosis of the Jaws (BRONJ). The importance of the consultation in between the medical doctors and the maxillofacial surgeons who experience the complications of bisphosphonates is emphasized. The practitioners who commonly prescribe bisphosphonates, should be aware of the complications of these drugs which may strongly diminish the quality of life of the patiens.

2. History and development of bisphosphonates

The bisphosphonates, in the past erroneously called diphosphonates, have been known to chemists since the middle of the 19th century, the first synthesis dating back to 1865 in Germany. Their use was industrial (mainly in the textile, fertilizer and oil industries) and, because of their property of inhibiting calcium carbonate precipitation, as preventors of scaling (1). Their use as 'water softeners'was based on their ability to act as sequestering agents for calcium, and in particular their ability to inhibit calcium carbonate precipitation, as do polyphosphates (2).

In the early 1960s, it is showed that body fluids such as plasma and urine contained inhibitors of calcification. Since it had been known since the 1930s that trace amounts of polyphosphates were capable of acting as water softeners by inhibiting the crystallization of calcium salts, such as calcium carbonate, they proposed that compounds of this type might be natural regulators of calcification under physiological conditions. Fleisch and his colleagues showed that inorganic pyrophosphate, a naturally occurring polyphosphate and a known by-product of many biosynthetic reactions in the body, was present in serum and urine and could prevent calcification by binding to newly forming crystals of hydroxyapatite. It was therefore postulated that pyrophosphate (PPi) might be the agent that normally prevents calcification of soft tissues, and regulates bone mineralization. Pathological disorders, such as the formation of kidney stones, might be linked to disturbances in PPi metabolism. The concentrations of pyrophosphate would be expected to be regulated by hydrolytic enzymes. Studies of the rare inherited disorder, hypophosphatasia, in which lack of alkaline phosphatase is associated with mineralization defects, showed that PPi levels were elevated in both plasma and urine, and verified that alkaline phosphatase was the key extracellular enzyme that hydrolyzes pyrophosphate. Attempts to exploit these concepts by using pyrophosphate and polyphosphates to inhibit ectopic calcification in blood vessels, skin, and kidneys in laboratory animals were successful only when the compounds were injected. Orally administered pyrophosphate and polyphosphates were inactive, due to the hydrolysis of pyrophosphate in the gastrointestinal tract, probably by mucosal brush border phosphatases. During the search for more stable analogues of pyrophosphate that might also have the antimineralization properties of pyrophosphate but that would be resistant to hydrolysis, several different chemical classes were studied. The bisphosphonates (at that time called diphosphonates) were among those studied. Like pyrophosphate, bisphosphonates had high affinity for bone mineral and were found to prevent calcification both in vitro and in vivo, but, unlike pyrophosphate, were also able to prevent pathological calcification when given orally to rats in vivo. This property of being active by mouth was key to their future use in humans. Perhaps the most important step towards the future use of bisphosphonates occurred when we found that bisphosphonates also had the novel property of being able to inhibit the dissolution of hydroxyapatite crystals. This led to studies to determine whether they might also inhibit bone resorption. Many studies using a variety of experimental systems showed that they were able to inhibit osteoclast-mediated bone resorption, both in organ cultures of bone in vitro, and in various animal models, e.g. thyroparathyroidectomized rats treated with parathyroid hormone to stimulate bone resorption in vivo (3).

3. Chemistry of bisphosphonates

Bisphosphonates are stable analogues of naturally-occurring inorganic pyrophosphate. Stability is conferred by a carbon atom replacing the oxygen atom that connects the two phosphates. This renders the molecule resistant to biological degradation. The BPs of clinical interest all have two phosphonate groups that share a common carbon atom (P-C-P). The P-C-P group is resistant not only to chemical but also to enzymatic hydrolysis. As a result, BPs are not converted to metabolites in the body and are excreted unaltered. The two phosphonate groups have a dual function. They are required both for binding to bone mineral and for cell-mediated antiresorptive activity. Modifications to one or both phosphonate groups can dramatically reduce the affinity of the BP for bone mineral, as well as reduce biochemical potency. The R1 and R2 side-chains attached to the carbon atom are responsible for the large range of activity observed among the BPs. R1 substituents such as hydroxyl or amino enhance chemisorption to mineral, while varying the R2 substituents results in differences in antiresorptive potency of several orders of magnitude. The increased antiresorptive potency observed with the different R2 groups is linked to the ability to affect biochemical activity, e.g., inhibition of the farnesyl pyrophosphate synthase (FPPS) enzyme (1, 4).

4. Classification

There are two classes of bisphosphonate regarding the presence or absence of Nitrogen. Non-Nitrogen containing bisphosphonates are; Etidronate (Didronel), Clodronate (Bonefos, Loron) and Tiludronate. The non-nitrogenous bisphosphonates(disphosphonates) are metabolised in the cell to compounds that replace the terminal pyrophosphate moiety of ATP, forming a nonfunctional molecule that competes with adenosine triphosphate (ATP) in the cellular energy metabolism. The osteoclast initiates apoptosis and dies, leading to an overall decrease in the breakdown of bone (5,6).

On the other hand, bisphosphonates can be classified into two groups regarding their administration routes as orally or intravenously. Orally administered bisphosphonates are; risedronate, alendronate, tiludronate and etidrontae. These are usually taken weekly Intravenously administered bisphosphonates are; pamidronate and zoledronic acid. These are usually administered monthly On the other hand ibandronate and clodronate can be administered as orally and intravenously (7,8,9).

Alendronate has a greater bone affinity than risedronate. The recommended weekly dose of alendronate at 70 mg weekly is almost double the potency of the recommended dose of 35 mg risedronate (10).

The duration of effect of bisphosphonates extends far beyond the duration of treatment. The effect of aledronate may be evident for more than five years after discontinuation of treatment and zoledronate has been shown to produce a sustained reduction in bone turnover for 12 months following administration of a single dose (8).

5. Pharmacology of bisphosphonates

Bisphosphonates can be given intravenously or orally. When taken orally, they must be taken after a prolonged fast (usually first thing in the morning), with water only, followed by 30–60 min with nothing else by mouth to allow for adequate absorption. Under ideal conditions, less than 1% of an orally administered dose is absorbed; taking a bisphosphonate with food or anything containing divalent cations will completely block its absorption. There is no systemic metabolism. The half-life in plasma is short. Fifty percent of the absorbed dose binds to bone surfaces, mostly avidly at sites of active remodeling. The skeletal capacity is large and the binding sites are virtually unsaturable. The 50% or so that does not bind to bone is excreted rapidly by the kidneys (11).

The renal/nonrenal clearance ratio differs significantly among bisphosphonates; the ratio is approximately 2 for clodronate and 0.3 for pamidronate. This may partly explain the higher dose of clodronate needed for a therapeutic effect. The distribution of the bisphosphonates within the skeleton is not homogeneous; the drug is targeted to sites of skeletal metabolism, where bone mineral is exposed to the surrounding fluids. The degree of skeletal uptake is dependent upon the rate of bone turnover. When the bisphosphonates are incorporated into bone, the half-life is extremely long, to over 10 years, relating to the turnover time of the active skeletal sites. After very high intravenous doses some bisphosphonates accumulate in liver, spleen, lung and kidney (9).

6. Mechanism of action

The mechanisms of action of the bisphosphonates in bone metabolism are complex and multifactorial. Although complex mechanisms are involved, the side chains influence the binding affinity (R1 side chain) and the antiresorptive potency (R2 side chain).They act almost exclusively on bone because of their specific affinity to bone where they are deposited in newly formed bone and close to osteoclasts. Although the time in the circulation is short, 30 to 180 minutes, once incorporated into bone they can persist for up to 10 years. Different types of bisphosphonates have differing affinities to bone with the rank order from greatest to least being zoledronate, alendronate, ibandronate, risedronate, etidronate and clodronate . Once in the bone they directly affect mononuclear activity, which is the parent cell of osteoclasts, they disrupt osteoclast mediated, bone resorption and increase apoptosis of osteoclasts. This in turn reduces bone deposition by osteoblasts. The net effect of this is to reduce bone resorption and bone turnover. Angiogenesis is reduced by depression of blood flow and a marked decrease in vascular endothelial growth factor. Epithelial keratinocytes are also inhibited. The net effect of these actions is to reduce healing capacity (10).

Treatment with bisphosphonates also results in a modest increase in bone mineral density (BMD). Non-nitrogen-containing bisphosphonates inhibit osteoclastic activity by producing toxic analogs of ATP that cause cell death. Nitrogen-containing bisphosphonates (*e.g.* alendronate, risedronate, ibandronate, and zoledronate) inhibit an enzyme called farnesyl pyrophosphate synthase, an enzyme in the 3-hydroxy-3- methylglutaryl coenzyme A reductase pathway. Inhibition of this enzyme interferes with a process called prenylation: preventing the addition of 15- and 20-carbon side chains that anchor GTP-binding proteins to the osteoclast cell membrane; this leads to reduced resorptive activity of osteoclasts and accelerated apoptosis (programmed cell death). The rank order of potency for inhibiting farnesyl pyrophosphate synthase is zoledronate _ risedronate __ ibandronate _ alendronate, with the more potent heterocyclic bisphosphonates (zoledronate and risedronate) having a more optimal fit than the compounds with an alkyl side chain (alendronate and ibandronate).

Each bisphosphonate has a unique profile of binding affinity and antiresorptive potency that likely results in clinically meaningful differences in the speed of onset and offset of effect, the degree of reduction of bone turnover, uptake in cortical *vs.* trabecular bone and types of antifracture effect (vertebral *vs.* nonvertebral) (11).

6.1 Effects of bisphosphonates on bone turnover

The degree of reduction of bone turnover achieved by each bisphosphonate, as well as the duration of action appears to be associated with their mineral-binding affinity and skeletal retention. Bisphosphonates with higher mineral-binding affinity and potential retention, such as alendronate and zoledronate, are associated with greater reduction of bone turnover and have a longer duration of effect after treatment is stopped. Bisphosphonates with lower mineral-binding affinity and retention, such as risedronate and etidronate, appear to reduce bone turnover less and this effect seems to be more readily reversible when therapy stops. In patients treated for 3 years or 7 years with risedronate, bone turnover markers returned to pretreatment levels within 1 year after discontinuation of treatment (12).

7. Clinical use of bisphosphonates

The most impressive clinical application of bisphosphonates has undoubtedly been as inhibitors of bone resorption, often for diseases where no effective treatment existed previously, but it took many years for them to become well established. However, the first clinical uses of bisphosphonates were as inhibitors of calcification. Etidronate was the only BP to be used in this way, first in fibrodysplasia ossicans progressiva (FOP, formerly known as myositis ossificans). Etidronate showed some promise in patients who had undergone total hip replacement surgery to prevent subsequent heterotopic ossification and to improve mobility. It was also used to prevent ectopic calcification and ossification, after spinal cord injury and in topical applications in toothpastes to prevent dental calculus. There is a recent and renewed interest in devising effective treatments for calcification in renal failure and vascular disease. One of the other early clinical uses of bisphosphonates was as agents for bone imaging, "bone scanning," for which they still remain outstandingly useful for detecting bone metastases and other bone lesions. The application of pyrophosphate and simple bisphosphonates as bone scanning agents depends on their strong affinity for bone mineral, particularly at sites of increased bone turnover, and their ability to be linked to a gamma-emitting technetiumisotope. Bisphosphonates have become the treatment of choice for a variety of bone diseases in which excessive osteoclast activity is an important pathological feature, including Paget's disease of bone, metastatic and osteolytic bone disease, and hypercalcaemia of malignancy, as well as osteoporosis.

Currently there are at least eleven bisphosphonates (etidronate, clodronate, tiludronate, pamidronate, alendronate, ibandronate, risedronate, and zoledronate, and also to a limited extent olpadronate, neridronate and minodronate) that have been registered for various clinical applications in various countries (2).

7.1 Bisphosphonates in oncology

Consensus guidance recommendations indicate that all patients with multiple myeloma and radiologically confirmed bone metastases from breast cancer should receive bisphosphonates from the time of diagnosis and continue indefinitel. Bisphosphonate treatment—specifically zoledronic acid—is also appropriate for patients with endocrine-resistant metastatic bone disease from prostate cancer. Patients with other tumours and symptomatic metastasis to bone should be considered for treatment with zoledronic acid if bone is the dominant site of metastasis, especially if the prognosis is reasonable. Patients with renal cell cancer particularly appear to benefit from treatment. There is extensive experience with intravenous bisphosphonates in breast cancer with zoledronic acid, pamidronate and ibandronate all showing useful clinical activity. For most patients with multiple myeloma intravenous bisphosphonates have become part of routine clinical management.

Over recent years great advances have been made in the development and use of bone-targeted therapy in oncology. The use of bisphosphonates in oncology has had a profound beneficial effect on the management of metastatic bone disease and the prevention of treatment-induced bone loss. Their use should be considered in all patients with bone metastases, especially those with symptoms and without immediately life-threatening extraskeletal disease. Guidelines for the use of the agents in preventing treatment-induced bone loss are evolving and trials investigating their potential role in the adjuvant setting to prevent metastasis are ongoing. If proven, the clinician will need to decide if the patient is at risk of bone loss, bone metastasis or both, as the dose and frequency of bisphosphonate may differ within each scenario. As a class the agents are well tolerated. Occasional serious toxicities in terms of renal impairment and osteonecrosis of the jawcan be largely avoided through adhering to the recommended dose and infusion times and good preventative dental care respectively (13).

7.2 Bisphosphonates in Paget's disease of bone

Paget's disease is characterised by focal abnormalities of increased bone turnover affecting one or more sites throughout the skeleton. The axial skeleton is preferentially affected, and common sites of involvement include the pelvis (70% of cases), femur (55%), lumbar spine (53%), skull (42%), and tibia (32%). Paget's disease was the first clinical disorder in which a dose dependent inhibition of bone resorption could be demonstrated using bisphosphonates in man, and was well established by the 1980s. The medical treatment of Paget's disease is now reliant almost exclusively on the use of the bisphosphonate class of drugs. There have been gradual improvements in the ability of these drugs to keep the disease under control, starting with etidronate in the 1970s, and progressing through the use of other BPs given by mouth, such as clodronate, tiludronate, alendronate, and risedronate. These days most patients are treated with BPs given by infusion, either as pamidronate or more recently as zoledronic acid (2, 14).

7.3 Bisphosphonates in osteoporosis

Osteoporosis is an emerging medical and socioeconomic threat characterised by a systemic impairment of bone mass, strength, and microarchitecture, which increases the propensity of fragility fractures. Bone mineral density (BMD) can be assessed with dual x-ray absorptiometry (DXA), and osteoporosis is defined by a T score of less than 2.5, ie, more than 2.5 standard deviations below the average of a young adult. About 40% of white postmenopausal women are affected by osteoporosis and, with an ageing population, this number is expected to steadily increase in the near future. The lifetime fracture risk of a patient with osteoporosis is as high as 40%, and fractures most commonly occur in the spine, hip, or wrist, but other bones such as the trochanter, humerus, or ribs can also be affected.

From a patient's perspective, a fracture and the subsequent loss of mobility and autonomy often represent a major drop in quality of life. Additionally, osteoporotic fractures of the hip and spine carry a 12-month excess mortality of up to 20%, because they require hospitalisation and they have subsequently enhanced risk of other complications, such as pneumonia or thromboembolic disease due to chronic immobilisation (15).

A number of bisphosphonates have been evaluated in postmenopausal osteoporosis and investigated in large clinical trials with fracture as an end-point. This has resulted in the licensing of alendronate, risedronate, ibandronate and zoledronic acid for the treatment of postmenopausal osteoporosis. Bisphosphonate therapy acts by lowering the activation frequency and so slows the deterioration in bone architecture. Bisphosphonates are effective in reducing bone turnover, with an earlier decrease in bone resorption than bone formation; there are differences in the time course and magnitude of response, depending on the type and route of administration of the bisphosphonate. There is an increase in BMD that results from filling in of the remodeling space and increasing mineralization of bone tissue. In consequence, there is a reduction in fracture risk in postmenopausal women with osteoporosis. The licensed bisphosphonates exhibit some differences in potency and speed of onset and offset of action. These differences mean that different agents may be more advantageous in different situations. Uncertainties remain around the optimum duration of treatment and treatment holidays, how best to use bisphosphonates with anabolic treatments, and the benefits of treatment in patients who do not have a BMD T-score below −2.5. (16).

7.4 Bisphosphonates in orthopedic interventions

The rationale for the potential use of bisphosphonates in orthopedics is similar to that of other uses to limit bone resorption. Recent years have seen a great many studies, both pre-clinical and clinical, exploring the potential application of the BPs to the problems of bone catabolism encountered in orthopedics. To date, the most promising roles for the BPs have been found in prevention of bone collapse following osteonecrosis and in enhancing implant fixation. Combination therapies that have both bone anti-resorptive and anabolic agents also show great promise for orthopedic applications. However, further large scale clinical trials are required to confirm whether these observations translate into a clinical benefit for patients and the development of robust indications for these therapies in orthopedic practice (17).

8. Side effects of bisphosphonates

The esophageal or gastric irritation caused by the oral preparations is an established adverse effect. However, osteonecrosis of the jaw (ONJ) and subtrochanteric fractures have attracted most of the attention mainly because their pathophysiology remains unclear.

8.1 Acute-phase reaction/response

Twenty four to seventy two hours or even several days after the first administration of an IV nitrogen-containing bisphosphonate, approximately 40% of the patients will experience influenza-like illness with pyrexia, chills, myalgia and arthralgia that tend to resolve within

3 days. This symptomatology can also occur after high oral doses and is associated with an acute-phase reaction. Supportive and symptomatic management with NSAIDs and acetaminophen is sufficient. The proportion of patients affected is decreased substantially following subsequent infusions (18).

8.2 Ocular inflammation

Nitrogen-containing bisphosphonates, usually IV pamidronate administration, have been associated with the development of ocular inflammation in the form of nonspecific conjunctivitis, uveitis, iritis, episcleritis and scleritis, with incidence ranging from 0.046% to 1%. Ocular inflammation can resolve after a short course of corticosteroid treatment and in cases of scleritis bisphosphonate administration must be discontinued. Also, avoidance of bisphosphonates or caution in their use (especially IV) for those with a history of inflammatory eye disease or uveitis is recommended (18).

8.3 Gastrointestinal side effects

Gastrointestinal (GI) problems are often considered to be an inevitable consequence associated with the oral use of bisphosphonates, which are currently extensively prescribed (alendronate, risedronate, and ibandronate) for the prevention and treatment of osteoporosis. However, the results from the major prospective RCTs assessing the reduction of fractures are notable in not showing an excess of GI problems. It is generally acknowledged that upper GI symptoms are very common in elderly patients whether or not bisphosphonates are given. In contrast, the more severe side effects associated with esophageal events such as ulceration are rare but potentially more serious, and were noted in particular after giving oral pamidronate or alendronate. In terms of practical management, the interference of absorption by food as well as these esophageal problems are minimized in patients taking oral bisphosphonates on an empty stomach, first thing in the morning, with sufficient plain water, while remaining in an upright position without eating or further drinking for at least 30 minutes (60 minutes in the case of ibandronate). Strict adherence to these instructions is thought to reduce the incidence of serious esophageal adverse events (12).

8.4 Atrial fibrillation

An international, multicenter, randomized, double-blind, placebo-controlled trial raised by the HORIZON found an increased incidence of serious atrial fibrillation in patients which use zoledronic-acid, as compared with the placebo group (19). While bisphosphonates are targeted to a patient group that is already at higher risk of atrial fibrillation than the background population, current studies from large health databases have identified either no increase or only a small increase in the risk of atrial fibrillation with oral bisphosphonate use, with no apparent added risk of thromboembolic complications (20). Despite the lack of a known biologically plausible explanation for bisphosphonate-induced atrial fibrilation, several potential mechanisms have been hypothesized. Given the absence of any proven mechanism for bisphosphonate-induced arrhythmia formation, continued reports of a possible association will justify the need for additional studies to more fully explore these and other potential mechanisms (21).

8.5 Atypical femoral fractures

Although bisphosphonates reduce the rates of fractures due to osteoporosis, recent reports suggested a link between bisphosphonate use and the development of atypical insufficiency fractures. This is thought to be due to long term oversuppression of bone turnover leading to impaired bone remodeling, accumulation of microdamage in bone and increased skeletal fragility (11).

Several publications demonstrated the occurrence of femoral fractures associated with long-term bisphosphonate use (22,23,24,25,26).

These fractures appear to be more common in patients who have been exposed to long-term BPs, usually for more than 3 years (median treatment 7 years). It must be emphasized that these fractures are rare, particularly when considered in the context of the millions of patients who have taken BPs and also when compared with typical and common femoral neck and intertrochanteric fractures. It also must be emphasized that BPs are important drugs for the prevention of common osteoporotic fractures. However, atypical femoral fractures are of concern, and more information is urgently needed both to assist in identifying patients at particular risk and to guide decision making about duration of BP therapy. Physicians and patients should be made aware of the possibility of atypical femoral fractures and of the potential for bilaterality through a change in labeling of BPs. Given the relative rarity of atypical femoral fractures, to facilitate future research, specific diagnostic and procedural codes should be created for cases of atypical femoral fractures, an international registry should be established,and the quality of case reporting should be improved. Research directions should include development of animal models, increased surveillance, and additional epidemiologic data to establish the true incidence of and risk factors for this condition and studies to address their surgical and medical management (27).

A position paper reported by Rizzoli et al, reviewed the evidence for an association between atypical subtrochanteric fractures and longterm bisphosphonate use. They demonstrated that the available evidence does not suggest that the well-known benefits of bisphosphonate treatment are outweighed by the risk of these rare, atypical, low-trauma subtrochanteric fractures. Nevertheless, it is recommended that physicians remain vigilant in assessing their patients treated with bisphosphonates for osteoporosis or associated conditions. They should continue to follow the recommendations on the drug label when prescribing bisphosphonates and advise patients of the potential risks. Patients with pain in the hips, thighs or femur should be radiologically assessed and, where a stress fracture is evident, the physician should decide whether bisphosphonate therapy should be discontinued pending a full evaluation, based on an individual benefit-risk assessment. The radiographic changes should be evaluated for orthopaedic intervention—since surgery prior to fracture completion might be advantageous—or be closely monitored (28).

8.6 Bone, joint, or muscle pain

In postmarketing experience, there are infrequent case reports describing severe and occasionally incapacitating bone, joint, and/or muscle pain in patients taking bisphosphonates. The pain could occur days, months, or even years after starting bisphosphonates. It is probably different or, at least, not only associated with the acute-phase response and presents within the first few days after the first treatment with an IV bisphosphonate. Most patients reported relief of symptoms after discontinuing therapy and a subset had recurrence of pain when restarting treatment with the same or a different bisphosphonate (12).

8.7 Bisphosphonate-related Osteonecrosis of the Jaws (BRONJ)

To distinguish BRONJ from other delayed healing conditions, the following working definition of BRONJ has been adopted by the American Association of Oral and Maxillofacial Surgeon. Patients may be considered to have BRONJ if all of the following 3 characteristics are present:Current or previous treatment with a bisphosphonate ; exposed bone in the maxillofacial region that has persisted for more than 8 weeks and no history of radiation therapy to the jaws. It is important to understand that patients at risk of, or with established, BRONJ can also present with other common clinical conditions not to be confused with BRONJ. Commonly misdiagnosed conditions can include, but are not limited to, alveolar osteitis, sinusitis, gingivitis/periodontitis, caries, periapical pathologic findings, and temporomandibular joint disorders (29,30).

A disease remarkably similar to the presentation of BRONJ was initially described in the match-making industry at the end of the 18th century. Considered by some to be the first identified instance of a disease caused by occupational exposure of a chemical (elemental phosphorus), "phossy jaw" was characterized by bone necrosis and infection that was isolated to the jaw. Recently, some reports have attempted to establish parallels with BRONJ and "phossy jaw." Although the clinical presentations of BRONJ and phossy jaw are quite similar, the chemical agents known to be the cause of these diseases are very different in structure and chemical properties. In reality, BRONJ is likely a disease entity that was no nexistent prior to the late 1990s, and is linked to the emergence of bisphosphonates as a popular mode of therapy for the treatment of osteolytic bone disease and osteoporosis (31).

BRONJ was first described by Marx and Stern in 2002. At that time it was only a curious finding of exposed, nonhealing bone when debridement was performed, the condition worsened and led to increased amounts of exposed bone. In 2003; Marx described 36 cases associated with intravenous bisphosphonates (pamidronate or zoledronate) in a medical alert published in the Journal of Oral and Maxillofacial Surgery (30,32). Since the original 2003 publication, more than 1,100 additional reports by over 4,500 authors and at least 14 position papers have been written about BRONJ (30).

8.8 Osteomyelitis, osteoradionecrosis and BRONJ

Microscopically, BRONJ presents a picture that may be either suppurative osteomyelitis or osteoradionecrosis. However representative central bone biopsy specimens identify distinct and unique histopathologies that underscore the separate mechanisms of each. Suppurative osteomyelitis shows inflammatory cells in the marrow space. It shows also necrotic bone and viable reactive bone. Osteoradionecrosis, similarly shows necrotic bone but without any marrow inflammation. Instead, the marrow space contains poorly cellular or acellular collagen consistent with marrow fibrosis and the well-documented hypocellular, hypovascular, hypoxic characteristics of radiated tissue. Microorganisms colonize on the bone surface but do not invade the tissue because osteoradionecrosis is an effect of radiation tissue damage and is not a primary bacterial process. BRONJ, in contrast, shows neither marrow inflammation nor marrow fibrosis. Instead, the marrow has empty acellular marrow spaces along with necrotic bone with numerous Howship lacunae. Surface microorganisms are frequently seen in associaton with necrotic bone and often prompt an inaccurate diagnosis of osteomyelitis. The clinical description and history remain the best tools available for distinguishing BRONJ from these other conditions of delayed bone and wound healing (30).

8.9 Comparison of long bone to alveolar bone and BRONJ

Alveolar bone exists to support the teeth. Its structure varies between individuals and generally it gets denser with age. Broadly, there is a dense bone wall near the gingivae and then the middle portion of the tooth root. There are larger marrow spaces near the tooth apex. The alveolar bone walls at the attachment of the periodontal membrane have a cribiform structure with open channels. The bone structure follows that of bone structure throughout the body with cortical bone containing osteons and Haversian systems. New bone is formed in a lamellar structure by osteoblasts with the osteocytes being incorporated within the bone. Older bone, or bone in the path of erupting or moving teeth is resorbed by osteoclasts. In keeping with all bone in the body, alveolar bone is a dynamic structure with the bone constantly remodelling and adapting to functional needs. The key question however, is whether alveolar bone is exactly the same as the long bones or whether it is subtly different. Alveolar bone develops as a membrane bone whereas the limbs and vertebrae develop as endochondral bones. The mandible is of neural crest origin whereas the limbs and vertebral column are of mesodermal origin. There are minor phenotypic differences between osteoblasts depending on their site of origin and anatomical location, which can be demonstrated biochemically. Membrane bone osteoblasts also have an increased rate of cell division as compared to iliac crest osteoblasts. Osteoclasts are derived from mononuclear precursor cells which migrate from the bone marrow via the vasculature to the bone site. Their function is dictated largely by interaction with the osteoblasts in the area. There are biochemical differences between osteoclasts of membrane bone origin and long bone origin. There are also differences in behaviour between giant cell tumours of the jaws and of the long bones. The long bone is deeply covered in soft tissue and they are not commonly exposed. On the other hand the alveolar bone is covered only mucoperiostally. The long bones are low vascular than the alveolar bone (10).

The alveolar crest remodels at 10 times greater than the rate of tibia, 5 times the rate of the mandible at the inferior border, and 3-5 times the rate of the mandible at the level of the mandibular canal. As a result, the alveolar bone of the jaws has a greater uptake of bisphosphonates and readily accumulates at higher concentrations. It is also reported that the alveolar bone depends more on osteoclastic bone resorption/remodeling and renewal than any other bone in the adult skeleton. The jaws are repeatedly traumatised by mastication and they expose to the oral environment and commensal micro-organisms more than the long bones. All these differences between the jaws and the other bones, explain why only the jaws are affected. To date it has not been reported in other skeletal sites as exposed bone; however, recent reports have identified femur fractures caused by long-term use of bisphosphonates (30).

8.10 Causality of BRONJ

Epidemiologic studies have established a compelling, albeit circumstantial, association between IV bisphosphonates and BRONJ in the setting of malignant disease. An association between IV bisphosphonate exposure and BRONJ may be hypothesised based on the following observations: (i) a positive correlation between bisphosphonate potency and risk for developing BRONJ; (ii) a negative correlation between bisphosphonate potency and duration of bisphosphonate exposure prior to developing BRONJ; and (iii) a positive correlation between duration of bisphosphonate exposure and developing BRONJ. However, the current level of evidence does not fully support a cause and effect relationship between bisphosphonate exposure and necrosis of the jaw. Although causality may never be proven, emerging iexperimental and epidemiologic studies have established a firm foundation for a strong association between monthly IV bisphosphonate therapy and BRONJ. The causal association between oral or IV bisphosphonates for treating osteoporosis and BRONJ is much more difficult to establish (29).

8.11 Incidence of BRONJ

IV bisphosphonate exposure in the setting of managing malignancy remains the major risk factor for BRONJ. According to case series, casecontrolled studies, and cohort studies, estimates of the cumulative incidence of BRONJ have ranged from 0.8% to 12%. Patients receiving oral bisphosphonate therapy are at a considerably lower risk of BRONJ than cancer patients treated with monthly IV bisphosphonates.

The clinical efficacy of oral bisphosphonates for the treatment of osteopenia/osteoporosis is well established and is reflected in the fact that over 190 million oral bisphosphonate prescriptions have been dispensed worldwide. Based on available data, the risk of BRONJ for patients receiving IV bisphosphonates is significantly greater than that for patients receiving oral bisphosphonates.Regardless, given the large number of patients receiving oral bisphosphonates for the treatment of osteoporosis/osteopenia, it is likely that most practitioners will encounter some patients with BRONJ. It is important to accurately determine the incidence of BRONJ in this population and to assess the risk associated with long-term use (ie, longer than 3 years) of oral bisphosphonates. The low prevalence of BRONJ in osteoporosis patients poses a significant challenge for future clinical trials aimed at establishing accurate incidence data (29).

8.12 Risk factors of BRONJ

BRONJ risks were categorized as drug-related, local, and demographic, systemic, genetic and preventative factors. Other medications, such as steroids and thalidomide, and other chemotherapeutic agents were thought to be risk factors, but no measurable associations were identified (29).

Drug-related risk factors include bisphosphonate potency and duration of therapy. Zoledronate (Zometa®) is more potent than pamidronate (Aredia®) and pamidronate (Aredia®) is more potent than the oral bisphosphonates; the IV route of administration results in a greater drug exposure than the oral route. Using a number of different risk measures, the BRONJ risk among cancer patients given IV bisphosphonate exposure ranged from 2.7 to 4.2, suggesting that cancer patients receiving IV bisphosphonates have a 2.7- to 4.2-fold increased risk for BRONJ than cancer patients not exposed to IV bisphosphonates. Longer duration od the use of bisphosphonates appears to be associated with increased risk.

Local risk factors include; dentoalveolar surgery, including, but not limited to extractions, dental implant placement, periapical surgery, periodontal surgery involving osseous injury. Patients receiving IV bisphosphonates and undergoing dentoalveolar surgery are at least seven times more likely to develop BRONJ than patients who are not having dentoalveolar surgery.

It has been observed that lesions are found more commonly in the mandible than the maxilla (2:1 ratio) and more commonly in areas with thin mucosa overlying bony prominences such as tori, bony exostoses and the mylohyoid. No data are available to provide risk estimates for anatomic structures and BRONJ.

Cancer patients exposed to IV bisphosphonates with a history of inflammatory dental disease, for example periodontal and dental abscesses, are at a sevenfold increased risk for developing BRONJ.

8.12.1 Demographic and systemic factors

Sex was not statistically associated with BRONJ. Race was reported in one study to be a risk factor, with Caucasians having an increased risk for BRONJ compared with blacks. Other systemic factors or conditions, that is renal dialysis, low haemoglobin, obesity and diabetes, were variably reported to increase the risk for BRONJ. Malignancy type was not statistically associated with an increased risk for BRONJ.

8.12.2 Genetic factors

It is reported that genetic perturbations, that is single nucleotide polymorphisms (SNPs), in the cytochrome P450-2C gene (CYP2C8) gene were associated with an increased risk for BRONJ among multiple myeloma patients treated with IV bisphosphonates.

8.12.3 Preventative factors

Alternative dosing schedules that reduce IV bisphosphonate exposure have comparable outcomes in terms of preventing a decreased risk of BRONJ.

The two largest risk factors for BRONJ are IV bisphosphonate exposure and dentoalveolar procedures. Recent studies suggest that manipulation of IV bisphosphonates dosing may be effective for minimising BRONJ risk. In addition, preventative dental interventions before initiating IV bisphosphonate treatment can also effectively reduce, but not eliminate, the risk of BRONJ (29).

8.13 Clinical management of BRONJ

The management of BRONJ currently is a dilemma. No effective treatment has yet been developed and interrupting bisphosphonate therapy does not seem to be beneficial because the drugs accumulate at high levels inside the bone matrix. However, cessation of bisphosphonate therapy can have severe problems, such as bone metastasis, multiple myeloma or hypercalcemia associated with tumors. In general all the guidelines related to the management of BRONJ recommended a nonsurgical approach consisting of a mix of medical therapies.

Treatment of BRONJ focuses on controlling pain, limiting secondary infection and extension of the exposed bone and maintaining function. These are achieved with the use of 0.12 % clorhexidine, 15 mL oral swish and spit three times daily. To control the pain of initial secondary infection Penicilin VK 500 mg by mouth four times daily can be used. If the patient is allergic to penicilin, alternatives are; doxycycline 100 mg once daily, levofloxacin 500 mg once daily, azithromycin 500 mg once daily. In patients who have a minimal response to these antibiotic regimens, adding metronidazole 500 mg three times daily for 10 days can resolve the secondary infection. More or less aggresive surgery is recommended only in advanced, nonresponsive cases. Surgical treatment, in accordance to AAOMS position paper, is reserved to patients affected by BRONJ lesions (30).

9. Clinical cases

The present chapter presents 3 clinical cases that were managed by the authors in Istanbul University, Dentistry Faculty, Department of Oral and Maxillofacial Surgery. The cases presented here show the importance of the clinical situation, to the all medical doctors which prescribe bisphosphonates. Theses cases presents also that the life quality of the patients can be very low because of this situation.

9.1 CASE 1

A 65-year-old woman has presented with a complaint of pain in the right side of the maxilla. Clinical examination of the patient showed a large necrotic mass of bone on the right half of the maxilla (Figure 1). The patients's medical history involved multiple myeloma disease resisting for more than 3 years. She informed that she had been using zoledronic acid for the last 1 year for the management of this disease. During this period, she had undergone multiple tooth extractions at the right side of the maxilla. MRI findings and orthopantomograph showed the necrotic bone (Figure 2, Figure 3). Clinical and radiological examinations, along with the medical anemnesis taken, revealed the diagnosis of ''BRONJ''.

Initially, a drug holiday has started for zoledronic acid after consultation with the patient's physician. Along with this, oral amoxicillin with clavulanic acid 1000 mg two times daily, combined with oral metronidazole 500 mg two times daily were prescribed. These were used for two months. 0.12% chlorhexidine oral rinsing 3 times daily was also used during this period for maintaining good oral hygiene. This type of treatment resolved the acute reactions and pain. Even though this treatment did not help the formation of a demarcation line of the necrotic bone, there wasn't either a progress in the enlargement of the necrotic area too. Bone resection was not permitted because of the severe multiple myeloma. The patient is still followed up continuously every three months.

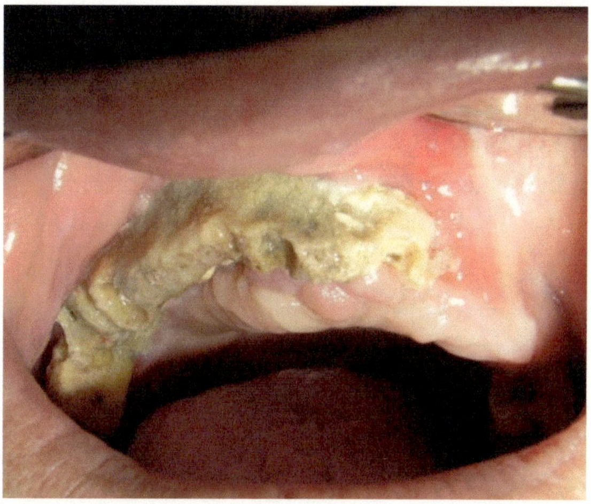

Fig. 1. Clinical view of the necrotic bone.

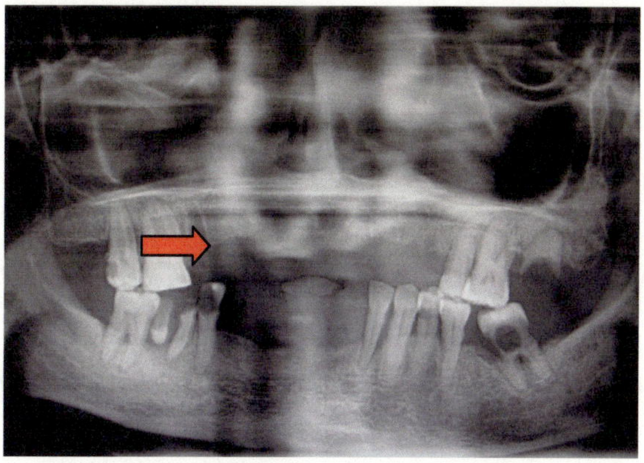

Fig. 2. Orthopantomograph showing the necrotic bone.

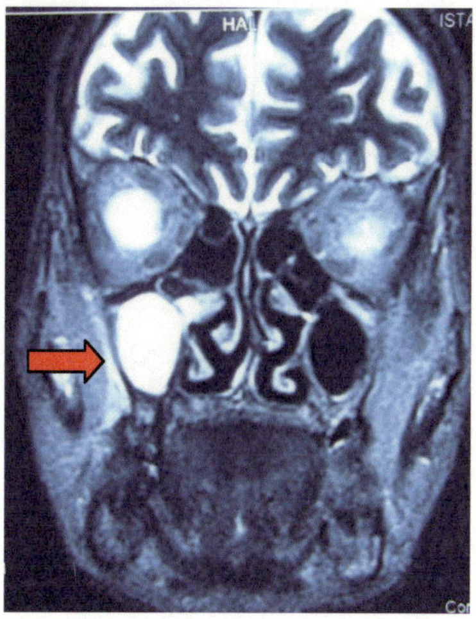

Fig. 3. MRI showing the infected right maxillary sinus.

9.2 CASE 2

A 75-year-old male patient has presented with a complaint of pain in the right side of the maxilla. Clinical examination has shown a large mass of exposed necrotic bone in the right side of the maxilla with the swelling of the palatal mucosa (Figure 4). The patient has been diagnosed with multiple myeloma for two years. He has informed that he had been using zoledronic acid since the beginning of his disease. Orthopantomograph has shown the necrotic area (Figure 5).

Initially, a drug holiday has started for zoledronic acid after consultation with the patient's physician. Along with this, oral amoxicillin with clavulanic acid 1000 mg two times daily, combined with oral metronidazole 500 mg two times daily were prescribed. These were used according to two months usage and one month holiday protocol. 0.12% chlorhexidine oral rinsing 3 times daily was also used during this period for maintaining good oral hygiene. This type of treatment resolved the acute reactions and pain. After one and a half years of conservative treatment, sequestrum formation was observed and it was peeled off by itself. (Figure 6 and Figure 7). The patient is followed up continuously every three months.

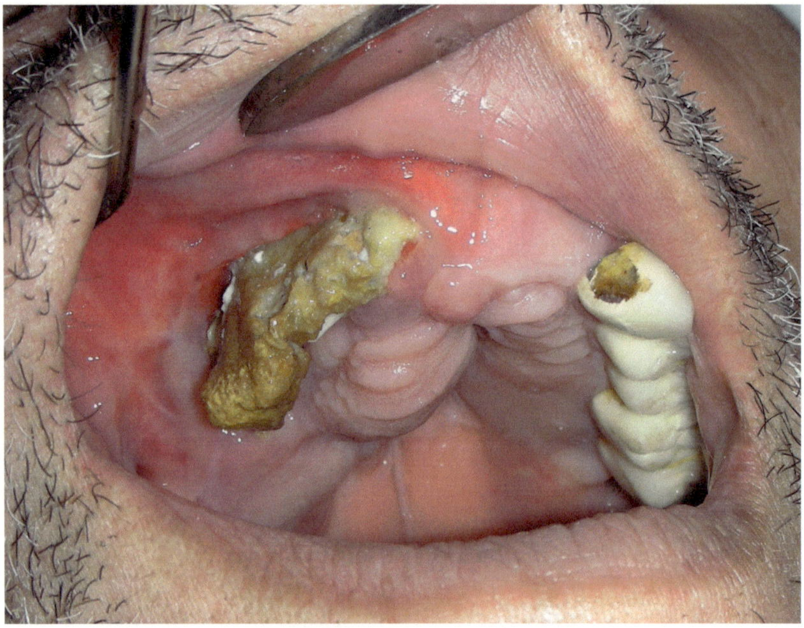

Fig. 4. Clinical view of the exposed bone.

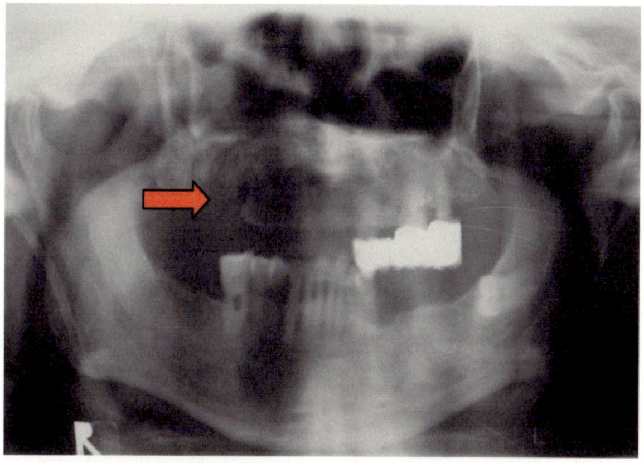

Fig. 5. Orthopantomograph showing the necrotic bone.

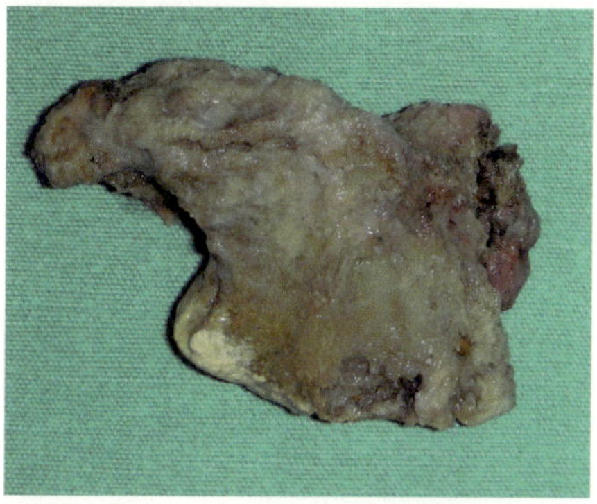

Fig. 6. **S**equestrum's clinical appearence at the right side of the mandible.

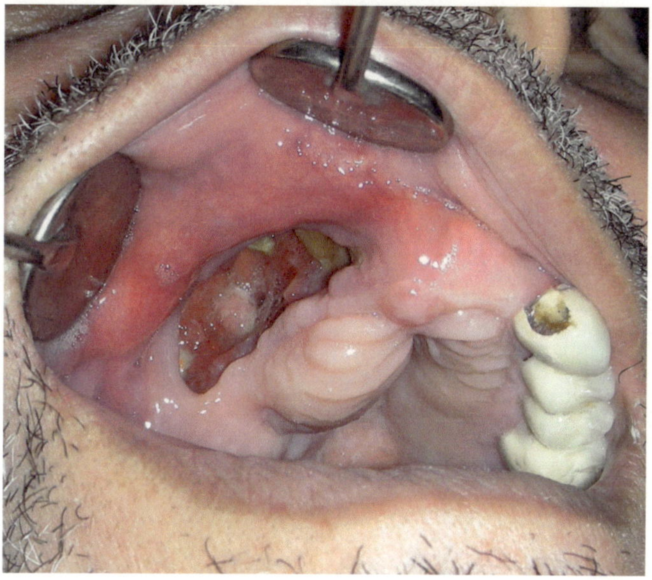

Fig. 7. Clinical view of the affected area after the removal of the sequestrum.

9.3 CASE 3

52-year-old woman was referred to our clinic with pain and exposed bone at the right mandibular posterior area (Figure 8). In 1997, she had undergone mastectomy for her breast cancer. In between the years 2001 and 2006, she had used zoledronic acid for her bone metastasis related with her breast cancer. In 2006, bisphosphonate related osteonecrosis of the right mandibular area was diagnosed in a private clinic. Her physician had decided to discontinue zoledronic acid and instead had prescribed ibandronat. A local curettage and debridement was performed in the private clinic before applying to our clinic. In the orthopantomograph, the necrotic bone was clearly observed (Figure 9). Amoxicillin with clavulonic acid combined with metronidazole was used to supress her infection. After a drug holiday of three month; in december 2010, we performed local curettage and debridement using Er,Cr: YSGG laser and the wound was closed primarily (Figure 10, Figure 11). Postoperative clinical and radiological examination did not reveal any sign of osteonecrosis or infection, 6 months after the operation (Figure 12, Figure 13) The patient is followed up continuously every three months.

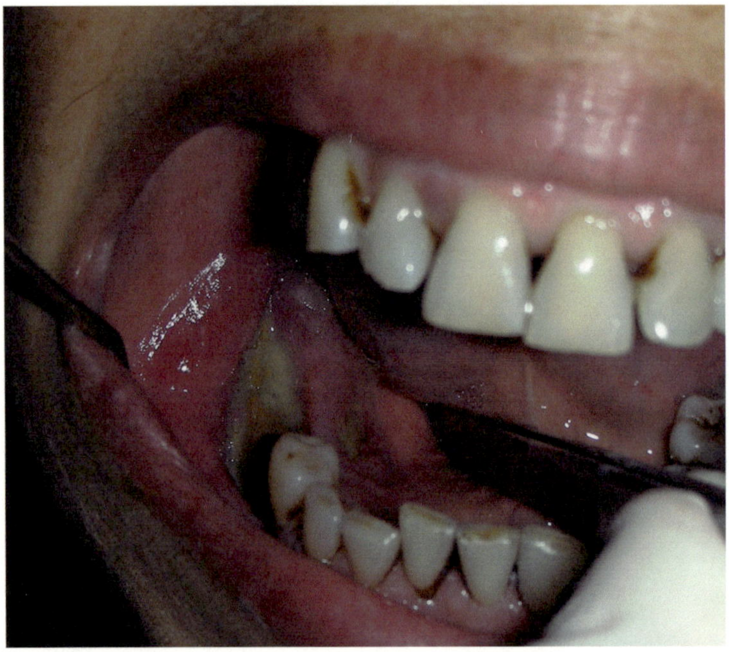

Fig. 8. Clinical view of the exposed bone at the vestibular and lingual part of the posterior right side of the mandible.

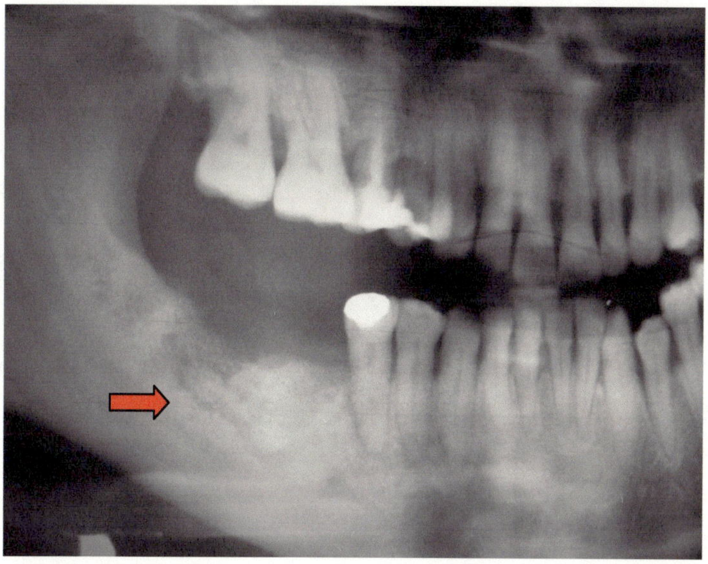

Fig. 9. Orthopantomograph showing the necrotic bone at the posterior right side of the mandible. Note the line of the demarcation.

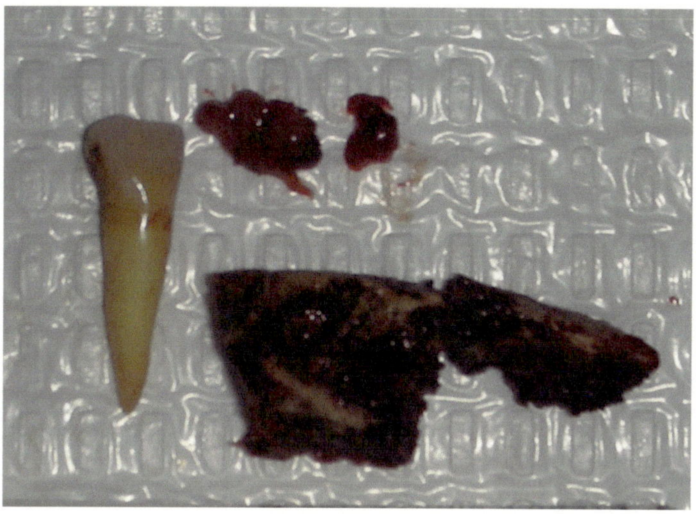

Fig. 10. Removed sequestrum and the associated teeth.

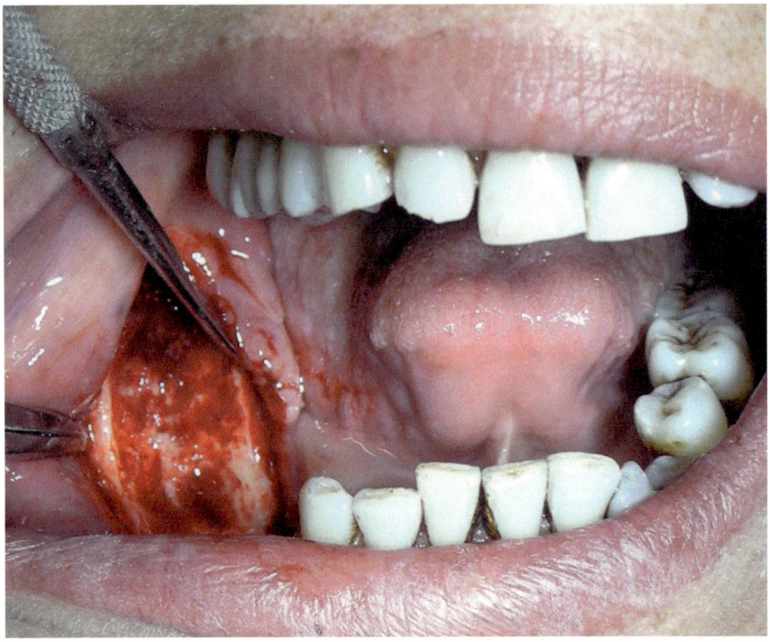

Fig. 11. Clinical view of the bone after the removal of the sequestrum and laser application.

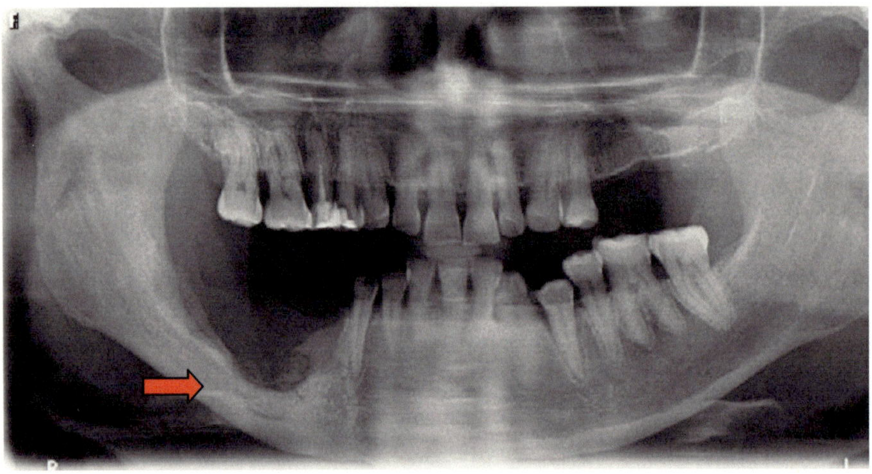

Fig. 12. Orthopantomograph showing the affected area 6 months after the operation.

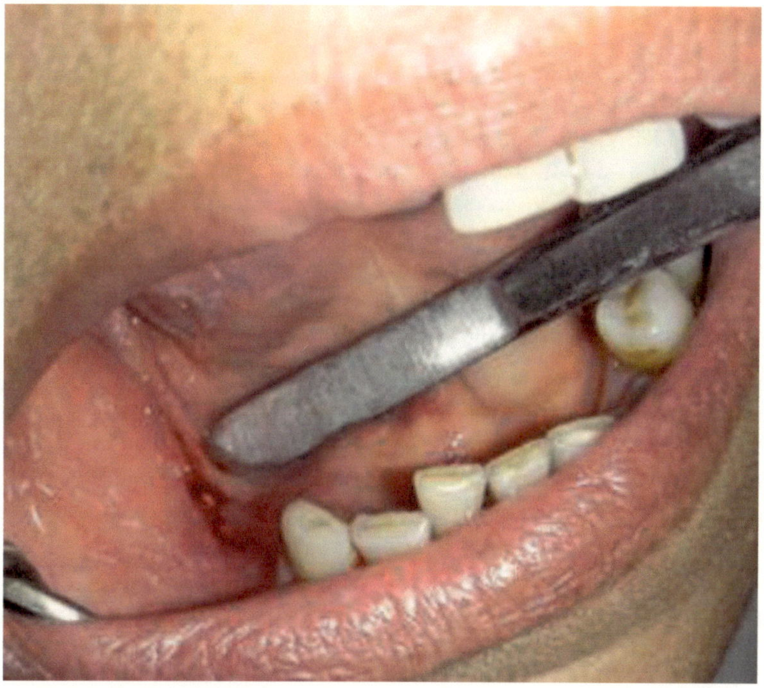

Fig. 13. Clinical appearence of the patient free of infection after 6 months post-operatively. Note that there's only a single small area of exposed bone.

10. Future research

Retrospective and prospective case studies have certainly established an association between bisphosphonates and jaw necrosis but the true incidence of this complication remains unknown. Clinical studies in the form of practitioner surveys or retrospective and prospective cohort investigations are needed to establish a more meaningful assessment of the associated risk factors and incidence of this problem in the population at risk. In addition, basic science research with the development of animal model system is needed to elucidate the cellular, molecular, and genetic mechanisms responsible for this process. Also, the development of an animal model for this disease process is important to establish treatment strategies that are evidenced based and associated with valid outcome data (33).

The effect of bisphosphonates on intraoral soft tissue wound healing; analysis of alveolar bone hemostasis and the response to bisphosphonate therapy; the antiangiogenic properties of bisphosphonates and their effects on jaw bone healing, pharmacogenetic research; and the development of valid BRONJ risk assessment tools should also be investigated in future. Continued governmental and institutional support is required to elucidate the underlying pathophysiologic mechanisms of BRONJ at the cellular and molecular level. Moreover, novel strategies for the prevention, risk reduction, and treatment of BRONJ need to be developed further so that more accurate judgments about risk, prognosis, treatment selection, and outcome can be established for patients with BRONJ (29).

11. Conclusions

All the medical doctors, who prescribe bisphosphonates, should strictly inform their patients about possible side effects of these drugs. One of the most important adverse effects of these drugs is BRONJ. This may occur spontaneously or following an oral surgical intervention such as a simple extraction, in patients with a history of bisphosphonate treatment. Prevention plays a crucial role since its management is difficult. Before prescribing these drugs, medical doctors should refer their patients to the dentists and maxillofacial surgeons in order to maintain optimum oral hygiene. All oral surgical operations should be completed prior to bisphosphonate therapy. Bisphosphonate therapy should only be started when the whole mucosal epithelization is formed.

BRONJ therapy has a more complicated management than the therapies for osteomyelitis and osteoradionecrosis. Its success rate is also less. These difficulties in the management of BRONJ leeds to a very diminished life quality for the patients. Therefore, consultation in between medical doctors and dentists and oral and maxillofacial surgeons gains importance. All medical allied personals must be careful in using these drugs which also have life saving properties.

12. References

[1] Fleisch H. Development of bisphosphonates. Breast Cancer Res. 2002; 4: 30-4.

[2] Russell RG. Bisphosphonates: The first 40 years. Bone. 2011; 49 :2-19.

[3] Russell RG, Rogers MJ. Bone. 1999;25: 97 -106. Bisphosphonates: from the laboratory to the clinic and back again.

[4] Russell RG, Watts NB, Ebetino FE, Rogers MJ· Mechanisms of action of bisphosphonates: similarities and differences and their potential influence on clinical efficacy Osteop Int 2008; 19: 6733-75.

[5] Frith JC, Mönkkönen J, Blackburn GM, Russell RG, Rogers MJ. Clodronate and liposome-encapsulated clodronate are metabolized to a toxic ATP analog, adenosine 5'-(beta, gamma-dichloromethylene) triphosphate, by mammalian cells in vitro. J Bone Miner Res. 1997; 12:1358-67.

[6] van Beek ER, Cohen LH, Leroy IM, Ebetino FH, Löwik CW, Papapoulos SE. Differentiating the mechanisms of antiresorptive action of nitrogen containing bisphosphonates. Bone. 2003; 33: 805-11.

[7] Papapetrou P. Bisphosphonate-associated adverse events. Hormones. 2009; 8: 96Y110.

[8] McLeod NM, Davies BJ, Brennan PA. Bisphosphonate osteonecrosis of the jaws; an increasing problem for the dental practitioner. Br Dent J. 2007; 8: :641-4.

[9] Sparidans RW, Twiss IM, Talbot S. Bisphosphonates in bone diseases. Pharm World Sci. 1998; 20: 206-13.

[10] Cheng A, Daly CG, Logan RM, Stein B, Goss AN. Alveolar bone and the bisphosphonates. Aust Dent J. 2009;54 Suppl 1:S51-61.

[11] Watts NB, Diab DL. Long-term use of bisphosphonates in osteoporosis. J Clin Endocrinol Metab. 2010; 95:1555-65.

[12] Pazianas M, Cooper C, Ebetino FH, Russell RG. Long-term treatment with bisphosphonates and their safety in postmenopausal osteoporosis. Ther Clin Risk Manag. 2010; 21: :325-43.

[13] Coleman RE, McCloskey EV. Bisphosphonates in oncology. Bone. 2011; 49: 71-6.
[14] Ralston SH, Langston AL, Reid IR. Lancet. Pathogenesis and management of Paget's disease of bone. 2008; 12: 155-63.
[15] Rachner TD, Khosla S, Hofbauer LC. Osteoporosis: now and the future. Lancet. 2011; 9: 1276-87.
[16] Eastell R, Walsh JS, Watts NB, Siris E. Bisphosphonates for postmenopausal osteoporosis. Bone. 2011; 49: 82-8.
[17] Bisphosphonates in orthopedic applications. Wilkinson JM, Little DG. Bone. 2011 ;49: 95-102.)
[18] Pazianas M, Abrahamsen B. Safety of bisphosphonates. Bone. 2011; 49 :103-10.
[19] Black DM, Delmas PD, Eastell R, Reid IR, Boonen S, Cauley JA, Cosman F, Lakatos P, Leung PC, Man Z, Mautalen C, Mesenbrink P, Hu H, Caminis J, Tong K, Rosario-Jansen T, Krasnow J, Hue TF, Sellmeyer D, Eriksen EF, Cummings SR; HORIZON Pivotal Fracture Trial. Once-yearly zoledronic acid for treatment of postmenopausal osteoporosis. N Engl J Med. 2007: 3: 1809-22.
[20] Abrahamsen B. Current Opinion in Rheumatology. 2010; 22: 404–409 Bisphosphonate adverse effects, lessons from large databases Bo Abrahamsen.
[21] Howard PA, Barnes BJ, Vacek JL, Chen W, Lai SM. Impact of bisphosphonates on the risk of atrial fibrillation. Am J Cardiovasc Drugs. 2010;10(6):359-67
[22] Capeci CM, Tejwani NC. Bilateral low-energy simultaneous or sequential femoral fractures in patients on long-term alendronate therapy. Journal of Bone and Joint Surgery. Series A. 2009;91: 2556–2561.
[23] Lenart BA, Lorich DG, Lane JM. Atypical fractures of the femoral diaphysis in postmenopausal women taking alendronate. New England Journal of Medicine. 2008;358: 1304–1306.
[24] Neviaser AS, Lane JM, Lenart BA, Edobor-Osula F, Lorich DG. Low-energy femoral shaft fractures associated with alendronate use. Journal of Orthopaedic Trauma. 2008;22: 346–350.
[25] Cheung RKH, Leung KK, Lee KC, Chow TC. Sequential non-traumatic femoral shaft fractures in a patient on long-term alendronate. Hong Kong Medical Journal. 2007;13: 485–489.
[26] Schneider JP. Should bisphosphonates be continued indefinitely? An unusual fracture in a healthy woman on long-term alendronate. Geriatrics. 2006; 61: 31–33.
[27] Shane E, Burr D, Ebeling PR, Abrahamsen B, Adler RA, Brown TD, Cheung AM, Cosman F, Curtis JR, Dell R, Dempster D, Einhorn TA, Genant HK, Geusens P, Klaushofer K, Koval K, Lane JM, McKiernan F, McKinney R, Ng A, Nieves J, O'Keefe R, Papapoulos S, Sen HT, van der Meulen MC, Weinstein RS, Whyte M; American Society for Bone and Mineral Research Atypical subtrochanteric and diaphyseal femoral fractures: report of a task force of the American Society for Bone and Mineral Research. J Bone Miner Res. 2010;25:2267-94.
[28] Rizzoli R, Akesson K, Bouxsein M, Kanis JA, Napoli N, Papapoulos S, Reginster JY, Cooper C. Subtrochanteric fractures after long-term treatment with bisphosphonates: a European Society on Clinical and Economic Aspects of Osteoporosis and Osteoarthritis, and International Osteoporosis Foundation Working Group Report. Osteoporos Int. 2011; 22: 373–390.

[29] Ruggiero SL, Dodson TB, Assael LA, Landesberg R, Marx RE, Mehrotra B; American Association of Oral and Maxillofacial Surgeons. American Association of Oral and Maxillofacial Surgeons position paper on bisphosphonate-related osteonecrosis of the jaws--2009 update. J Oral Maxillofac Surg. 2009;67(5 Suppl):2-12.
[30] Oral and Intravenous Bisphosphonate-Induced Osteonecrosis of the Jaws. History, Etiology, Prevention, and Treatment, Second Edition. Marx RE, 2011.
[31] Ruggiero SL. Bisphosphonate-related osteonecrosis of the jaw (BRONJ): initial discovery and subsequent development. J Oral Maxillofac Surg. 2009;67 (5 Suppl):13-8.
[32] Marx R E. Pamidronate (Aredia) and Zoledronate (Zometa) induced avascular necrosis of the jaws: a growing epidemic. J Oral Maxillofac Surg 2003; 61: 115-118.
[33] Ruggiero SL. Bisphosphonate-related osteonecrosis of the jaw: an overview. Ann N Y Acad Sci. 2011; 1218: 38-46.

9

Biochemical Measurement of Injury and Inflammation in Musculoskeletal Surgeries

Dinesh Kumbhare, William Parkinson,
R. Brett Dunlop and Anthony Adili
McMaster University
Canada

1. Introduction

Sufficient tissue trauma produces a temporary rise in circulating concentrations of various tissue proteins including creatine kinase (CK), myoglobin (Mb), myosin heavy chain (MHC), and collagen metabolites, as well as acute phase inflammation related analytes such as C-reactive protein (CRP), and the cytokines, interleukin-6 (IL-6) and interleukin-8 (IL-8) that mark the presence or absence of an injury or inflammatory response. Chronic, or late, elevations in biomarkers may also correlate with surgical complications. Measurement of biomarkers in orthopedic surgeries has been undertaken for 2 purposes: 1) to evaluate surgeries per se for improvement of surgical techniques and reducing adverse consequences, and 2) to examine measurement properties of biomarkers, using surgeries as models of musculoskeletal trauma and inflammation. In this chapter, some of the findings are described to illustrate both research objectives and their inter-relatedness, and to a degree, to capture aspects of the state of development of the overall biomarker research paradigm for surgical musculoskeletal injuries. The cytokine, interleukin-6 and the muscle cytoplasmic protein, creatine kinase, are emphasized partly because of known physiology and the relatively greater volume of research on these biomarkers over other candidates. However, some available research comparing these biomarkers with others is shown which has provided early evidence to substantiate better measurement characteristics for at least some applications. The survey is largely restricted to circulating blood concentrations over other possibilities (e.g. urine, joint synovial fluid, saliva) to allow comparison across studies, and given the potential for easier research and clinical application with venipuncture in comparison to joint fluid analysis, but not out of a lesser importance of investigations of other body fluids. Joint arthroplasty and lumbar surgery are the main focus since other surgeries (e.g. arthroscopy) produce much less tissue disruption and might be better studied by local tissue or fluid sampling, and because surgeries in emergency settings (e.g. fracture reduction) involve a more complex biochemical response post-surgery created by the combination of the original injury and the surgical injury. Findings from orthopedic surgeries are given priority but findings from non-orthopedic surgeries are shown when there is a difference in measurement principles or when measurement properties or clinical implications have been made clearer.

2. Measurement properties

2.1 Basic physiology

Historically, basic and applied physiology studies implicated a large number of proteins as potential markers of tissue injury, injury related inflammation, and inflammation created during injury by secondary causes such as infection or stress responses (Bauman 1994; Febarraio & Pederson 2005; Fong et al 1990; Jakab & Kalabay 1998; Wu & Perryman 1992).

In the early, pro-inflammatory, stages of the response to trauma, monocytes and macrophages release IL-6, TNF-alpha, and IL-1beta. TNF-alpha and IL-1beta have feed forward effects on endothelial cells and fibroblasts to also release IL-6, which is produced in these cells. While all 3 proteins could be markers of trauma, IL-6 was found to be the most potent inducer of the liver acute phase proteins including CRP and has captured much of the interest in injury research since that time (Heinrich et al 1990). IL-6 was named in 1987 based on studies aimed at isolating a hepatocyte stimulating factor (Poupart et al 1987; Yasukawa et al 1987).

CK is found in the muscle cytoplasm and is involved in the conversion of adenosine triphosphate to adenosine diphosphate during the energy transfer process. Separate isoforms exist for skeletal muscle (CK-MM), cardiac muscle (CK-MB) and brain (CK-BB). This specificity for skeletal muscle has advantages over other analytes such as MB and MHC which do not have separate cardiac and skeletal muscle isomers. Musculoskeletal trauma studies have measured either the total CK or CK-MM but the total circulating CK has invariably been found to consist almost exclusively of CK-MM (Kawaguchi 1996, 1997; Strecker et al. 1999; Kumbhare et al. 2007) in non-cardiac research.

Given the large number of biomarkers being measured in clinical studies, short-listing to a manageable number of analytes that are most typically effective would be useful. Apart from the kinetics of biomarkers in circulation, other factors affecting the usefulness of biomarkers include the relative stabilities of proteins at room temperature, when frozen, and after repeated freeze thaws, as well as all of the measurement properties characteristic of the chemistry assays such as upper and lower detection limits, coefficients of variation, and the ability of the assay to recover/capture the true protein concentrations in the sample.

Studies of the rapidly changing acute stage biochemical markers have reported differences in the magnitudes of peak concentrations, the statistical significance of a protein change, and the timing of the peak. Such differences require careful analysis to establish what is consistent, as part of the development of the biomarker paradigm.

2.2 Response sensitivity

Many pioneering studies have focused partly on the simple question as to whether a reliable biochemical response is achievable with one or more proteins. The sensitivity of a response, while relevant to diagnostic accuracy, is not the same thing, the latter requiring accurate placement of patients in the clinically positive group, and the clinically negative group.

Two very early studies on lumbar surgery without fusion or instrumentation, found a serum mean CK-MM response of just over 500 U/L for single level posterior surgery, which was over 4 times the baseline CK-MM levels (Kawaguchi et al. 1996, 1997).

Injury responses to lumbar decompression with spinal instrumentation were studied including CRP and the cytokines IL-1ra, IL-6, IL-8, IL-10, TNF-RI, TNF-RII (Takahashi et al., 2001). With sampling 1, 2, and 7 days following lumbar surgeries, IL-6, IL-8, and IL-10 were elevated only in a decompression plus spinal instrumentation group (n = 7) and not in groups having decompression only (n = 7) or decompression plus fusion (n = 6) although there appeared to be trends towards increases in these biomarkers in these less invasive surgeries. Given the likelihood that the biochemical responses are smaller to less invasive surgeries, small sample sizes may have prevented injury detection. In a subsequent study, involving 12 subjects and more serial measures, a significant increase in mean IL-6 was obtained at 6 hours following lumbar decompression (Kumbhare et al., 2009) with trends toward significant elevations at 12 and 24 hours. The IL-6 response was weaker than CK, consistent with the previous research showing an easily detected CK response but more difficult to detect rise in IL-6 in the lumbar decompression model. A similar study on CK showed excellent separation of the distributions of proteins for baseline to peak, versus baseline fluctuations (Kumbhare et al., 2007) showing sensitivity to lumbar decompression. The reduced sensitivity of IL-6 to muscle trauma, in comparison to CK could be related to the degree to which IL-6 is inducible in muscle. Examination of tissue homogenates found greatest concentrations of IL-6 in bone and lung, lower concentrations in skin and adipose tissue, and lowest concentrations in skeletal muscle (Perl et al. 2003).

In the instrumentation research (Takahashi et al., 2001, 2002), IL-8 and IL-10 were found to peak earlier than IL-6 such that the injury response was largely absent by the next day, whereas IL-6 remained elevated the day after surgery and had not resolved by day 2 post-surgery. This suggested narrow diagnostic windows for IL-8 and IL-10, which could make these proteins more difficult to capture in sampling.

Myosin heavy chain (MHC) has the advantage of a wider diagnostic window than CK or the pro-inflammatory cytokines. Yet, it has been studied very little in orthopedic research. MHC is a component of the contractile apparatus of muscle. Onuoha and coworkers (2001) measured serum MHC concentrations before fracture reduction and serially after the operation in a heterogenous group having various types of fracture surgeries. Twenty-four hours post surgery, group mean (n = 12) MHC concentrations showed an approximate 3-fold increase over mean baseline concentration which was about 100 ug/L. This amounted to an effect size of about 3 standard deviations. MHC was argued to be a better marker than the traditional use of CK or myoglobin because the latter can increase in circulation with a leaky membrane only, whereas elevated MHC reflects destruction of the contractile mechanism and therefore, is more consistent with the concept of injury. In short, CK-MM has the advantage of skeletal muscle specificity, whereas MHC of specificity to the state of injury may be more specific to the state of injury.

Munoz et al (2005) compared biomarker responses following spinal instrumentation surgery with serial measures at pre-operation, post-operation, 1 day, 2 days, and 7 days. They measured a wide range of potential biomarkers including CRP and IL-6 as well as IL1b, IL-2, IL-4, IL-5, IL-8, IL-10, IL-12, TNF-alpha, and interfeuron-gamma. Only CRP and IL-6 showed sensitivity to the surgical trauma. Similarly, a study of total knee replacement (TKR) in Britain, found no serum injury responses for TNF-alpha (Andres et al., 2003) at 6, 24, or 48 hours following total knee arthroplasty and IL-1beta was elevated at the 24 hour time point only. This team did obtain stronger elevations in these proteins in joint drain fluid. Given that TKR produces biochemical changes that are quite large in comparison to other surgeries, analysis of circulating TNF-alpha and IL-1beta have not been supported as general indices of the pro-inflammatory response with the current chemistry assays when circulating concentrations are used. TNF-alpha and IL-1beta may be useful for analyses on joint fluid. TNF-alpha was found to be elevated in circulation for short bursts among patients hospitalized for sepsis (Damas et al., 1992). IL-1 beta was not. However, even in that study, persisting IL-6 elevations were not only easier to measure by virtue of their longer time course in fluctuations, but allowed greater prediction of shock than TNF-alpha.

In a British study (Hall et al., 2000) a factor analysis was used to examine the temporal pattern of a number of proteins including IL-6, CRP, and cortisol. The cortisol response started earliest and had returned to baseline by about 48 hours and was only about 50% higher than baseline at 24 hours showing less response magnitude and a shorter time course than IL-6 or CRP. Separate independent factors were created by the distinctly different time x magnitude profiles for these 3 proteins. This contrasted with the use of epinephrine and norephineprine, which were inter-correlated implying redundancy in measurement. The findings demonstrated a need for separate time series protocols when studying these different proteins.

The routine availability of a biomarker is a practical advantage and must be weighed against measurement properties of proteins that might be expensive to measure or measurable only in specialty laboratories. For example, IL-6 has frequently been considered to be preferable to CRP for measurement of early phase inflammation. However, while this seems more evident for some applications, a more general superiority of IL-6 over other candidates cannot yet be concluded. The fact that CRP is routinely available in many clinical laboratories, whereas IL-6 requires purchasing or developing immunological assays forces a need for evidence of sufficient superiority. The fact that clinical research might become applied more quickly and easily in the case of CRP is relevant. One example is a study on post-surgery infection (DiCesare et al., 2005) following TKR and THR. The statistical effect size for group differences were just over 1 standard deviation for all 3 significantly elevated proteins (Il-6, CRP, ESR) showing no relative advantage of IL-6 for separating the infected and non-infected distributions with the exception of a slightly weaker group separation by CRP in the THR patients created by a high standard deviation in the infected group. In an earlier study, that also involved hip and knee arthroplasties, the acute phase responses for IL-6 and CRP had similar effect sizes, amounting to roughly 2.5 standard deviation increases over baseline (Wirtz et al., 2000).

Outside of orthopedic surgery research, superiority of IL-6 over CRP has been reported. For example, IL-6 and procalcitonin levels were higher in the presence of episodes of bacteremia in neutropenic patients with hematological malignancies. CRP was elevated in the population but showed no correlation with the presence of bacteremia (von Lilianfield-Toll et al., 2004). The quicker return to baseline by IL-6 over CRP is a particular advantage in such situations, where the clinical condition fluctuates over time.

2.3 Time course

Surgery models offer the advantage of a pre-surgery baseline. In knee and hip arthroplasty, typical periods of hospitalization allow for control while sampling in the sensitive time windows for most of the biomarkers studied to date.

Evaluation of biomarker time courses requires multiple serial measures. Studies differ substantially on serial measurement, ranging from a single post-injury sample, to many time points, and all studies do not include pre-surgery or late enough time points to establish baselines and return to baseline. Therefore, there has been a limited ability to clarify the sensitive time windows and more precision is required.

Two early studies provided multiple serial measures to capture biomarker time-sensitive windows for inflammation related proteins. Wirtz et al (2000) included pre-operative and post-operative sampling at 6 and 12 hours and at daily intervals to 1 week following hip (n = 20) and knee (n = 10) arthroplasties. They compared the IL-6 time course with CRP. This revealed a slower rise in CRP relative to IL-6 and a much slower decline such that group peak CRP was reached between 1 to 2 days after surgery and remained about two-thirds of peak at 4 days and had not returned to baseline by day 7. IL-6 showed re-established baseline by about 3 days. The authors noted that other research showed the return to baseline for CRP is about 3 weeks, and ESR requires about 3 months. Therefore, an unusual persistent post-surgical elevation would be evident sooner with IL-6.

A second study (Hall et al 2000) included many serial data points and a relatively large sample (n = 158) of subjects who had either TKR or THR. Samples were taken before and after surgery prior to tourniquet release, and at 2, 4, 8, 12, and 24 hours and then daily to 7 days. Peak IL-6 occurred at 24 hours, whereas the CRP peak occurred at 48 hours. IL-6 returned to baseline more quickly than CRP. However, smaller but significant elevations in both proteins were still present on day 7. In other words, the pattern of relative changes in IL-6 and CRP were consistent with other research.

However, these 2 studies showed outcome differences of potential importance. First, the mean protein concentrations do not coincide. Wirtz et al obtained a peak IL-6 of about 400 pg/ml in each of the TKR and THR groups. Peak CRP was about 150 mg/L in each group. In the Hall study, peak IL- 6 was 125 pg/ml after THR and 175 pg/ml after TKR. The teams used different chemistry assays for both proteins. Whether these dramatic differences are related to assay sensitivities, differences in drugs used in the different study locations, or other factors is not known. The use of different assays and different clinical protocols in different jurisdictions may be sources of variability in biochemical studies.

Comparisons between proteins on peak timing need to take individual differences into account. In a protocol aimed at defining the time course for CK and IL-6, serial measures were made before and immediately after lumbar decompression surgery and at 6, 12, 24, 48, at and 72 to 96 hours, and at 7 days (Kumbhare et al., 2007, 2009). The highest CK concentration occurred at different time points between 12 to 48 hours across subjects and the highest IL-6 concentration had a range of 6 to 24 hours. Time related individual differences create enough variance that this could affect various conclusions. For example, differences between 2 equally effective biomarkers on their prediction of clinical outcomes could be created by how closely sampling is done to the average peaks for each protein, or variability in peak timing within proteins in the subject sample.

2.4 Validity

The search for validity has been somewhat of a challenge because of the difficulty finding criterion measures. Some research suggests that biomarker responses might largely be all or none. For example, unaccustomed exercise produces a well documented rise in CK (Critz & Cunningham 1972) and IL-6 (Petersen & Pederson 2005; Steensberg 2003). Bicep curls with both arms produced no greater change in CK than exercise at the same weight load, in one arm (Nosaka et al., 1992, 2002). Such findings could reflect a relative lack of biomarker sensitivity to injuries of different magnitude. Findings from some orthopedic studies involving direct validity quantification have produced more promising results. In a similar demonstration (Kugisaki et al., 2011), unilateral TKR was compared with bilateral TKR. The serum peak IL-6 for bilateral TKR was 246% of the peak for unilateral TKR. While a perfect outcome would be 200% difference, the design was between subjects by necessity and therefore individual differences might account for the relatively greater than double biochemical response in the bilaterals. Bilateral TKR produced only a 146% increase in CRP compared to unilateral TKR providing some evidence that CRP may be less sensitive creating less validity for detecting varying amounts of injury.

In studies of orthopedic and non-orthopedic surgeries, circulating IL-6 concentration was correlated with length of operation (Sakamoto 1994), amount of blood loss (Sakamoto 1994), and patients with higher blood loss requiring transfusions had higher IL-6 as a group in comparison to those with blood loss under 400ml and not requiring transfusions (Avall et al 1999). Studies described later in this chapter showing correlation of IL-6 responses with body temperature and post-operative pain provide further convergent type validity evidence (Lisowska et al. 2006).

In lumbar surgery, 7 patients with decompression plus instrumentation had higher post-surgery biomarker concentrations in comparison to 7 subjects who had decompression alone. Decompression plus fusion (n = 6) showed an intermediate biochemical response (Demura et al., 2006). In an older study (Kawaguchi et al., 1996), the CK-MM response was higher in patients with multiple level surgery (n = 14) in comparison to single level (n = 10). In the same study, dividing the group into greater retraction forces (retraction pressure x retraction time) and lesser forces revealed a higher CK-MM in the greater force subgroup. However, this could have been related to a higher proportion of multilevel surgeries in the greater force group given longer surgery times. Accordingly, in this team's subsequent report on a larger sample (n = 47) multilevel surgery continued to produce a higher CK-mm response than single level, but separate analysis of surgery time showed no increased CK-MM in the subgroup having longer surgery times compared to shorter duration of muscle strain (Kawaguchi et al., 1997). They also found no difference between 2 subgroups separated on the basis of the length of the incision.

To further explore the potential for developing a criterion measure in lumbar surgery, the length and depth of the muscle isolated and retracted (i.e. surface area) was used as a criterion measure for validity examination in 18 subjects who underwent lumbar decompression (Kumbhare et al., 2008). Rather than divide the sample into subgroups, the correlation was examined continuously against individual peak serum CK. Muscle surface area and peak CK response had a Pearson r correlation of .60, falling in a moderate range.

2.5 Summary

Studies of basic measurement properties have largely involved relatively small samples. This is partly related to the need for many serial samples creating many data points.

Therefore, the extent to which the findings on kinetics of biomarkers generalize across subjects partly remains to be determined. Practical barriers make it impossible to sample precisely time-wise. Data presentations frequently use such increments as "Day 1, Day 2", acknowledging such imprecision. It is therefore difficult to know exactly when samples were taken, and therefore difficult to extract the true time course. Muscle proteins have been studied less often than inflammation proteins and with smaller sample sizes, so relatively less is known about measurement properties in application to surgeries. Use of some proteins as general markers is weakened by relatively low sensitivity or short time courses. CK appears to be quite sensitive to surgical muscle trauma being consistently elevated even with low trauma surgery. Among the inflammation related markers, IL-6 and CRP have shown robustness in comparison to other proteins, in that they consistently are elevated. Some evidence suggests that CRP is less sensitive than IL-6 as a general proinflammation marker but the differences between IL-6 and CRP have not been large. Time courses have not been entirely consistent across studies. This could be related to difficulties timing sampling or to individual differences in time to peak. It seems likely that validity is in a moderate rather than high range in general. This could be related to variance created by: i. variability in sample timing within and between studies, or ii. the choice of criterion measures which may only approximate the construct of interest. Not discussed in this chapter are confounds and patient characteristics that may vary across individuals such as gender, age, body mass, anesthetics and other pharmacological agents, comorbidity, dehydration, activity levels, and other lifestyle factors. In fact, it may be unrealistic to expect better than moderate correlations between biomarkers and clinical outcomes.

These basic measurement issues must be kept in mind when one is considering the reasons for various findings of studies that examine clinical applications of the biomarker paradigm, and the challenges faced when attempting to obtain precise prediction.

3. Surgery evaluation, complications, and outcomes

Non-orthopedic studies have included a range of surgeries including: cardiac (Antunes et al., 2008; Booth et al., 2010), aortic (Baigrie), stomach (Aguilar-Nascimento et al., 2007; Herrera et al., 2010), bowel (Herroeder et al., 2007), liver (Gravante et al., 2010; Sato et al., 1996), hernias (Correla et al., 2001), cholesystemctomy (Chambrier et al., 1996; Kristiansson et al, 1999) and various cancers (Veenhof et al., 2011). Among orthopedic studies, there are now a large number of reports involving the use of biochemical injury measures for risk screening including their use in attempts to identify post-operative fever, and infection. Smaller literatures focus on technique comparisons for amount of tissue disruption or amount of inflammation, application in predicting hardware failure, and shorter term post-surgical recovery and hospital stay.

3.1 Post-operative fever

Post-operative fever has been of some interest in the biomarker paradigm. This is despite uncertainty about its clinical significance, leading to claims that it may simply be a normal response to surgeries (Andres et al., 2003, Pile 2006; Shaw & Chung 1999,). It has been argued that unusually high or prolonged post-operative fever is a risk factor for complications (Munoz et al 2004; Pile 2006). There are numerous previously suggested causes (Fanning et al., 1998) including: urinary tract infections, pneumonia, blood transfusions, infections at the wound, surgical site, intravenous catheter or created by the prosthesis, deep venous thrombosis, and C-deficile related to peri-operative antibiotics.

Andres and coworkers (2003) sought to provide evidence that post-operative fever was caused by the acute phase inflammatory response after arthroplasty. Half of their sample of 20 had early (first 3 days) post-operative temperatures in the febrile range (>38.5C). The mean IL-6 concentration was higher in this group than the afebrile group at 24 and 48 hours, supporting the hypothesis that fever reflects an unusually high inflammatory biochemical response in the post-surgery phase. This separation based on fever, was not evident in circulating measurements of TNF-alpha or IL-1beta. Positive correlations between IL-6 and post-operative fever were also reported by others (Frank et al., 2000; Miyawaki et al., 1998). However, none of the febrile patients in the Andres et al study had complications, implying that IL-6 levels might correlate with fever, but neither IL-6 nor fever is specific for complications. Moreover, Andres et al. (2003) cite studies showing poor associations between fever and various post-operative complications. Fever may not have sufficient risk stratification potential on its own. One idea is that the fever is more typically related to extravasated blood and cellular debris (Shaw & Chung 1999) following arthroplasty. These early findings suggested that a correlation between IL-6 in the early post-operative phase and complications might exist, but prove not to be very strong.

3.2 Post-operative pain

The inflammatory response has been thought to contribute to pain in the early post-operative period leading to the hypothesis that treatment by antiinflammatories will reduce the acute phase response, reduce pain, and possibly improve return to functioning. There has been a consistent improvement in post-operative pain when various antiinflammatories are administered prior to operations. For example, intravenous diclofenac reduced post-operative pain and use of analgesics in a heterogenous sample having various surgeries (Claeys et al.1992). Naproxen reduced postoperative pain following knee arthroscopy (Code et al., 1994) and following spinal surgery (Munoz et al, 2004).

In contrast, the effect of anti-inflammatories on the biochemical acute phase response has not been consistent. Using spinal surgery as a model, patients undergoing spinal fusion with instrumentation were assigned alternately to 2 groups of 20 subjects each, one that received 500 mg/day of naproxen combined with 40 mg/day famotidine in an attempt to blunt the inflammatory response, or to a no anti-inflammatory treatment control (Munoz et al. 2004). Following the operation, patients who received the anti-inflammatory treatment had lower body temperatures and requested less analgesic. CRP was reduced substantially from a group peak of 18.2 mg/ml to 6.7 mg/ml. This pattern was similar to that found in a study with spinal surgery without instrumentation (Takahashi et al. 2001). However, there was no significant difference between the groups on the IL-6 response, despite the anti-inflammatory pre-treatment. This contrasts with the finding of a reduction in the IL-6 response, with no reduction in CRP, to peri-operative administration of ibuprofen in cholecystectomy (Chambrier et al., 1996). Finally, Diclofenic produced no reduction in the CRP response despite pre-treatment and 24 hours continuous infusion of the drug in their sample having various major surgeries (Claeys et al., 1992).

3.3 Infection, osteolysis and hardware loosening

Studies examining the relationship between post-operative fever and infection have been reviewed for non-orthopedic surgeries (Fanning et al., 1998) and studies on knee and hip surgeries (Shaw & Chung 1999). The consistent result is that fever is an insufficient predictor of infection in non-orthopedic studies, which may be at least partly related to the high incidence of fever yet low rate of infection (Pile 2003). This has prompted the question as to whether biomarkers measured in the acute, early post-operative period, will generate the desired prediction.

Studies on chronically elevated biomarkers, typically measured at the time of resection arthroplasty, have had some success. Serum IL-6 has been evaluated for association with periprosthetic infection specifically. Recent studies have included sensitivity and specificity evaluations, which become important if there is to be a clinical application. For example, DiCesare and coworkers(2005) compared the predictive relationships of IL-6, C-reactive protein (CRP), white blood cell count (WBC), and erythrocyte sedimentation rate (ESR). Fifty-eight patients requiring re-operation were separated into 2 groups, those with, and those without infection confirmed histologically. Blood sampling was done at a mean of 84 months after the 1st operation, well after the acute elevations related to surgical injury would have resolved and baseline would be restored. Those with infection (n = 17) had higher concentrations of all 4 markers although WBC was not statistically significant. Using 10 pg/ml or higher as the cut-off/criterion, IL-6 had perfect sensitivity (1.0) and close to perfect specificity (.95) meaning 1 subject was misclassified as infected who was not. CRP had poorer performance with a sensitivity of 94 specificity of .78. In the second study, Bottner and coworkers (2007) studied a larger sample of 78 subjects. Using a cut-off score of 12 pg/ml (which is remarkably close to the cut-off in the previous study) IL-6 had a sensitivity of .95 but had a specificity of .87. CRP had the same sensitivity and .96 specificity. The combination of IL-6 > 12 pg/ml and CRP > 3.2 pg/ml correctly classified all patients. Such impressive accuracy has not always been obtained. In another study, IL-6 had a specificity of 1.0 when the cut-off was set to minimize false positives, but sensitivity was only modest at .57 (Buttaro et al, 2009).

A recent review has focused on the association between biomarkers measured at clinical follow-ups following arthroplasty (Mertens& Singh 2001) and the incidence of hardware loosening, osteolysis, and infection at the site of prosthesis. In general, synovial fluid analyses produced stronger and more consistent separation of those with and without complications. In serum analyses, prosthesis loosening had the lowest potential for prediction. IL-6 showed no significant relationship in 2 studies. TNF-alpha and IL-1beta showed significant prediction in 1 of 2 and 1 of 3 studies respectively. Collagen I had better than chance prediction in 2 of 5 studies, with the suggestion that this might have been related to the different assays used. In osteolysis, serum collagen I was significantly higher in the affected group in 1 of 2 studies. No significant relationship was obtained for IL-6, CRP, TNF-alpha, or IL-1b in any of the studies. Performance of serum biochemistry was best, in general, in the case of infected prostheses. Significant correlations were obtained for IL-6 in 2 of the 2 available studies described individually earlier, CRP in 3 of 3 studies, ESR in 3 of 3 studies, and TNF-alpha in 1 of 1 study. Analyses on the degree of sensitivity and specificity for complication versus no complication were not attempted.

In a second review, sensitivity and specificity analyses were performed on data from multiple studies (Berbari et al., 2010) creating a pooled sensitivity, with focus on circulating protein concentrations. The review included three studies in which IL-6 was measured, and 23 on CRP, 25 with ESR measurements, and 15 having measured WBC. Pooled sensitivity and specificity were as follows: WBC .45 and .87, ESR .75 and .70, CRP .88 and .74, and IL-6 .97 and .91, suggesting that IL-6 produces the best association with infection. However, as described earlier, examination of individual studies, revealed that IL-6 had modest sensitivity in 1 study (Buttaro 200) in the presence of high specificity, and CRP had better specificity than IL-6 in another study despite equal sensitivity (Bottner et al. 2007). Sensitivity and specificity are influenced by the effect size of a group difference, which is a ratio of group mean differences to standard deviation. In small sample sizes, standard deviations can vary substantially from one study to another. Therefore, it is somewhat premature to conclude a superiority of IL-6 over CRP in the identification of infection.

The possibility that biomarkers could help to time staged surgeries has been of recent interest. One model is repeat TKR following infection associated with the first procedure, whereby a 2nd surgery is performed to remove the hardware and cement, debride tissue, and insert a spacer block. The infection is then treated and re-implantation is performed when the infection is resolved. Given the promising evidence for an association between inflammation markers and infection, the question is raised as to whether these proteins could be used to judge when inflammation has been sufficiently controlled. Ghanem et al (2009) found no accurate relationship between either serum or joint fluid concentrations of C-reactive protein or erythrocyte sedimentation prior to re-implantation, and the rate of persisting infection following re-implantation. Investigation of other biomarkers was suggested. In a summary of conditions for re-implant timing, the authors do recommend including a return to normal CRP, which persists after discontinuing antibiotics, as one criterion for re-implanation. They also emphasize that this is insufficient and that other criteria should be used including, effective treatment of the potential source of the infections including resolution of urinary tract infections, cellulitis, poor dentition, or skin ulceration. Treatment of otherwise unwell patients (e.g. immunocompromised, malnourished) should be optimized before re-implantation, and there should be good healing of the soft tissues and resolution of erythema.

3.4 Relative tissue disruption

It has been argued that biomarkers may help to evaluate minimally invasive techniques against more traditional surgical approaches (Cohen et al., 2009 ; Hartzband et al., 2004) or against varying minimal trauma approaches under development.

Chimento and coworkers (2005) compared their minimally invasive total hip arthroplasty procedure to the standard posterolateral approach. With the minimally invasive technique, the incision was 8 cm instead of 15 and smaller retractors were used. The technique also spared the quadratus femoris and the femoral insertion of the gluteus maximus. Circulating IL-6 concentrations did not differ between the 2 groups after surgery. However, the exact post-surgical time point was not reported. Given that the peak IL-6 concentrations were very low falling between about 5 pg/ml to 6.5 pg/ml in both the minimally invasive and traditional surgery groups, the assay may have had low sensitivity or the sampling time may not have been near peak concentrations.

In another study, a minimally invasive posterior approach that spared the quadrates femoris was compared to standard posterolateral approach to total hip arthroplasty (Fink et al., 2010). There were no differences in circulating CK or Mb at 24 or 48 hours post-surgery, indicating that these proteins may not be sufficiently sensitive to the amount of affected muscle.

Cohen and coworkers (2009) compared 3 approaches for hip arthroplasty, 1. minimally invasive Watson Jones technique, 2. miniposterior transmuscular approach, and 3. minimally invasive -II (MIS-II) incision. The first technique involves an anterior approach with no muscle detachment but muscle is retracted creating strain forces. The posterior technique involves a small incision and minimizes, but does not eliminate, muscle detachment. In MIS-II there is an anterior incision to access the acetabulum, and a posterior incision for passage of instruments. Muscle is separated or bypassed, but not cut or detached. The 3 techniques had mean incision lengths of about 10 cm, 9cm and 9cm (combined anterior + posterior) respectively. Serum Mb and CK showed injury responses in the first 24 hours that were just over double and 4 times the normal respectively. The 3 techniques were not different in the magnitude of the biochemical response. However, group sizes of 10 were compared leading to the question as to whether larger samples could reveal subtle differences.

3.5 Other adverse effects

In their study described earlier, Cohen et al. found only 1 case in 30 of an elevated cardiac troponin following their minimally invasive hip replacement procedure. Cytokine responses were higher in patients who developed pancreatitis associated with spinal fusion surgery (He et al 2004). In a very recent study on mortality risk after hip fracture (Sun et al., 2011) IL-6, TNF-alpha, and IL-10 were measured before surgical repair, 1hour after the operation, and at 1, 3 and 5 days. Thirty-one of the 127 patients had died by the 6 or 12 month follow-ups. All 3 biomarkers showed significantly higher concentrations in the early post-surgical period in non-survivors. The best separation of the outcome groups was with IL-6 at 1 day post-surgery. Sensitivity and specificity analyses found IL-6 to be the best predictor. Setting the cut-off to minimize false negatives, IL-6 had a sensitivity of .935, but lower specificity at .635. This moderate level of prediction was also evident by the fact that the effect size of the group difference was about 1 standard deviation. This would imply a sizeable overlap in distributions. Nevertheless, the findings suggest that almost all of those who died could be predicted from the acute biochemical response while still reducing the total sample to a smaller high risk group that might be followed clinically.

3.6 Early post surgical status and hospital length of stay

Among non-orthopedic surgery studies, IL-6 on the day of haemopoietic stem cell transplantation predicted hospital length of stay (Tegg et al., 2001). Peri-operative lidocaine has been found to affect hospital length of stay for some abdominal surgeries. McCarthy (2010) reviewed studies in bowel surgery involving a total 395 treated patients and 369 controls. Lidocaine suppressed IL-6, improved post-operative pain, and reduced length of stay by an average 1.1 days. In contrast, lidocaine had no effect on length of stay following hysterectomy (Bryson et al., 2010).

In a very recent study with 68 subjects having hip or knee arthroplasty (Koppensteiner et al., 2001), both CRP and IL-6 in the acute phase, predicted the absence of complications during hospital stay. However, because IL-6 normalized faster, it provided the better criterion for safe discharge.

3.7 Summary

In general, circulating levels of biomarkers have been found to have considerably less sensitivity than measurement of these proteins in joint or drain fluids. Circulating chronic elevations in IL-6 and CRP have been found to be correlated with the development of infections with some promising sensitivity and specificity findings. There is some promising evidence for a predictive relationship between acute phase protein elevations and complications during hospitalization outside of orthopedic surgeries with an implication that proteins might be helpful in discharge decisions. The potential for affecting length of stay in orthopedic surgeries needs to be explored. Biomarker changes in the acute or chronic period have not been sufficiently sensitive to identify loosening of surgical hardware. However, a biomarker could increase in a similar manner to a range of pathologies, or increase only to some complications thereby helping with differential diagnosis. Accordingly, lower IL-6 might rule out infection leaving hardware loosening as a possibility thereby providing useful information. The potential for sensitivity to osteolysis has met with equivocal results but has not been ruled out.

4. Summary and future directions

The study of biomarker measurement properties with surgery models and their applications in surgery issues can be argued to be a relatively young paradigm, with the introduction of IL-6 occurring only just over 20 years ago. Commercially available assays have taken time to develop but are now available for many biomarkers, allowing an expansion of this research in recent years. Early research often involved small samples and there was a need to compare proteins and establish time courses for the rapidly changing concentrations in the early post-surgery phase. Nevertheless basic measurement properties have not been sufficiently worked out. The reasons for some differences in time courses in studies on the same proteins remain unknown. The reasons why response magnitudes vary across studies are also not known. In research on muscle injury, advantages and disadvantages of cytoplasmic versus contractile apparatus proteins have been argued but need to be studied. There are a large number of patient characteristics and potential confounds including various drugs that could influence the different proteins in different ways. All of these issues require future research. Insufficient understanding of these variables could be creating weaker associations with clinical criterion variables than might be achievable.

In applying biomarkers to clinical issues, the most promising findings have been in identifying risk of infection with many studies on CRP but few studies of IL-6. While it is tempting to conclude that IL-6 is the superior infection marker, more research is needed comparing IL-6 to CRP and on the possibility of their combination to improve risk stratification. Further improvement in assays might reveal applications for osteolysis and hardware failure but diagnostic accuracy has not been evident thus far. It seems unlikely that improvement in blood sampling will change this given that chronic levels are measured which should be much less variable than protein concentrations in the early post-surgery period. Nevertheless, adjustment for within subject fluctuations to improve baseline estimation could be attempted.

In the early post-operative period, the rapidly changing nature of biomarker concentrations is a major challenge. This becomes quite relevant in application to identifying early complications that affect length of stay. Given the paucity of research on this issue, there is a need for further research. A caveat is that insufficient understanding of the time courses or reasons for differences in time courses across studies, and the sources of variance outside of injury and inflammation, will reduce the efficiency of that line of research. This probably forces such studies to make many serial measures and measure a wide range of potential confounds or covariates before simpler models can be trusted. What appears to be emerging from the drug research is that there are substantial differences in the effects of different pharmacological agents on different proteins. Different antiinflammatories do not affect inflammation biomarkers equally. This is worthy of investigation itself, but becomes a problem when the absence of a change in a biomarker is interpreted to reflect no clinical effect. The use of multiple biomarkers and multiple clinical outcomes will continue to be necessary in this line of research.

5. References

Aguilar-Nascimento JE, Marra JG, Slhessarenko N, Fontes CJ. (2007). Efficacy of National Nosocomial Infection Surveillance score, acute-phase proteins, and interleukin-6 for predicting postoperative infections following major gastrointestinal surgery. *Sao Paulo Med J*, Vol. 125(1), pp. 34-41.

Andres BM, Taub DD, Gurkan I, Wenz JF. (2002). Postoperative fever after total knee arthroplasty: The role of cytokines. *Clin Orthop Relat Res* Vol. 415, pp. 221-31.

Antunes N, Dragosavc D, Petrucci Junior O, Oliveira PP, Kosour C, Blotta MH, Braile DM, Vieira RW. (2008). The use of ultrafiltration for inflammatory mediators removal during cardiopulmonary bypass in coronary artery bypass graf surgery. *Rev Bras Cir Cardiovasc* Vol. 23(2), pp.175-82.

Baumann H, Gauldie J. (1994). The acute phase response. *Immunol Today* Vol. 15, pp. 74-80.

Berbari E, Mabry T, Tsaras G, Spangehl M, Erwin PJ, Murad MH, Steckelberg J, Osmon D. (2010). Inflammatory Blood Laboratory Levels as Markers of Prosthetic Joint Infection: A Systematic Review and Meta-Analysis. *J Bone Joint Surg* Vol. 92A(11), pp. 2102-9.

Booth AJ, Bishop DK. (2010). TGF-beta, IL-6, IL-17 and CTGF direct multiple pathologies of chronic cardiac allograft rejection. *Immunotherapy*, Vol. 2(4), pp. 511-20.

Bottner F, Wegner A, Winkelmann W, Becker K, Erren M, Gotze C. (2007). Interleukin-6, procalcitonin and TNF-Markers of peri-prosthetic infection following total joint replacement. *J Bone Joint Surg*, Vol. 89-B (1), pp 94-99.

Buttaro MA, Tanoira I, Comba F, Piccaluga F. (2009). Combining C-reactive protein and interleukin-6 may be useful to detect periprosthetic hip infection. *Clin Orthoped Rel Res*, Vol. 468(12), pp. 3263-67.

Chambrier C, Chassard D, Bienvenu J, Sudin F, Parurel B, Garrigue C, et al. (1996). Cytokine and hormonal changes after cholecystectomy. Effect of ibuprofen pretreatment. *Ann Surg* Vol. 224, pp. 178-182.

Chimento GF, Pavone V, Sharrock N, Kahn B, Cahill J, Sculco TP. (2005). Minimally invasive total hip arthroplasty: A prospective randomized study *J Arthroplasty*, Vol. 20 (2), pp.139-144.

Claeys MA, camu F, Maes V. (1992). Prophylactic diclofenac infusions in major orthopedic surgery: effects on analgesia and acute phase proteins. *Acta Anaesthesiol Scand*, Vol. 36:270-5.

Code WE, Yip RW, Rooney ME, Browne PM, Hertz T. (1994). Preoperatiove naproxen sodium reduces postoperative pain following arthoscopic knee surgery. *Can J Anaesth* Vol. 41, pp. 98-101.

Cohen RG, Katz JA, Skrepnik NV. (2009). The relationship between skeletal muscle serum markers and primary THA: a pilot study. *Clin Orthoped Rel Res* 2009 Jul, Vol. 467(7), pp. 1747-52.

Correia MI, Caiaffa WT, da Silva AL, Waitzberg DL. (2001). Risk factors for malnutrition in patients undergoing gastroenterological and hernia surgery: an analysis of 374 patients. *Nutr Hosp* Vol. 16(2), pp. 59-64.

Cruikshank AM, Fraser WD, Biurns HJG, Damme JV, Shenkin A. (1990). Response of serum interleukin- 6 in patients undergoing elective surgery of varying severity. *Clin Sci*, Vol. 79, pp. 161-5.

Damas P, Ledoux D, Nys M, Vrindts Y, De Groote D, Franchimont P, Lamy M. (1992). Cytokine serum level during severe sepsis in human IL-6 as a marker of severity. *Ann Surg*, Vol. 215, pp. 356-62.

Demura S, Takahashi K, Kawahara N, Watanabe Y, Tomita K. (2006). Serum interleukin-6 response after spinal surgery: estimation of surgical magnitude. *J Orthop Sci* Vol. 11, pp. 241-7.

Di Cesare PE, Chang E, Preston CF, Lui CJ. (2005). Serum interleukin-6 as a marker of periprosthetic infection following total hip and knee arthroplasty. *J Bone Joint Surg* Vol. 87A(9), pp. 1921-7.

Fanning J, Neuhoff RA, Brewer JE, Castaneda T, Marcotte MP,Jacobson RL. (1998). Frequency and yield of postoperative fever evaluation. *Infect Dis Obstet Gynecol*, Vol. 6, pp. 252–5.

Febbraio MA, Pedersen BK. (2005). Contraction-induced myokine production and release: is skeletal muscle an endocrine organ? *Exerc Sport Sci Rev*, Vol. 33, pp. 114-9.

Fink B, Mittelstaedt A, Schulz MS, Sebena P, Singer J. (2010). Comparison of a minimally invasive posterior approach and the standard posterior approach for total hip arthroplasty: A prospective and comparative study *J Orthoped Surg Res*, Vol. 5, pp 46.

Fong Y, Mokdawer LL, Shires GT, Lowry SF. (1990). The biological characteristics of cytokines and their implications in surgical injury. *Surg Gynecol Obstet*, Vol. 170, pp.363-78.

Frank SM, Kluger MJ, Kunkel SL. (2000). Elevated thermostatic setpoint in postoperative patients. *Anesthesiology*, Vol. 93, pp. 1426-31.

Ghanem E, Azzam K, Seeley M, Joshi A, Parvizi J. Staged revision for knee arthoplasty infection: What is the role of serologic tests before reimplantation? Clin Orthop Relat Res 2009;467(7):1699-1705.

Gravante G, Knowles T, Ong SL, Al-Taan O, Metcalfe M, Dennison AR, Lloyd DM. (2010).Bile changes after liver surgery: experimental and clinical lessons for future applications. *Dig Surg* Vol. 27(6), pp. 450-60.

Hall GM, Peerbhov D, Shenkin A, Parker CJ, Salmon P. (2000). Hip and knee arthroplasty: a comparison and the endocrine, metabolic and inflammatory responses. *Clin Sci* Vol. 98(1), pp. 71-9.

Handel M, Winkler J, Hornlein RF, Northoff H, Heeg P, Sell S. (2001). Time-related changes of collected shed blood in autologous retransfusion after total knee arthroplasty. *Arch Orthop Trauma Surg,* Vol. 121(10), pp. 557-60.

Hartzband MA. (2004). Posterolateral minimal incision for total hip replacement: technique and early results. *Orthop Clin North Am.,*Vol. 35, pp. 119–129.

He Z, Tonb DJF, Dabney KW, et al. (2004). Cytokine release, pancreatic injury, and risk of acute pancreatitis after spinal fusion surgery. *Dig Dis Sci* Vol. 49(1), pp. 143-9.

Heinrich PC, Castell JV, Andus T. (1990). Interleukin-6 and the acute phase response. *Biochem J* Vol. 265, pp. 621-36.

Herrera MF, Pantoja JP, Velázquez-Fernández D, Cabiedes J, Aguilar-Salinas C, García-García E, Rivas A, Villeda C, Hernández-Ramírez DF, Dávila A, Zaraín A. (2010). Potential additional effect of omentectomy on metabolic syndrome, acute-phase reactants, and inflammatory mediators in grade III obese patients undergoing laparoscopic Roux-en-Y gastric bypass: a randomized trial. *Diabetes Care* Vol. 33(7), pp. 1413-8.

Herroeder S, Pecher S, Schönherr ME, Kaulitz G, Hahnenkamp K, Friess H, Böttiger BW, Bauer H, Dijkgraaf MG, Durieux ME, Hollmann MW. (2007). Systemic lidocaine shortens length of hospital stay after colorectal surgery: a double-blinded, randomized, placebo-controlled trial. Vol. 246(2), pp. 192-200.

Hogevold HE, Lyberg T, Kahler H, Haug E, Reikeras O. (2000). Changes in plasma IL-1beta, TNF-alpha and IL-6 after total hip replacement surgery in general or regional anaesthesia. *Cytokine* Vol. 12(7), pp. 1156-9.

Jakab L, Kalabay L. (1998). The acute phase reaction syndrome: the acute phase reactants (a review). *Acta Microbiol Immunol Hung,* Vol. 45(3-4), pp.409-18.

Kawaguchi Y, Matsui H, Tsuji H. (1996). Back muscle injury after posterior lumbar spine surgery: a histologic and enzymatic analysis. *Spine* Vol. 21(8), pp. 941-4.

Kawaguchi Y, Matsui H, Tsuji H. (1997). Changes in serum creatine phosphokinase isoenzyme after lumbar spine surgery. *Spine* Vol. 22(9), pp. 1018-23.

Koppensteiner W, Auersperg V, Halwachs-Baumann G. (2011). The use of inflammatory markers as a method for discharging patients post hip or knee arthroplasty. *Clin Chem Lab Med* Jun 24.

Kristiansson M, Saraste I, Soop M, Sundqvist KG, Thorne A. Diminished interleukin-6 and C-reactive protein responses to laparoscopic versus open cholecystectomy. *Acta Anaesthesiol Scand* 1999;43:146-52.

Kugisaki H, Sonohata M, Komine M, Tsunoda K, Shinsuke S, Honke H, Mawatari M, Hotokebuchi T. (2011). Serum concentrations of interleukin-6 in patients following unilateral versus bilateral total knee arthroplasty. *J Orthopaed Sci,* Vol. 14(4), pp. 437-42.

Kumbhare D, Parkinson W, Dunlop R, et al. (2007). Biochemical measurement of muscle injury created by lumbar surgery. *Clin Invest Med,* Vol. 30(1), pp. 12-20.

Kumbhare D, Parkinson W, Dunlop R. (2008). Validity of serum creatine kinase as a measure of muscle injury produced by lumbar surgery. *J Spine Dis Techniq,* Vol. 21(1), pp. 49-54.

Kumbhare D, Parkinson W, Dunlop RB, Richards C, Kerr C, Buckley N, Adachi J. (2009). Injury measurement properties of serum interleukin-6 following lumbar decompression surgery. *J Surg Res,* Vol. 157 (2), pp. 161-7.

Lisowska B, Maldyk P, Kontny E, Michalak C, Jung L, Cwiek R. (2006). Postoperative evaluation of plasma interleukin-6 concentration in patients after total hip arthroplasty. *Ortop Tramatol Rehabil* Vol. 8(5), pp. 547-4.

Martin F, Cherif K, Gentili ME, et al. (2008). Lack of impact of intravenous lidocaine on analgesia, functional recovery,and nociceptive pain threshold after total hip arthroplasty. *Anesthesiolog,* Jul; 109 (1), pp. 118.

McCarthy GC, Megalla SA, Habib AS.(2010). Impact of intravenous lidocaine infusion on postoperative analgesia and recovery from surgery: a systematic review of randomized controlled trials. *Drugs,* Vol. 70(9), pp.1149-63.

Mertens MM, Singh JA. (2011). Biomarkers in Arthroplasty: A Systematic Review. *Open Orthopaedics Journal,* Vol. 5, pp. 92-105.

Miyawaki T, Maeda S, Koyama Y, Fukuoka R, Shimada M. (1998). Elevation of plasma interleukin-6 level is involved in postoperative fever following major oral and maxillofacial surgery. *Oral Surg Oral Med Oral Pathol Oral Radiol Endod,* Vol. 85, pp. 146-52.

Munoz M, Garcia-Vallejo JJ, Semper JM, Romero R, Olalla E, Sebastian C. (2004). Acute phase response in patients undergoing lumbar spinal surgery: modulation by perioperative treatment with naproxen and famotidine. *Eur Spine J,* Vol. 13, pp. 367-73.

Munoz M, Cobos A, Campos A, Ariza D, Munoz E, Gomez A. (2005). Impact of postoperative shed blood transfusion, with or without leucocyte reduction, on acute-phase response to surgery for total knee replacement. *Acta Anesthesiol Scand,* Vol. 49(8), pp. 1182.

Nosaka K, Clarkson PM, (1992). Relationship between post-exercise plasma CK elevation and muscle mass involved in exercise. *Intern J Sports Med,* Vol. 13(6), pp. 471-5.

Nosaka K, Newton M. (2002). Difference in the magnitude of muscle damage between maximal and submaximal eccentric loading. *J Strength Condition Res,* Vol. 16(2), pp. 202-8.

Onuoha GN, Alpar EK, Laprade M, Rama D, Pau G. (2001). Levels of myosin heavy chain fragment in patients with tissue damage. *Arch Med Res,* Vol. 32, pp.27-9.

Perl M, Gehbard F, Knoferl MW, Bachem M, Gross H-J, Kinzl L, Strecker W. (2003). The pattern of preformed cytokines in tissues frequently affected by blunt trauma. *Shock,* Vol. 19(4), pp.299- 304.

Petersen AM, Pedersen BK. (2005). The anti-inflammatory effect of exercise. *J Appl Physiol*, Vol. 98(4), pp. 1154-62.

Pile JC.(2006). Evaluating post-operative fever: a focused approach. *Cleveland Clinic J Med*, Vol. 73(Supplement 1), S62-6.

Poupart P, Vandenabeele P, Cayphas S, Van Snick J, Haegemann G, Cruys V, Fiers W, Content J. (1987). B-cell growth modulating and differentiating activity of recombinant human 26kd protein (BSF-2, HuIFN-beta2, HPGF) EMBO J Vol. 6, pp. 1219-24.

Sakamoto K, Arakawa H, Mita S, Ishiko T, Ikei S, Egami H, et al. (1994). Elevation of circulating interleukin-6 after surgery: factors influencing the serum level. *Cytokine*, Vol. 6, pp. 181-6.

Sato T, Asanuma Y, Masaki Y, et al. (1996). Changes in tumor necrosis factor-alpha and interleukin-1 beta production following liver surgery on cirrhotic patients. *Hepatogastroenterology*, Vol. 43, pp. 1148-53.

Shaw JA, Chung R. (1999). Febril response after knee and hip arthroplasty. *Clin Orthop*, Vol. 367, pp. 181-9.

Steensberg A. (2003). The role of IL-6 in exercise-induced immune changes and metabolism. *Exerc Immunol Rev*, Vol. 9, pp. 40-7.

Strecker W, Gebhard F, Rager J, Bruckner UB, Steinbach G, Lothar K. (1999). Early biochemical characterization of soft-tissue trauma and fracture trauma. *J Trauma*, Vol. 47(2), pp. 358-64.

Sudhoff T, Giagounidis A, Karthaus M. (2000). Serum and plasma parameters in clinical evaluation of neutropenic fever. *Antibiot Chemother*, Vol. 50, pp. 10–19.

Takahashi J, Ebara S, Kamimura M, Kinoshita T, Itoh H, Yuzawa et al. (2001). Early-phase enhanced inflammatory reaction after spinal instrumentation surgery. *Spine*, Vol. 26, pp. 1698-1704.

Takahashi J, Ebara S, Kamimura M, Kinoshita T, Misawa H, Shimogata M, Tozuka M, Takaoka K. (2002). Pro-inflammatory and anti-inflammatory cytokine increases after spinal instrumentation surgery. *J Spinal Dis Techniq*, Vol. 15(4), pp. 294-300.

Tegg EM, Griffiths AE, Lowenthal RM, Tuck DM, Harrup R, Marsden KA, Jupe DML, Ragg S and J P Matthews JP. (2001). Association between high interleukin-6 levels and adverse outcome after autologous haemopoietic stem cell transplantation. *Bone Marrow Transplantation* Vol. 28(10), pp. 929-33.

Sun T,Wang X,Lui Z, Chen X, Zhang J. (2011). Plasma concentrations of pro- and anti-inflammatory cytokines and outcome prediction in elderly hip fracture patients. *Int. J. Care Injured*, Vol. 42, pp. 707–13.

Veenhof AA, Sietses C, von Blomberg BM, van Hoogstraten IM, vd Pas MH, Meijerink WJ, vd Peet DL, Tol MP, Bonjer HJ, Cuesta MA. (2011). The surgical stress response and postoperative immune function after laparoscopic or conventional total mesorectal excision in rectal cancer: a randomized trial. *Int J Colorect Dis*, Jan;26(1):53-9.

von Lilienfeld-Toal M, Dietrich MP, Glasmacher A, et al. (2004). Markers of bacteremia in febrile neutropenic patients with hematological malignancies: procalcitonin and IL-6 are more reliable than C-reactive protein. *Eur J Clin Microbiol Infect Dis*, Vol. 23(7), pp. 539-44.

Wirtz DC, Heller KD, Miltner O, Zilkens KW, Wolff JM. (2000). Interleukin-6: a potential inflammatory marker after total joint replacement. *Internat Orthoped,* Vol. 24 (4), pp. 194-6.

Wu AHB, Perryman G. (1992). Clinical applications of muscle enzymes and proteins. *Curr Opin Rheumatol,* Vol. 4, pp. 815-20.

Yasukawa K, Hirano T, Watanabe Y, Muratani K, Matsuda T, Nakai S, Kishimoto T. (1987). Structure and expression of human B cell stimulatory factor-2 (BSF-2/IL-6) gene. EMBO J Vol. 6, pp. 2939-45.

Part 5

Anesthesia Considerations for Orthopaedic Trauma Surgery

10

Anesthesia for Orthopedic Trauma

Jessica A. Lovich-Sapola and Charles E. Smith
Case Western Reserve University School of Medicine
Department of Anesthesia, MetroHealth Medical Center, Cleveland
USA

1. Introduction

Orthopedic trauma surgeons realize the tremendous importance of coordinated care at trauma centers and by trauma systems. The anesthesiologist is an important link in the coordinated approach to orthopedic trauma care. "Musculoskeletal injuries are the most frequent indication for operative management in most trauma centers." Trauma management of a multiply-injured patient includes early stabilization of long-bone, pelvic, and acetabular fractures, provided that the patient has been adequately resuscitated. (Miller, 2009) Early stabilization leads to reduced pain and improved outcomes. (Smith, 2008) Studies have shown that failure to stabilize these fractures leads to increased morbidity, pulmonary complications, and increased length of hospital stay. (Miller, 2009) "Life threatening and limb-threatening musculoskeletal injuries should be addressed emergently." (Smith, 2008)

The chapter will discuss the following orthopedic trauma anesthesia issues:

- Pre-operative evaluation
- Airway management including difficult airways and cervical spine precautions
- Intra-operative monitoring
- Anesthetic agents and techniques (regional vs general anesthesia)
- Intra-operative complications (hypotension, blood loss, hypothermia, fat embolism syndrome)
- Post-operative pain management

2. Pre-operative evaluation

Orthopedic trauma patients can be challenging for Anesthesiologists. These patients can range in age from young to the elderly, may have multiple co-morbid medical conditions, and even a previously healthy patient may have trauma-associated injuries that may have a significant impact on the anesthetic plan. The Anesthesiologist's role is to evaluate the entire patient, with particular focus on the cardiovascular, respiratory, and other major organ system function. All patients undergoing anesthesia for an orthopedic surgery require pre-operative evaluation. (Miller, 2009) The goal of pre-operative evaluation is to obtain pertinent information that may alter the response to anesthetic drugs and increase the risk of complications due to impaired tissue oxygen delivery. Medical complexity, as assessed by the American Society of Anesthesiologists (ASA) physical status, correlates with perioperative morbidity and mortality.

Class	Description
Class I	Normally healthy
Class II	Patient with mild systemic disease (e.g. hypertension)
Class III	Patient with severe systemic disease (e.g. heart failure,), non-decompensated
Class IV	Patient with severe systemic disease, decompensated (e.g., decompensated heart failure, respiratory failure, unstable angina, hepatic encephalopathy)
Class V	Moribund patient, survival unlikely with or without surgery

Table 1. American Society of Anesthesiologists Physical Status (Miller, 2009)

2.1 Major organ systems

Age and functional status are useful in evaluating organ system reserves, and in determining sensitivity to anesthetic drugs. Patients with severe cardiac, pulmonary, hepatic, renal or neurologic disease are at increased risk for developing complications related to anesthesia, as are those with substance abuse and pregnant patients. (Miller, 2009)

2.1.1 Cardiovascular disease

Cardiovascular diseases including uncontrolled hypertension, ischemic heart disease, congestive heart failure, heart block, and arrhythmia increase the risk of anesthesia. Associated cardiac trauma may lead to low cardiac output due to tamponade, myocardial contusion, valvular disruption, and aortic dissection. Ischemic hypoxia and insufficient blood flow leads to cardiogenic shock and inadequate delivery of oxygen to the tissues. Any condition characterized by low cardiac output such as poor heart function, intense vasoconstriction, hypovolemia, or severe obstruction to blood flow should be optimized prior to surgery. Congenital heart disease may lead to intra-cardiac shunt and hypoxia.

Condition	Clinical Characteristics
Rhythm Disturbances	Significant, severe, or new onset arrhythmia, heart block, supraventricular tachycardia, ventricular arrhythmia or tachycardia
Coronary Artery Disease	Severe or unstable coronary syndromes, recent myocardial infarction
Valvular Heart Disease	Severe valvular disease, e.g., aortic stenosis and mitral valve disease
Congestive Heart Failure	Decompensated, worsening, or new heart failure

Table 2. Cardiac conditions requiring evaluation and treatment prior to orthopedic surgery (Fleisher, 2007)

2.1.2 Pacemakers and Internal Cardiac Defibrillators (ICDs)

If electrocautery is used in close proximity to an ICD or pacemaker, the electrical current generated can inhibit the pacemaker resulting in cardiogenic shock if the patient is pacemaker dependent. With an ICD device, use of the cautery may activate the ICD resulting in multiple shocks to the patient. The device itself may be damaged by electrocautery. Injury to cardiac tissue from current induced in leads imbedded in cardiac muscle may occur, leading to device failure. These patients deserve a cardiology consultation to properly manage the device. The ASA practice advisory recommends changing the conventional pacing function to an asynchronous pacing mode in pacemaker-dependent patients. The anti-tachyarrhythmia functions of ICDs, including the ability to provide defibrillation, should be suspended for the duration of surgery, assuming that electrocautery is required. After surgery, the device needs to be reprogrammed and function confirmed.

2.1.3 Respiratory disease

Patients with significant respiratory disease are at increased risk for pulmonary complications because of limited pulmonary reserve and because anesthetic drugs decrease the respiratory response to hypoxia and hypercarbia. This patient population develops hypoxia sooner than patients with normal respiratory function due to lower airway obstruction, lung tissue disease, inadequate alveolar-capillary transfer or intrapulmonary shunt. Respiratory failure may ensue, requiring post-operative mechanical ventilation. Chest trauma including pulmonary contusion, hemothorax, and pneumothorax may contribute to respiratory insufficiency. Pneumothorax may lead to shock if under tension, especially in the presence of positive pressure ventilation. Hemothorax may result in hemorrhagic shock (Smith, 2008)

Hypoxemia- Decreased arterial oxygen tension
Ventilation-Perfusion (V/Q) mismatch Diffusion impairment Hypoventilation
Hypercarbia - Increased arterial carbon dioxide (CO2) tension
Increased Dead Space Increased CO_2 production Disease affecting respiratory control centers Respiratory muscle weakness Increased respiratory muscle load

Table 3. Causes of respiratory failure

Causes of V/Q mismatch include interstitial lung disease, acute lung injury (ALI) or acute respiratory distress syndrome (ARDS), pneumonia, pulmonary edema, and pleural effusion. Causes of hypoventilation include depression of the central nervous system by drugs, diseases affecting the brainstem, neuromuscular disease resulting in respiratory muscle weakness, and chest wall abnormalities.

Increased dead space occurs in conditions such as pulmonary embolus or emphysema. Increased work of breathing due to impaired pulmonary compliance and increased pulmonary resistance may also contribute to respiratory failure. Increased resistance is due to bronchoconstriction, airway inflammation, or secretions in the airway. Decreased lung compliance may be due to pulmonary edema, pneumonia, fibrosis, or atelectasis. Decreased compliance can also be due to muscle or skeletal abnormalities of the chest wall or from intra-abdominal processes such as ascites, distended bowel, or abdominal compartment syndrome.

2.1.4 Morbid obesity

Obesity has become epidemic in industrialized countries and is an important contributor to early death. Patients with a body mass index (BMI) > 40 are considered morbidly obese. The pathophysiologic consequences of obesity impact every major organ system, and increases both morbidity and mortality. (Miller, 2009)

Factor	Considerations
Increased Prevalence of Obstructive Sleep Apnea (OSA) and Obesity-Hypoventilation Syndrome	Risk of hypoventilation, hypercarbia, apnea, hypoxia, arrhythmias, and cardiopulmonary arrest
Decreased Functional Residual Capacity	Decreased oxygen reservoir following period of apnea; Increased right-to-left trans-pulmonary shunt and atelectasis
Increased Work of Breathing	Increased oxygen consumption, increased weight of chest wall, decreased chest wall compliance
Difficult Airway Management	Large head and face makes mask placement difficult; Increased fat infiltration into oropharynx and peri-glottic structures interferes with glottic visualization during laryngoscopy; Increased airway obstruction during bag-mask ventilation; decreased head/neck movement.

Table 4. Respiratory system considerations in morbid obesity

OSA predisposes patients to airway obstruction, especially when sedated. Opioids are especially worrisome due to the potential for impaired control of breathing, post-operative apnea, and hypopneic episodes. OSA patients may require prolonged recovery in a monitored setting. The classic symptoms include daytime somnolence, a history of snoring, and apneic episodes while sleeping. Screening for OSA is routine. The apneic-hypopneic index is a useful measure of OSA severity and is obtained from polysomnography. Pulmonary hypertension, right ventricular failure and arrhythmias are not uncommon.

S. Snoring – "Do you snore loudly (louder than talking or loud enough to be heard through closed doors)?"
T. Tiredness during daytime – "Do you often feel tired, fatigued, or sleepy during daytime?"
O. Stop breathing during sleep – "Has anyone observed you stop breathing during your sleep?"
P. High blood pressure – "Do you have or are you being treated for high blood pressure?"
B. BMI – greater than 35 kg/m^2
A. Age – older than 50 years old
N. Neck circumference – greater than 40 cm (15.75 inches)
G. Gender – male

Table 5. STOP-BANG screening for OSA. High risk if positive for 3 or more of these 8 (Chung, 2008)

2.1.5 Liver disease

The liver is responsible for protein synthesis (albumin, coagulation factors, acute phase reactants), metabolism of carbohydrates, lipids, and amino acids, and drugs. The liver also has a role in immunity endocrine functions, red blood cell degradation and bilirubin excretion. The liver influences the plasma concentration and systemic availability of most drugs. The ability to metabolize and excrete IV anesthetic drugs may be significantly impaired in patients with severe hepatic disease. Common lab abnormalities include anemia, thrombocytopenia, elevated AST, ALT, alkaline phosphatase, increased PT and INR, and decreased albumin. (Miller, 2009)

2.1.6 Renal disease

Patients with kidney failure have multisystem abnormalities including neurological, cardiovascular, pulmonary, gastrointestinal, hematological, and musculoskeletal disease. Serum creatinine and blood urea nitrogen (BUN) are simple routine tests that are helpful as screening guides in management of patients with kidney impairment and provide a rough measure of glomerular filtration rate. The ability to excrete drugs may be significantly impaired in patients with end stage kidney disease. Anemia due to chronic disease, may contribute to hypoxia. Timing of dialysis and protection of dialysis access sites are important prior to surgery. (Miller, 2009)

2.1.7 Neurologic disease

Etiologies include traumatic brain injury, intracranial hypertension, infection, seizure disorder and neuromuscular disease. Dementia, delirium, confusion, poisoning, drug overdose, substance abuse, and metabolic disorders alter the clinical picture of neurologic disease. Neurologic disease can result in a disordered control of breathing, abnormal respiratory patterns, decreased minute ventilation and increased risk of hypoxemia. Patients with acute spinal cord injury may have impaired respiratory and cardiovascular function and present with neurogenic shock. Autonomic dysreflexia occurs in patients with chronic spinal cord injury. In these patients, stimuli below the level of spinal cord transection elicit increased reflex sympathetic activity over the splanchnic outflow tract without the normal descending inhibitory modulatory impulses due to blockade at the level of injury. The response is severe vasoconstriction below the level of transection, but vasodilation and bradycardia above the injury. The syndrome occurs most commonly when the lesion is above the T6 level. Stimuli such as bladder or intestinal distention can cause persistent hypertension, headache, visual changes, sweating, bradycardia and arrhythmias. If untreated, autonomic dysreflexia may cause stroke, seizure and death.

2.1.8 Elderly

Elderly patients have limited physiologic reserves. Illnesses tend to accumulate in both frequency and severity with age. Coronary artery disease, hypertension, and heart failure are more prevalent. There is a decreased heart rate response to hypovolemia due to decreased beta-adrenergic activity. The prevalence of atrial fibrillation is increased. Ventilatory responses to hypoxia and hypercarbia are reduced. The lungs lose their elastic recoil with aging and there is an age-related reduction in vital capacity and minute ventilation. Respiratory muscle strength consistently declines with age. Decreased chest wall compliance and increased alveolar dead space increase the work of breathing. There is an increase in V/Q mismatching, alveolar dead space, and right-to-left transpulmonary shunt. Cough is less vigorous and there may be impaired swallowing reflexes, decreased secretion clearance, and increased incidence of pneumonia. Age-related central nervous system changes predispose the elderly to delirium and ICU psychosis. There is increased vulnerability to cerebral ischemia associated with hypotension. Renal and hepatic functions are reduced. The aging kidney has a decreased ability to dilute and concentrate urine and is vulnerable to nephrotoxins. The volume of distribution for anesthetic drugs is altered due to decreased lean body muscle mass. Serum protein production, including albumin, is decreased. Malnutrition and anemia are common.

2.1.9 Pediatrics

The pediatric age group covers a broad range of physiology and sizes, from newborn infants to adolescents. Infants are more dependent on heart rate to maintain an adequate cardiac output. They are unable to increase their stroke volume to the same extent as adults. Pediatric patients also have relatively high vagal tone and may develop bradycardia in response to vagal stimulation or hypoxia. Children have a higher incidence of upper respiratory tract infections and asthma which may contribute to increased risk of laryngospasm and bronchospasm. History of latex allergy or sensitivity should be specifically obtained since there is a large cohort of potentially latex allergic pediatric patients. Congenital heart disease and specific syndromes need to be documented and appropriately managed.

2.2 Previous anesthetics

Previous adverse experience with regional, general and nerve block anesthesia should be documented, especially with regards to cardiac arrest during anesthesia, unplanned ICU admission and difficult airway management. Malignant hyperthermia (MH) is a life-threatening pharmacogenetic disease resulting from exposure of a susceptible patient to a trigger agent. It is characterized by rapidly increasing temperature (as much as 1°C every 5 minutes), extreme acidosis, exaggerated CO_2 production, and muscle rigidity. The most common triggering drugs are succinylcholine and inhalation agents (halothane, isoflurane, desflurane, and sevoflurane).

2.3 Medications

Chronic medications should be continued with few exceptions (Table 6). Abrupt cessation of beta-blockers can produce undesirable effects such as rebound hypertension and arrhythmias. Patients on beta-blockers will not show the same degree of cardiovascular response to stress. Abrupt withdrawal of the alpha-2 agonist clonidine may result in severe rebound hypertension.

Long-acting oral agents for diabetes may lead to symptomatic hypoglycemia in a fasting patient. Oral diabetic medication should be discontinued prior to surgery and a finger stick glucose measurement should be obtained prior to initiating anesthesia. There are multiple types of insulin with differing half-lives, time and level of peak effect.

Patients with coronary artery drug-eluting stents should continue on dual antiplatelet therapy (i.e. clopidogrel, and aspirin) for at least one year following placement, and then continue indefinitely with at least one of those drugs thereafter. The risk of bleeding is increased. Individualized patient management is required to determine if the risk of coronary artery stent thrombosis and myocardial infarction is greater than the risk of perioperative bleeding.

Medication	Interactions with Anesthesia
Beta Blockers	Decreased heart rate response to hypovolemia; exaggerated hypotension with hypovolemia and anemia
Insulin/ Hypoglycemics	Risk of hypoglycemia during fasting
Antipsychotics	May increase sedative effects
Anxiolytics	May increase sedative effects
Seizure Medications	May increase sedative effects
Alpha Adrenergic Blockers	May increase possibility of hypotension
Calcium Channel Blockers	Risk of hypotension and blunted heart rate response
Antidepressants	Anti-cholinergic induced impairment of sweating
Anticoagulants	Increased risk of bleeding

Table 6. Medications and interactions with anesthesia

2.4 Substance abuse

Substance abuse is frequently encountered in trauma patients and can affect the pulmonary, cardiovascular, nervous, renal and hepatic systems.

Substance	Considerations
Alcohol	Risk of alcoholic hepatitis, cirrhosis, portal hypertension, cardiomyopathy, arrhythmias, seizures, neuropathies, dementia, Wernicke-Korsakoff syndrome (ataxia, cognitive dysfunction) Anemia from vitamin deficiencies Delirium tremens Pneumonia Gastrointestinal bleeding Coagulopathies due to hepatic dysfunction or vitamin K deficiency. Life-threatening withdrawal with autonomic instability and hyperpyrexia
Cocaine/ Amphetamine	Risk of hemodynamic instability, cerebrovascular accidents, cardiomyopathy, arrhythmias, coronary artery vasoconstriction, angina, myocardial infarction, pulmonary edema, paranoia, anxiety, and seizures Long-term use: ventricular hypertrophy, myocardial necrosis, nasal septal perforation
Ecstasy	Excessive thirst, hyponatremia; pulmonary or cerebral edema
Marijuana	Tachycardia, dysrhythmias, EKG abnormalities, increased cardiac output
Opioids	Tolerance to opioids Acute use: decreased respiratory rate and cause lethargy and pinpoint pupils Methadone: prolonged QT interval. IV use: hepatitis, HIV, endocarditis, limited IV access

Table 7. Anesthesia considerations for patients with substance abuse

2.5 Pre-operative testing

2.5.1 Laboratory tests

For all emergency orthopedic cases, certain laboratory tests should be ordered as soon as possible: (Miller, 2009)

- Complete blood count (CBC): for baseline hemoglobin, hematocrit, and platelet levels
- Type and screen
- Coagulation panel
- Basic metabolic panel (BMP)
- Consider a toxicology screen
- Consider a hepatic panel
- Further lab work should be performed based on the patients past medical history and mechanism of injury

2.5.2 Electrocardiogram (EKG)

The American College of Cardiology / American Heart Association guidelines recommend pre-operative cardiac testing in patients that are at increased cardiac risk, based on their clinical risk profile, functional capacity, and type of surgery. (Miller, 2009) According to the ACC/AHA guidelines, every patient undergoing a high risk surgery (emergency surgery), especially those ≥ 50 years of age should have an EKG unless time does not allow this. For an emergent surgery, the patient should have continued peri-operative cardiac surveillance, post-operative risk stratification, and risk factor management. Patients undergoing an intermediate risk surgery (orthopedic) and have known coronary artery disease, peripheral arterial disease, cerebrovascular disease, or one clinical risk factor require an EKG prior to surgery. (Fleisher, 2007)

2.5.3 Chest X-ray

A chest X-ray is recommended for patients with: significant chest trauma, significant debilitating pulmonary disease history with no recent chest X-ray (within one year), significant change in pulmonary status within the past 6 months, or a recent pneumonia/ COPD exacerbation. (Fleisher, 2007) Computed tomography (CT) may also be indicated in patients with suspected aortic trauma. Smith, 2008)

2.5.4 Urine BHCG

Trauma in a pregnant patient is associated with a high risk of spontaneous abortion, pre-term labor, and/ or premature delivery. The best treatment for the fetus is rapid and complete resuscitation of the mother. Serious trauma occurring in the first trimester of gestation can lead to birth defects or miscarriage secondary to the hemorrhagic shock with uterine ischemia, pelvic irradiation, or medication effects. A urine BHCG pregnancy test should be performed on all female orthopedic trauma patients of child-bearing age. (Miller, 2009) Trauma occurring in the second or third trimester of pregnancy requires an ultrasound evaluation. Fetal heart monitoring is indicated in the operating room if the fetus would be viable if delivered. Consider left lateral uterine displacement if possible for all patients in their third trimester to alleviate the compression on the inferior vena cava and resulting impaired venous return to the heart and hypotension. The obstetrician should be consulted immediately if it is determined that the patient is pregnant. (Miller, 2009)

2.6 NPO guidelines

The pre-operative fasting guidelines are written for healthy patients undergoing elective procedures requiring general anesthesia, regional anesthesia, and sedation. These guidelines do not apply for trauma patients, women in labor, or emergent surgeries, and do not guarantee complete gastric emptying. A trauma patient presenting for emergency surgery is considered to be a "full stomach" and is at risk for pulmonary aspiration of gastric contents with resultant pneumonia. (ASA Practice Guidelines, 2011) Reasons include ingestion of food or liquids less than 8 hours prior to the injury, swallowed blood from nasal or oral injuries, delayed gastric emptying associated with stress of trauma, and administration of oral contrast for CT.

Type of Food/Drink	Fasting Hours Required
Clear Liquids	• 2 hours • Examples: water, fruit juice without pulp, carbonated beverages, clear tea, and black coffee • Excludes alcohol • Volume of liquid is less important than the type ingested
Breast Milk	• 4 hours
Infant Formula	• 6 hours
Light Meal and Nonhuman Milk	• 6 hours • Example: plain toast and a clear liquid • The volume of nonhuman milk is important in determining the fasting time
Fried or Fatty Foods and Meat	• 8 hours

Table. 8. Pre-operative fasting guidelines (ASA Practice Guidelines, 2011)

3. Airway management

"Advanced trauma life support (ATLS) emphasizes the importance of the ABCDE mnemonic: airway, breathing, circulation, disability, and exposure." Verification of an open airway and acceptable respiratory mechanics are of primary importance, because hypoxia is the trauma patient's most immediate threat to life. The inability to oxygenate a person can lead to permanent brain injury and death within 5-10 minutes. Airway obstruction in a trauma patient can be secondary to: direct facial or neck trauma, hemorrhage of the nose, mouth, or upper airway, decreased consciousness, or aspiration of gastric contents/foreign body. Poor ventilation may be due to decreased respiratory drive, direct injury to the trachea or bronchi, pneumothorax, chest wall injury, pulmonary contusion, aspiration, cervical spine injury, or bronchospasm. (Miller, 2009)

3.1 Basic airway management

Airway management for any patient requires the proper equipment and medications. This becomes especially important in an emergency case. (Smith, 2008)

Equipment Required for Intubation
• Oxygen source • Ventilation: bag-valve-mask device, soft nasal airway, rigid oral airway, laryngeal mask airway (LMA) • Intubation: Laryngoscope (multiple sizes), endotracheal tubes (multiple sizes), gum-elastic bougie (Eschmann tracheal tube introducer), flexible fiberoptic scope, video-laryngoscope (e.g., Glidescope), tape to secure the airway • Suction • Monitor: End tidal CO_2, pulse oximeter • Medications: sedative/hypnotic, neuromuscular relaxant (paralytic), local anesthetics (for airway anesthesia), resuscitation medications • Functioning intravenous (IV) access • Miscellaneous: syringes, needles, IV tubing, emergency tracheotomy/ cricothyroidotomy kit

Table 9. Equipment required for intubation. (Smith, 2008)

Airway management begins with the proper positioning of the patient. Mask ventilation is usually the first technique used to ventilate a patient. Proper mask ventilation can be life saving. The face mask should be applied firmly to the face to ensure an adequate seal. A jaw-thrust maneuver (instead of the chin lift) should be used in any patient with a suspected cervical injury to help facilitate ventilation. The most common cause of airway obstruction during mask ventilation is when the tongue and epiglottis fall back in the supine/ unconscious patient. An oral airway or nasal airway (if not contraindicated) can help to open the airway. The rigid oral airway can cause gagging in a conscious patient resulting in vomiting and increased intracranial pressure. The nasal airway is usually better tolerated in an awake or semiconscious patient, but is contraindicated in certain facial fractures and basal skull injuries. (Smith, 2008)

If the patient's airway exam is not predictive of difficult intubation, rapid sequence induction and intubation (RSI) is preferred following 3-5 minutes of preoxygenation with 100% oxygen. Cricoid pressure has been routine for most Anesthesiologists in an attempt to decrease passive regurgitation of gastric contents after sedation and paralysis. Recently, the value of cricoid pressure has been questioned due to its ability to distort the airway, displace the esophagus, and worsen the laryngeal view during intubation. In a traditional RSI, no attempts to manually ventilate the patient's lungs should be made until the endotracheal tube is secured in the trachea. If preoxygenation is insufficient (uncooperative patient, respiratory distress) or laryngoscopy proves difficult and oxygen desaturation occurs, mask ventilation should be done. Ventilation and oxygenation is the main priority. (Smith, 2008)

Time (min)	Action
-3 min to 0	Preoxygenation is a critical step for RSI
-1 min (optional)	Small dose opioid
0 min	Induction agent (propofol, thiopental, etomidate, or ketamine)
At loss of consciousness	Cricoid pressure (controversial) Neuromuscular blocking agent: • succinylcholine, 1 mg/kg or • rocuronium, 1 mg/kg No manual ventilation (unless inadequate preoxygenation or at risk of hypoxia)
+ 0.75 to 1.5 min (When blockade complete)	Laryngoscopy and tracheal intubation
After tracheal intubation	Confirm end-tidal carbon dioxide & bilateral breath sounds

Table 10. Timing for Rapid Sequence Induction and Intubation (RSI). (Smith, 2008)

When performing RSI in a patient with hemorrhagic shock, etomidate and ketamine are preferred over propofol and thiopental due to less hypotension. Succinylcholine is the gold standard for paralysis due to its rapid onset and short duration. Undesirable side effects of succinylcholine include increased intragastric pressure, intraocular pressure, and intracranial pressure (ICP). Succinylcholine is associated with exaggerated potassium release in patients with certain neuromuscular disorders and burns and is contraindicated in patients with malignant hyperthermia. If succinylcholine is contraindicated, longer acting agents like rocuronium or vecuronium can be used to induce paralysis. The laryngeal mask airway (LMA) should be used whenever bag-mask ventilation is difficult. The LMA can alleviate ventilatory obstruction above the vocal cords. The LMA is not an effective device for periglottic or subglottic pathology, such as laryngospasm. The LMA is not a definitive airway and does not prevent aspiration in a trauma patient with a presumed "full stomach". (Smith, 2008)

Rigid direct laryngoscopy is the most common technique used to place an endotracheal tube. If this technique is unsuccessful, then video laryngoscopy (e.g., Glidescope), flexible fiberoptic scope, or a surgical airway may be indicated. Help should be summoned as soon as the airway management plan is recognized as being difficult. (Smith, 2008)

3.2 Difficult airways

Common predictors of a difficult airway include: facial dissymmetry (trauma), tracheal deviation, cervical fractures, small mouth opening, inability to visualize the faucial pillars and uvula (Mallampati), limited neck range of motion, prominent incisors, distance between the thyroid cartilage and mandible < 6 cm, and a narrow maxillary arch. (Miller, 2009) If after performing an airway exam there is doubt about the ability to intubate the trachea following induction of anesthesia, consideration should be given towards securing the airway with topical anesthesia and mild sedation; induction agents and neuromuscular relaxants should be avoided before the airway is secured. If there is concern of airway injury (stridor, hoarseness, subcutaneous emphysema), spontaneous ventilation is maintained provided the patient is cooperative, stable, and is not in respiratory distress. A surgical airway or rapid sequence fiberoptic intubation may be necessary in these situations. If time permits, lateral neck radiographs, CT scanning, and endoscopy can be used to better define airway anatomy. In patients with difficult or compromised airways, choice of intubation technique is ultimately determined by skills, judgment, experience, available equipment, and urgency of the situation. (Smith, 2008)

3.3 Cervical spine precautions

Blunt trauma patients are assumed to have cervical spine injury until proven otherwise. Distracting injuries, intoxication, and altered mental status can make clearing the cervical spine difficult prior to proceeding to the OR for surgical management. The incidence of cervical spine injury is roughly 2% in patients with a closed-head injury and 2-6% for all blunt trauma patients. During direct laryngoscopy, the primary force applied is the extension of the occiput on C1 combined with flexion of the lower vertebrae. It is therefore possible to aggravate or worsen a cervical injury with the standard direct laryngoscopy approach. (Lovich-Sapola, 2010) Manipulation of the airway can exacerbate a spinal cord injury. Imaging studies of the patient's cervical spine should be reviewed prior to induction of anesthesia, if time permits. In patients with a known spinal cord injury and/or neurological symptoms, awake fiberoptic intubation is a prudent choice provided the patient is cooperative and adequate airway anesthesia can be achieved. A key advantage of a well performed awake fiberoptic intubation is the ability to document neurologic integrity after intubation, before inducing general anesthesia. In other patients, RSI with in-line cervical stabilization is preferred. (Smith, 2008)

3.3.1 How to clear a cervical spine

In an alert patient without intoxication, neck pain, decreased level of consciousness, distracting injury, or neurologic abnormalities, the patient's cervical spine can be cleared clinically. The patient's cervical spine can not be cleared even with the appropriate radiographs if they have a "distracting injury". A normal cervical spine X-ray does not rule out a cervical injury, because ligamentous injuries may not be recognized on an X-ray. A CT scan/MRI may be required to rule out the cervical ligament injury, and there is often no time to do this testing in a trauma situation prior to going to the operating room. (Lovich-Sapola, 2010)

3.3.2 Indications for cervical spine precautions

Indications for Cervical Spine Precautions
• All acute trauma patients with a depressed level of consciousness • Patients reporting neck pain • Patients with midline cervical spine tenderness • Upper extremity paresthesia • Focal motor deficits • Pain from other injuries that would be likely to mask neck pain • Specific mechanisms of injury: falls, diving accidents, high-speed motor vehicle accidents

Table 11. Indications for cervical spine precautions (Lovich-Sapola, 2010)

3.3.3 In-line stabilization

The patient's occiput should be held firmly on the backboard or operating table to limit the amount of "sniff". Immobilization of the spine can be accomplished by an assistant providing manual in-line stabilization. A semi-rigid collar or sandbag placed on both sides of the neck and head can also help in maintaining the proper neck position. A well-fitted hard collar can make an intubation almost impossible and should be removed prior to any intubation attempt. Hold the patient's head in-line with the cervical spine to prevent any cervical twisting. Laryngoscopy will always be more difficult with cervical stabilization. While the cervical neck is immobilized, multiple different techniques can be used to improve the success of intubation, including the McCoy blade, Wu/ Bullard scope, Glidescope, and flexible fiberoptic scope. (Lovich-Sapola, 2010) The use of a Glidescope with in-line stabilization has been shown to provide better glottic visualization, but does not significantly decrease the movement of the cervical spine when compared to direct laryngoscopy. (Robitaille, 2008) If the cervical collar was removed during intubation, it should be replaced immediately after the intubation is confirmed. (Lovich-Sapola, 2010)

4. Intra-operative monitoring

Every anesthetic no matter the location requires standard ASA monitors. These include a person qualified to monitor, evaluate, and care for the patient present in the room at all times and a way to monitor the patient's oxygenation, ventilation, circulation, and body temperature. (Lovich-Sapola, 2010)

Standard ASA Monitor Classifications	Specific Monitors
Oxygenation	• Oxygen analyzer: measures the oxygenation of the inspired gas • Pulse oximeter: measures the oxygenation of the patients blood • Observation: patient color
Ventilation	• Monitor the expired carbon dioxide ($EtCO_2$) • Measure the respiratory volumes • Disconnect alarms on the mechanical ventilator • Observation: clinical signs of chest rise, reservoir bag movement, and auscultation of breath sounds
Circulation	• Electrocardiogram • Blood pressure monitor (at least every 5 minutes) • Heart rate monitor • Observation: pulse palpation, auscultation of heart sounds
Body Temperature	• Continuous body temperature monitoring

Table 12. Standard ASA Monitors (Lovich-Sapola, 2010; Smith, 2008)

4.1 Pulse oximetry

The pulse oximeter uses two wavelengths of light: red (660 nm) and infrared (940 nm). The light is transmitted from one side of the sensor to the photodetector on the opposite side, through pulsatile tissue. Oxy- and deoxyhemoglobin vary in light absorption at different wavelengths. The measured wavelength absorption ratio is converted to percent oxygen saturation. (Smith, 2008)

4.2 Electrocardiogram

The electrocardiogram (EKG) is a measurement of the electrical activity of the heart. Whenever a patient is undergoing anesthesia they must have continuous EKG monitoring. Limb lead II is used to monitor for arrhythmias and chest lead V5 is used to watch for ischemia. (Lovich-Sapola, 2010)

There are multiple EKG changes that are common in a trauma patient. The EKG changes can be a result of metabolic derangements from hemorrhage and resuscitation, structural injury to the heart itself, or central nervous system injury. Trauma patients are also at risk for cardiac ischemia due to high circulating catecholamines in the potential presence of existing coronary disease. (Smith, 2008)

Electrical activity to the heart does not guarantee perfusion, as seen in pulseless electrical activity (PEA). In PEA there is electrical activity to the heart, but no myocardial contraction. PEA can occur in multiple trauma scenarios including, cardiac tamponade, tension pneumothorax, hypovolemia, hyperkalemia, and hypothermia. (Smith, 2008)

4.3 Blood pressure monitoring

Blood pressure should be monitored at least every five minutes while a patient is undergoing anesthesia. Blood pressure can be monitored non-invasively or invasively. Non-invasive blood pressure monitoring requires the use of a manual or automatic blood pressure cuff. This technique is the one most commonly used. Complications of a non-invasive blood pressure cuff include compartment syndrome from overuse of the cuff and inappropriate treatment of erroneous blood pressure readings from the improper positioning/ placement of the cuff. (Lovich-Sapola, 2010)

Indications for the Placement of an Arterial Line
• Continuous, real-time blood pressure monitoring
• Planned pharmacologic or mechanical cardiovascular manipulation
• Repeat blood sampling: arterial blood gas, hematocrit, glucose
• Failure of non-invasive blood pressure monitor: patient obesity, patient positioning
• Supplementary diagnostic information from the arterial waveform: arterial pulse contour analysis (systolic pressure variation, pulse pressure variation)
• Patient with end organ disease
• Patient with large fluid shifts

Table 13. Indications for the placement of an arterial line. (Lovich-Sapola, 2010)

Invasive arterial blood pressure monitoring requires the placement of a catheter into an artery, usually the radial, brachial, or femoral artery. The placement of an arterial line is not without risk. The complications of an arterial line include distal ischemia secondary to thrombosis, proximal emboli, or prolonged shock, pseudoaneurysm, arteriovenous fistula, hemorrhage, hematoma, infection, skin necrosis, peripheral neuropathy, misinterpretation of data, and cerebral air embolism secondary to retrograde flushing of the catheter. (Lovich-Sapola, 2010)

4.4 Temperature monitoring

The patient's core temperature should be monitored for any case requiring anesthesia for longer than 20-30 minutes. Every effort should be made to maintain normothermia throughout the case. (Lovch-Sapola, 2010) Maintaining euthermia can be very challenging in a trauma case secondary to the large volumes of fluid resuscitation and multiple areas of patient exposure. (Smith, 2008) The normal body temperature is 36.7 °C to 37.0 °C ±0.2 ° C to 0.4 ° C. Continuous monitoring is recommended, but 15 minute intervals is acceptable. Core temperature sites for measurement include the pulmonary artery, distal esophagus, tympanic membrane, and nasopharynx. Intermediate sites include the mouth, axilla, bladder, and rectum. (Lovich-Sapola, 2010)

Hypothermia must be avoided in all cases, but especially trauma cases secondary to the resulting coagulation disturbances, cardiac arrhythmias, inappropriate diuresis, delayed drug metabolism, and increased risk of infection caused by prolonged hypothermia. The operating room should be heated for all trauma cases to >24 °C to help prevent further hypothermia. (Smith, 2008)

4.5 Central Venous Pressure (CVP) monitor

CVP is usually obtained by venous access in the internal jugular vein, subclavian vein, or femoral vein. The CVP is an indicator of preload, although there is wide variability due to compliance of the venous system and right atrium. Fluid status can be monitored by following CVP trends. (Smith, 2008)

Indication for Central Venous Access and Central Venous Monitoring
• CVP monitoring • Transvenous cardiac pacing • Required for the insertion of a pulmonary artery catheter • Temporary hemodialysis • Drug administration: vasoactive drugs, hyperalimentation, chemotherapy, prolonged antibiotic treatment • Rapid infusion of fluids: trauma, major surgery • Aspiration of a venous air embolism • Inadequate peripheral access • Sampling site for repeated blood testing

Table 14. Indications for central venous access and central venous monitoring (Lovich-Sapola, 2010)

Complications of Central Venous Access and Central Venous Monitoring
• Mechanical injury: arterial, venous, nerve, and cardiac tamponade • Respiratory compromise: airway compression by hematoma, pneumothorax • Arrhythmias • Thromboembolic event • Infection • Misinterpretation of data

Table 15. Complications of central venous access and central venous monitoring (Lovich-Sapola, 2010)

4.6 Pulmonary Artery Catheter (PAC)

Pulmonary Artery Catheter Measurements	Pulmonary Artery Catheter Indications
• Cardiac output (CO)/ cardiac index (CI) • RV pressure • Pulmonary artery pressure (PAP) • Central venous pressure (CVP) • Calculation of oxygen delivery • Assessment of cardiac work • Mixed venous oxygen saturation (MVO_2) • Pulmonary capillary wedge pressure (PCWP) • Systemic vascular resistance (SVR)	• Cardiac: congestive heart failure, low ejection fraction, left sided valvular heart disease, CABG, aortic cross clamp • Pulmonary: COPD and ARDS • Complex fluid management: shock, burns, acute renal failure • Surgical: high risk for venous air embolism

Table 16. Pulmonary artery catheter measurements and indications (Lovich-Sapola, 2010 & Smith, 2008)

Pulmonary Artery Catheter Complications
• Injury: arterial, venous, nerve • Arrhythmias: Right bundle branch block, complete heart block, ventricular fibrillation, tachycardia • Pulmonary: pneumothorax • Air embolism • Misinterpretation of data • Catheter: pulmonary artery rupture, valve injury, endocarditis, infections

Table 17. Pulmonary artery catheter complications (Lovich-Sapola, 2010)

4.7 Transesophageal Echocardiography (TEE)

TEE has become the preferred method for assessing hemodynamics in trauma patients. TEE is an excellent monitor of ventricular performance and volume. TEE in a trauma patient can be used to asses left and right ventricular function, wall motion abnormalities, valvular disease, pericardial effusion, cardiac tamponade, aortic injury, diastolic function, and pulmonary embolism. TEE can be used to estimate the pulmonary artery systolic pressure, left ventricular end-diastolic pressure, and CVP. In the 2010 practice guidelines update for perioperative TEE, the consultants and ASA members:

- Agree that TEE should be used for noncardiac surgical patients when the patient has known or suspected cardiovascular pathology that might result in hemodynamic, pulmonary, or neurologic compromise.
- Strongly agree that TEE should be used during unexplained persistent hypotension.
- Agree that TEE should be used when persistent unexplained hypoxemia occurs.
- Strongly agree that TEE should be used when life-threatening hypotension is anticipated.
- Agree that TEE should be used during major abdominal or thoracic trauma.
- Disagree that TEE should be used during orthopedic surgery.

Category 1 Indications: • Intra-operative evaluation of acute, persistent, and life-threatening hypotension • Pre-operative use in unstable patients with suspected thoracic aortic injury • Peri-operative use in unstable patients with unexplained hypotension, suspected acute valve lesions or any cardiac emergency
Category 2 Indications: • Peri-operative use in trauma with increased risk of myocardial ischemia or infarction • Peri-operative use with increased risk of hemodynamic disturbance • Pre-operative assessment of suspected acute thoracic aortic injury • Intra-operative use during repair of descending thoracic aortic injury
Category 3 Indications: • Intra-operative monitoring for pulmonary emboli • Intra-operative assessment of thoracic aortic repair • Intra-operative evaluation of pleural effusion • Right ventricular function assessment during lung surgery

Table 18: Indications for use of perioperative TEE in trauma patients, excluding cardiac surgical procedures (Fayad, 2011)

TEE should not be done in patients with known or suspected esophageal disease.

Contraindications
• Esophageal or oropharyngeal trauma • Unprotected airway • Active upper gastrointestinal bleeding • Patient refusal • Esophageal stricture or history of dysphagia • Post-esophageal or gastric surgery • Esophageal or gastric tumor

Table 19. Contraindications to the performance of TEE (Fayad, 2011)

4.8 Urine output

Urine output is a traditional tool used to guide fluid resuscitation in a trauma patient. Urine output is a reflection of organ perfusion. Approximately 0.5 mL/kg/hr is desired for urine production. Trauma patients should all be catheterized for accurate urine output evaluation. If there is a concern of significant bladder injury from the trauma, a Urologist should be consulted. (Smith, 2008)

5. Anesthetic agents and techniques in the operating room

Many orthopedic cases are well suited for regional anesthetic techniques, but there is controversy over whether regional anesthesia has an advantage over general anesthesia. For many orthopedic trauma cases a combined regional and general anesthetic approach is optimal to incorporate the hemodynamic, analgesic, and anxiolytic benefits of each. (Miller, 2009)

5.1 General anesthesia in an orthopedic trauma patient

Advantages	Disadvantages
• Rapid speed of onset • Duration: can last as long as required • Allows multiple procedures on different sites of injury • Greater patient acceptance • Allows for positive pressure ventilation	• Unable to do a global neural examination • Requires airway instrumentation • Hemodynamic management may be more complex • Increased risk of barotrauma to the lungs

Table 20. Advantages and disadvantages of general anesthesia in an orthopedic trauma patient (Miller, 2009)

5.1.1 Goals of general anesthesia

Goals of general anesthesia consist of re-establishing and maintaining normal hemodynamics, maximizing surgical exposure, and minimizing complications. Hypotension is initially treated with fluids. Vasopressors may be required afterwards. Frequent evaluation of acid-base status, hematocrit, and urinary output is routine during major orthopedic trauma. Titration of additional anesthetics can be done if satisfactory hemodynamics. (Bassett, 2011)

Goals of General Anesthesia
• Maximize surgical exposure • Optimize neuromuscular blockade and surgical relaxation • Limit hypothermia and coagulopathy • Warm IV fluids and blood, Keep patient covered with convective warming blanket • If hypothermic: warm the operating room warm (> 24 °C) • If coagulopathic, administer plasma, platelets, cryoprecipitate, fibrinogen, factor concentrates as clinically indicated • Limit complications to other systems: if head injury, monitor intracranial pressure, maintain cerebral perfusion pressure >70 mmHg • Monitor peak airway pressure and tidal volume. Be vigilant for pneumothorax

Table 21. Goals of general anesthesia for orthopedic trauma (Bassett, 2011)

Nonvolatile IV anesthetic agents include propofol, etomidate, ketamine, thiopental, and midazolam. Volatile anesthetics include isoflurane, sevoflurane, desflurane, and nitrous oxide. Nitrous oxide is generally avoided in trauma due to its ability to diffuse into air containing cavities, especially in patients with pneumothorax, intestinal obstruction, intracranial air, and air embolism (Bassett, 2011). Most anesthetic agents have direct cardiovascular depressant effects and inhibit compensatory hemodynamic reflexes such as central catecholamine output and baroreceptor reflexes. Baroreceptor depression is typically greater for the volatile agents compared to IV agents. In hypotensive patients, etomidate or ketamine are the preferred induction Etomidate offers greater cardiovascular stability compared to propofol or thiopental. Heart rate, cardiac output, and cardiac contractility usually remain unchanged. Ketamine typically increases blood pressure, heart rate, and cardiac output, making it favorable for hypovolemic patients. Isoflurane, sevoflurane, and desflurane all decrease blood pressure through reductions in systemic vascular resistance and depression of myocardial contractility. Isoflurane and desflurane both cause an increased heart rate to compensate for the fall in blood pressure. Sevoflurane is nonpungent which makes it a good choice for inhalational induction. Emergence delirium after sevoflurane occurs in pediatric patients. Desflurane is associated with fast wakeup times due to its low blood gas solubility. (Bassett, 2011)

Effect	Made worse by	Comments
Common side effects Fasciculations & Myalgia		Especially in muscular individuals
Hyperkalemia	Burns, spinal cord trauma, crush injuries	Previously hyperkalemic patients might be at risk. Increased risk with acidosis
Bradycardia, asystole	More common in children or after 2nd dose	Prevented by atropine
Catecholamine release		
Increased intra-ocular pressure	Light anesthesia, inadequate paralysis	
Increased intracranial pressure	Light anesthesia, inadequate paralysis	Not clinically significant after head trauma
Rare side effects Malignant hyperthermia		Life threatening condition
Masseter spasm		May prevent jaw opening & intubation
Prolonged blockade		In patients with atypical plasma cholinesterase activity
Rhabdomyolysis	Muscle dystrophy, corticosteroid therapy	Risk of hyperkalemic cardiac arrest
Anaphylaxis		

Table 22. Side effects of succinylcholine (Smith, 2008)

Hypotension produced by anesthetic agents can contribute to the development of cerebral ischemia. Thiopental, propofol, midazolam, and etomidate produce dose dependent reductions in cerebral spinal fluid formation, cerebrovascular constriction causing decreased cerebral blood flow, and decreased cerebral metabolic requirement for oxygen ($CMRO_2$). Ketamine increases $CMRO_2$ and causes increased intracranial pressure. Agents for neuromuscular blockade include depolarizers (succinylcholine) and non-depolarizers (all others). Despite its numerous side effects, succinylcholine is commonly used for rapid sequence induction and intubation (RSI). Rocuronium and vecuronium are also used for neuromuscular blockade. (Bassett, 2011)

5.2 Regional anesthesia in an orthopedic trauma patient

Advantages	Disadvantages
• Able to assess mental status (although patients usually require sedation which may limit this evaluation) • Improved post-operative mental status and pain management • Decreased: blood loss and incidence of deep venous thrombosis • Increased: vascular flow • Avoidance of airway instrumentation • Early mobilization	• Difficult to assess nerve function • Not helpful if the patient has multiple sites of injury • Patient refusal is common • Block may wear off before the surgery is completed • May take longer to place the block than to induce a general anesthetic • Patient will still likely require additional sedation • Hemodynamic instability may occur with an epidural/spinal anesthetic • Venous thromboembolism prophylaxis may limit the ability to safely perform the technique • Unknown patient anticoagulation status in a trauma patient may limit the ability to safely perform this technique • Placement may be difficult secondary to restrictions in positioning of a poly-trauma patient

Table 23. Advantages and disadvantages of regional anesthesia in an orthopedic trauma patient (Miller, 2009)

6. Specific orthopedic injury management

Life-threatening Injuries	Limb-threatening Injuries
• Pelvic ring injuries with hemorrhage • Long bone fractures with hemorrhage	• Traumatic amputation • Vascular injury • Compartment syndrome

Table 24. Life and limb threatening injuries (Smith, 2008)

Surgery is Recommended Within 6-8 Hours	Surgery is Recommended within 24 Hours
• Open fracture • Traumatic arthrotomy • Dislocated joint • Displaced femoral neck fracture in a young adult	• Unstable pelvis/acetabulum fracture • Unstable femur fracture • Proximal fracture in the elderly

Table 25. Orthopedic injuries requiring urgent surgical treatment (Smith, 2008)

6.1 Femur fracture

Femur fractures carry a mortality rate as high as 25%. "Life threatening hemorrhage can occur with bilateral femur fractures or multiple long-bone fractures." The average blood loss from a femur fracture can be as high as 1,500 cc. Secure venous access is mandatory (e.g., two large bore peripheral IV catheters). (Smith, 2008)

Early definitive stabilization of the femur fracture (within 24 hours of the injury) has been shown to be safe in most patients. This includes patients with multiple injuries such as severe abdominal, chest, or head injuries as long as adequate attention has been paid to resuscitation and medical optimization prior to surgery. (Nahm, 2011) This optimization should include fluid resuscitation with crystalloid, colloid, and blood products as needed. The patient should be followed with serial arterial blood gas samples to follow the lactate levels and pH levels to show if the resuscitation is effective. Early consultation with other services including Neurosurgery, General Surgery, Cardiology, Pulmonary, Renal, may be life saving for the patient. (Miller, 2009)

Benefits of Early Definitive Stabilization of a Femur Fracture (< 24 hours)
• Fewer pulmonary complications • Fewer ventilator days • Fewer deep venous thromboses (DVT) • Shorter hospital stay • Lower health care costs

Table 26. Benefits of early definitive stabilization of a femur fracture (Nahm, 2011)

6.2 Pelvic fracture

Pelvic fractures are often caused by a significant trauma to the lower trunk and are "often accompanied by chest (21%), head (16%), and liver/spleen (8%) injuries". The three-month mortality of a pelvic fracture is around 14%. (Miller, 2009)

The bleeding from a pelvic fracture is often into a closed space and therefore not immediately obvious to an examiner. Pelvic fractures can be associated with several liters of blood loss. Urgent resuscitation and early stabilization of the pelvic fracture can minimize the morbidity and mortality. (Smith, 2008) An arterial line and multiple large gauge venous catheters are recommended. (Miller, 2009)

Pelvic ring fractures require immediate recognition and management by the trauma team. Patients with a pelvic ring fracture are at a high risk for hemorrhage. Bleeding often occurs at multiple disrupted venous beds in the pelvis, and if the pelvis is unstable, there is no anatomic barrier to the continued expansion of this retroperitoneal bleed. Pelvic fractures can result in fatal retroperitoneal bleeding. Surgical exploration is usually not the required treatment. Successful treatment often includes volume resuscitation, external fixation of the unstable pelvis, and angiography. Intubation and anesthesia involvement is often required secondary to the associated hypotension and need for active fluid resuscitation. (Miller, 2009)

Treating an unstable pelvic arterial bleed in angiography is not without risks. Angiography is often performed in remote locations in the hospital. The unstable patient would require transport to the angiography suite and then potentially to the operating rooms. An anesthesia team is often requested to accompany the patient in the angiography suite to perform continued monitoring, airway management, and resuscitation. The anesthesia equipment and monitors used in the remote location should meet the same standards as those used in the operating room. The Anesthesiologist must also have a reliable way to communicate for help if needed. (Smith, 2008)

Most reports suggest that the optimal time for stabilization of a pelvic fracture is within one week of the injury. (Miller, 2009) Recent studies have shown that there are benefits associated with an early (within 24 hours of injury) stabilization or reduction and definitive fixation of an unstable pelvic fracture. These benefits include: control of bleeding, assist with resuscitation, pain relief, ability to mobilize the patient, ease of reduction, improved reduction quality, elimination of traction, elimination of recumbency, reduced risk of pulmonary, septic, and thromboembolic complications, less organ failure, reduced morbidity and mortality, decreased length of stay in the intensive care unit, and shorter overall hospital stay. (Vallier, 2010)

6.3 Hip dislocation

A hip dislocation is a medical emergency, often resulting from a high impact trauma. Failure to quickly diagnose and treat this injury can result in avascular necrosis of the femoral head and significant neurologic injury. A hip dislocation usually requires a very deep level of anesthesia to facilitate a successful reduction. While occasionally the hip dislocation can be reduced in a spontaneously breathing patient with a combination of midazolam, fentanyl, ketamine, and/or propofol, often they require a nondepolarizing muscle relaxant. If a trauma patient requires complete relaxation with a nondepolaring muscle relaxant, then the procedure should be performed in the operating room with full ASA monitors and an endotracheal tube secondary to the trauma patients increased risk of aspiration. Patients that present to the hospital and are inebriated, uncooperative, confused, hemodynamically unstable, or have pulmonary dysfunction, should also be intubated prior to a hip reduction. (Miller, 2009)

6.4 Hip fracture (femoral neck fracture)

Hip fractures are most common in the elderly. They are associated with a significantly high morbidity and one-year mortality (30%). These patients often present in considerable pain, high stress states, and possibly exhibiting symptoms of myocardial ischemia. Early surgery (<12 hours) has resulted in: lower pain scores, decreased length of hospital stay, and reduced peri-operative complications. Compared with delayed surgery, there is no association with increased survival. Early surgery should be the goal for stable patients, combined with early mobilization, rehabilitation, and aggressive medical care. (Miller, 2009)

Hip fractures can result in significant blood loss. The patients are often dehydrated and anemic. A normal intravascular blood volume should be restored prior to anesthesia and surgery. Placement of a central venous catheter and arterial line can guide the fluid management and help prevent congestive heart failure from over-resuscitation. (Miller, 2009)

Peri-operative Complications of Hip Fractures
• Cardiac complications: myocardial ischemia
• Pulmonary complications: fat embolism, pulmonary embolism
• Deep venous thrombosis
• Delirium: secondary to dehydration and electrolyte abnormalities

Table 27. Peri-operative complications of hip fractures (Miller, 2009)

Patients undergoing a hip fracture surgery have the highest risk of death from a pulmonary embolism. A spinal anesthetic is recommended for the actual surgery, but an epidural is rarely indicated for post-operative pain management secondary to the aggressive post-operative anticoagulation that will be initiated. (Miller, 2009)

6.5 Open fracture

Open fractures are surgical emergencies. The infection rate increases after a delay of 6-8 hours. Debridement and irrigation in the operating room plus provisional or definitive fixation of the fracture should happen as soon as it is safely possible. Open fractures require cleaning, pulse lavage, and debridement as soon as possible to minimize the risk of infectious complications. If the patient is not stable enough to go to the operating room, this should be done at the bedside. (Smith, 2008)

6.6 Traumatic amputation

A traumatic amputation requires immediate treatment with pressure, control of the bleeding, early intravenous antibiotics, and tetanus prophylaxis. Emergent surgery is often necessary to control the bleeding and perform surgical debridement. (Smith, 2008)

6.7 Vascular injury

"Injury to the major arterial flow of a limb is a surgical emergency." It is most common after a penetrating trauma, but can be seen with blunt injuries. Traumatic knee dislocations are the most common etiology for a vascular injury in a blunt trauma. A major arterial injury should be suspected in a patient that presents with pallor, coolness, and decreased pulses of the extremity. The patient may also present with an expanding hematoma or massive bleeding. Blood and fluid replacement by the anesthesia team is critical for the patient's survival. (Smith, 2008)

7. Intra-operative complications

7.1 Hypotension

Hypotension can occur during any case in the operating room. In a trauma situation, it is especially important to consider a wide differential so that the true cause of the hypotension is not missed. Hypotension may be caused by hypovolemia: undetected or underestimated blood loss, insensible losses, gastrointestinal loss, renal loss, excessive venodilation, and redistribution of fluid to an extravascular space. All forms of shock including obstructive, cardiogenic, and vasodilated shock should be ruled out. (Smith, 2008)

Type of shock	Differential Diagnoses
Obstructive	• Tension pneumothorax • Pericardial tamponade • Massive pleural effusion • Hemothorax • Abdominal compartment syndrome • Arterial or venous occlusion: air emboli, thrombus, tumor • Pregnancy: aortocaval compression
Cardiogenic	• Blunt cardiac injury: myocardial contusion • Preexisting cardiac disease • Myocardial infarction
Vasodilated	• Spinal cord injury • Anaphylaxis • Adrenal insufficiency • Arteriovenous fistula • Sepsis • Systemic inflammatory disease • Hepatic failure

Table 28. Types of shock (Smith, 2008)

Resuscitation from shock refers to the restoration of normal physiology after injury. Resuscitation after a hemorrhagic shock requires the restoration of a normal circulating blood volume, normal vascular tone, and normal tissue perfusion. (Miller, 2009)

Early resuscitation occurs while active bleeding is still ongoing. The goals in early resuscitation are to maintain the systolic blood pressure at 80 to 100 mmHg, maintain the hematocrit at 25-30%, maintain the coagulation panel and ionized calcium level within a normal range, keep the platelet count > 50,000, maintain the core temperature at > 35 °C, and prevent worsening acidosis. Late resuscitation is defined as after the bleeding is controlled and has separate goals that include maintaining the systolic blood pressure > 100 mmHg, maintaining a normal hematocrit, normalizing the coagulation status, electrolytes, temperature, and urine output, and maximizing the cardiac output. (Miller, 2009)

7.2 Significant blood loss

Patients with orthopedic injury and poly-trauma including orthopedic injury may present with a significant blood loss. Massive transfusion protocols (MTP) have been designed and implemented in many large urban trauma centers to provide a rapidly bleeding patient with automatic regular shipments of blood products to facilitate fluid resuscitation during an emergency surgery. The goal of the design ratio of packed red blood cells, plasma, and platelets built into the protocol are based on the need for volume support, oxygen delivery, and coagulation support required at each stage of the resuscitation. (Smith, 2008)

When should the MTP be initiated? This is often a judgment call made by the Surgeon or Anesthesiologist. It can be guided by these criteria: 5-unit blood loss in one hour, or 10-unit blood loss anticipated for the entire case or within 12-24 hours of observation, or hypovolemic hypotension uncorrected by crystalloid and/or packed red blood cell resuscitation during an ongoing hemorrhage. (Smith, 2008)

During the MTP, a cooler containing blood products is brought one at a time to the operating room as each is finished or until the MTP is terminated. The MTP will vary from hospital to hospital. See below for a sample MTP. (Smith, 2008)

Cooler	Packed Red Blood Cells	Thawed Plasma	5 Pack of Platelets	Cryoprecipitate	Recombinant factor VIIa
1a (No type and screen available.)	5 (O negative)	2 (AB)			
1b (Type and Crossed)	5	2			
2	5	2	1		
3	5	2		10	1
4	5	2	1		

Table 29. Sample massive transfusion protocol (MTP) (Smith, 2008)

7.3 Hypothermia

Hypothermia is defined as a core temperature less than 36 °C. Hypothermia is usually caused by prolonged exposures to cold temperatures. Many trauma patients present to the operating room very cold secondary to prolonged exposure to the elements after the initial trauma. Mild hypothermia, about 1-2 °C below normal triples the incidence of morbid cardiac outcomes, triples the incidence of wound infections, directly impairs immune function, prolongs hospitalization by up to 20%, significantly increases surgical blood loss, and can lead to cold-induced platelet dysfunction. (Lovich-Sapola, 2010)

Trauma patients may enter the operating room already cold, but even if they are normothermic, the patients' core temperatures usually decrease by 0.5-1.5 °C in the first 30 minutes after the induction of anesthesia secondary to the internal redistribution of heat. Mechanisms for heat loss include radiation loss, convection loss, conduction loss, and evaporative loss. (Lovich-Sapola, 2010)

Temperature	Physiologic Effect
33 °C	• Hypertension, tachycardia, and increased cardiac output • Increased oxygen consumption • Hyperventilation • Shivering • Piloerection • Muscle mis-coordination • Confusion
30 °C	• Metabolism is reduced by 50% • Significant neural and organ depression • Loss of consciousness • Body loses its ability to generate heat by shivering. • Prolonged bleeding and clotting times; usually reversible with re-warming
28 °C	• Hyperglycemia: plasma fall in insulin and increased catecholamines from the stress of hypothermia • Hypovolemia: cold diuresis; physiologic increase in hematocrit and hypotension • Cardiac arrhythmias: bradycardia, nodal rhythm, premature ventricular contractions, atrio-ventricular block, ventricular fibrillation • EKG changes: prolonged PR interval, widening of the QRS complex, prolonged QT interval, ST segment elevation, J wave • Oxy-hemoglobin dissociation curve shift to the left • Decreased oxygen consumption • Thrombocytopenia • Metabolic acidosis • Prolonged drug metabolism
<25°C	• Metabolism is reduced by 60% • Ventricular fibrillation • Cessation of respiration • Acid-base disturbances, unless ventilation is maintained

Table 30. Physiologic effects of hypothermia. (Lovich-Sapola, 2010)

Treatment of Hypothermia
• Surface re-warming: warmed blankets, forced air heating blankets, gel pad warming system • Heated (humidified) inspired gases • Fluid warmers • Warming the operating room • Warm body cavity lavage: bladder, stomach, chest, and abdominal cavity • Extracorporeal: hemodialysis, hemofiltration, continuous arteriovenous re-warming, cardiopulmonary bypass

Table 31. Treatment of hypothermia (Lovich-Sapola, 2010 and Smith, 2008)

During the active re-warming of a patient, the following monitors are routine: continuous core temperature monitor and bladder catheterization to monitor the urine output and therefore the adequacy of the intravascular volume and organ perfusion. Arterial line for continuous blood pressure monitoring and frequent blood gas draws is also valuable. On occasion, a pulmonary artery catheter may be useful to follow the cardiac output (Lovich-Sapola, 2010)

7.4 Fat embolism syndrome

Fat embolism syndrome (FES) occurs when microembolism of fat and marrow from the patients long-bones result in clinically significant symptoms. Intra-operative transesophageal echocardiography (TEE) has shown that most patients undergoing long-bone fracture manipulation experience this microembolization, but most patients do not have any clinical impact. Clinically significant FES occurs in about 3-10% of patients having a long-bone repair with the higher incidence if the patient has multiple long-bone fractures. "The presentation of FES can be gradual, developing over 12 to 72 hours, or fulminate leading to acute respiratory distress and cardiac arrest." (Miller, 2009)

Clinical Manifestations of Fat Embolism Syndrome (FES)
Hypoxia
Tachycardia
Mental status change: drowsiness, confusion, obtundation, coma
Petechial rash of the upper body: conjunctiva, oral mucosa, skin folds of the neck, shoulders, axilla, upper arms, and chest
Elevated pulmonary artery pressure
Decreased cardiac index
Lab results: fat microglobulinemia, anemia, thrombocytopenia, high ESR, fat globules in the urine
Chest X-ray: bilateral alveolar infiltrates

Table 32. Clinical manifestation for FES (Miller, 2009; Smith, 2008)

Treatment for Fat Embolism Syndrome (FES)
• Early recognition • Ventilation management: oxygen, higher PEEP, and possible long-term mechanical ventilatory support • Judicious fluid management

Table 33. Treatment for FES (Miller, 2009)

7.5 Acute compartment syndrome

Acute compartment syndrome is defined as a "condition in which increased pressure within a limited space compromises the circulation and function of the tissues within that space." The most common fractures associated with compartment syndrome are the tibial shaft and forearm. The most common cause of compartment syndrome with orthopedic trauma patients is edema secondary to muscle injury and associated hematoma formation. (Miller, 2009)

The diagnosis of acute compartment syndrome is primarily clinical. (Olsen, 2005) The earliest symptoms are often "pain out of proportion to the injury", pain with passive motion, and tense swelling of the affected area. (Miller, 2009; Smith, 2008) Decreased distal sensation and loss of proprioception are seen next, followed by complete anesthesia and muscle weakness. (Smith, 2008) The late-onset "classic"symptoms of pulselessness, pallor, paralysis, and paresthesia often do not present until irreversible loss of function has occurred. (Miller, 2009; Olsen, 2005; Smith, 2008))

The Surgeon and the Anesthesiologist must be careful because certain anesthetic techniques such as nerve blocks and epidural anesthesia can mask these symptoms and lead to a delay in diagnosis. This delay can be limb-threatening. (Olsen, 2005) These same symptoms can also be masked by an altered level of consciousness, deep sedation, or large doses of pain medication; therefore a high index for suspicion is required along with serial physical examinations so that the compartment syndrome is not missed. (Miller, 2009; Smith, 2008)

The treatment for compartment syndrome is a fasciotomy of all involved compartments. To be effective, the fasciotomy must be performed as early as possible to prevent irreversible damage. (Miller, 2009)

Conditions That Can Result in Acute Compartment Syndrome
Trauma: • Fractures: tibial shaft, radius, ulna • Gunshot wounds • Crush injury • Burns • Snake bites
Iatrogenic: • Infiltration form venous or arterial puncture sites • Extravasation of fluids with pulsatile lavage • Pressurized infusions • Casts and circular dressings • Intraosseous fluid replacement in a child/infant
Bleeding disorders
Vascular: • Post-ischemic swelling • Reperfusion injury • Hemorrhage with hematoma formation • Contusions
Drug overdoes: prolonged immobile state
Prolonged limb compression

Table 34. Conditions that can result in acute compartment syndrome (Miller, 2009; Olsen, 2005)

7.6 Crush injury

Crush syndrome is defined as rhabdomyolisis secondary to the associated hypovolemia and toxin exposure after a crush injury with resultant skeletal muscle compression. Rhabdomyolysis occurs when the components of the damaged skeletal muscle enter the patient's circulation. Serum creatinine kinase (CK) levels correlate with the degree of muscle injury, and can be used to assess the severity of the rhabdomyolysis. Acute renal failure (ARF) is the most serious consequence of rhabdomyolysis. ARF "occurs in 4-33% of the cases"and has a "mortality rate of 3-50%". (Malinoski, 2004)

Common Mechanisms of a Crush Injury
• Blunt trauma • Electrical injuries: lightning strikes, high-voltage power lines • Sudden automobile deceleration • Alcohol intoxication: fall, immobility, coma • Earthquakes, landslides, building collapses • Trapped in one position for an extended period of time • Improper intra-operative positioning: extended lithotomy, lateral decubitus • Prolonged tourniquet use • Vascular compromise: arterial thrombosis, embolus, traumatic injury • Soft tissue infections • Medications: steroids, neuromuscular blocking drugs

Table 35. Crush injury mechanisms (Malinoski, 2004; Miller, 2009)

Clinical Symptoms of a Crush Injury
• Shock • Swollen extremities • Rhabdomyolysis • Dark urine secondary to myoglobinuria • Acute renal failure • Electrolyte abnormalities

Table 36. Clinical symptoms of a crush injury (Malinoski, 2004; Miller, 2009)

Treatment and Prevention of Renal Failure after a Crush Injury
Early and vigorous volume replacement: crystalloid • Treat the hypovolemic shock • Treat the hyperkalemia • The total body deficit may be up to 15 L
Confirm the urine flow prior to forced mannitol-alkaline diuresis (controversial treatment) • Mannitol • Alkalization of the urine with sodium bicarbonate • Goal: prevent the precipitation of myoglobin in the renal tubules
Closely monitor the urine output
Closely monitor the electrolytes
Daily hemodialysis or continuous hemodialysis/hemofiltration

Table 37. Treatment and prevention of renal failure after a crush injury (Malinoski, 2004)

8. Post-operative pain management

Managing a patient's pain is always challenging, but it can be especially difficult in a poly-trauma/multiple orthopedic injury patient. Pain management in these patients will require a multimodal approach. Inadequate analgesia can lead to complications with healing, immune function, and autonomic dysfunction. Prolonged untreated pain can lead to the development of a chronic pain state that can be very difficult to treat and may lead to lifelong problems. The goal of pain management in a trauma patient is to reduce the stress response, and provide the patient with pain relief while maintaining cardiovascular stability and tissue homeostasis. (Smith, 2008)

The initial pain management after an orthopedic surgery case usually begins in the recovery room. The administration of rapidly acting intravenous agents in small doses at frequent intervals under continuous monitoring should be continued until adequate pain relief is attained. The total dose of medication required to relieve the patient's pain can then be used to determine the patient's basal requirements before starting a long-acting medication or patient-controlled analgesia (PCA). (Miller, 2009)

Post-operative physical therapy after an orthopedic injury can have a significant impact on the pain medication requirements. It is important to consider the physical therapy schedule and plan the pain medication dosing appropriately. The goal of the dosing is to allow for enough pain relief to successfully perform the physical therapy but not so much that they are too sedated to participate. Physical therapy and activity after an orthopedic trauma is very important because it lowers the risk of pulmonary embolism, venous thrombosus, and decubitus ulcers. While physical therapy is more painful in the short term, the sooner the patient is mobilized, the lower the analgesic doses will be in the long term. (Miller, 2009)

Neuropathic pain occurs when there is direct injury to a major sensory nerve. This type of injury is common after spinal cord trauma, traumatic amputations, and major crush injuries. Neuropathic pain presents with a burning sensation, intermittent electrical shocks, and dysthesia in the affected dermatomal distribution. Neuropathic pain often responds poorly to narcotic analgesics used for somatic pain. The first line of treatment should be with gabapentin, 200 mg three times per day, with daily titration up to a maximum of 2-3 g/day. Persistent neuropathic pain may require selective regional anesthesia to "break the cycle" of spinal cord receptor recruitment. (Miller, 2009)

8.1 Pharmacologic measures

Acetaminophen is an analgesic/ antipyretic drug. It is popular because it is relatively safe compared with other anti-inflammatory medications. Acetaminophen is an important adjuvant to opioid analgesia because it decreases the total amount of opioid required and therefore decreases the adverse effects of excess opioids. The ceiling effect of oral acetaminophen is 1g/dose. (Smith, 2008)

Nonsteroidal anti-inflammatory drugs (NSAIDs) are powerful COX inhibitors and the first line treatment for many pain conditions. NSAIDs are effective for moderate to severe pain. The use of NSAIDs is often limited by their side effect profile: gastric ulcers, renal and platelet dysfunction, and decreased bone fusion and healing which is particularly troublesome in orthopedic trauma patients. (Smith, 2008)

Opioids are the cornerstone of acute pain management. The most commonly used types of opioids include: morphine, meperidine, codeine, fentanyl, hydromorphone, oxycodone, methadone, and buprenorphine. Opioids significantly decrease pain score ratings in trauma patients. Carefully titrated opioids are used as the most common treatment method in trauma cases. The opioids are usually given by a fixed dosing schedule or PCA technique. Opioids can be administered by several routes (oral, intravenous, subcutaneous, intramuscular, intrathecal, epidural, transmucosal, transdermal, inhaled, intra-articular, and local injection into the wound) thus making them very versatile in clinical applications. Side effects of opioids include nausea, vomiting, constipation, sedation, altered sensorium, and respiratory depression. (Smith, 2008)

Ketamine, a phencyclidine derivative, is a noncompetitive inhibitor at the NMDA receptor. Ketamine is unique in that it produces a dissociative state that causes amnesia and an intense analgesia, while maintaining the vital brain stem functions and hemodynamic stability. It provides profound amnesia and analgesia. Ketamine has been shown to decrease opioid requirements. Ketamine is a very useful drug for frequent dressing changes, treating burn patients, and minor trauma procedures. The drawbacks of ketamine include resulting excessive secretions, agitation on recovery, hallucinations, and increase in intracranial and intraocular pressure. The hallucinations can be decreased by giving a benzodiazepine. Ketamine should be avoided in any patient with an associated head trauma. (Smith, 2008)

Tricyclic antidepressants (TCAs) are useful in the treatment of neuropathic pain conditions. TCAs are especially helpful in trauma patients because they can reduce pain, facilitate sleep, and alleviate depression. TCAs have a delayed onset of action; the patient must be educated that it may take days to see results. Recommended TCAs include amitriptyline, nortriptyline, imiprimine, and desipramine. Side effects can include: prolonged QT interval, arrhythmia, and paralytic ileus. (Smith, 2008)

Gabapentin and pregabalin are anticonvulsants used to treat neuropathic, postsurgical, and posttraumatic pain. These medications can only be given in the oral form, so they can not be started until the patient is tolerating food. Side effects may include sedation, dizziness, confusion, and headache. (Smith, 2008)

Multimodal analgesia is the key to the treatment of pain in a poly-trauma patient. The goal is an optimal balance of multiple medications. In addition to pharmacologic methods, non-pharmacologic approaches such as psychologic support, counseling, hypnosis, relaxation techniques, biofeedback, and acupuncture should be considered. (Smith, 2008)

8.2 Regional anesthesia

Regional analgesia from an epidural or continuous catheter should be considered in any orthopedic trauma patient if possible secondary to the resultant sparing of narcotics, high level of patient satisfaction, improved pulmonary function (with associated thoraco-abdominal injury), and facilitated early mobilization. (Miller, 2009) Localized and regional pain can be treated with local, regional, or neuraxial analgesia. Regional blocks provide selective pain relief with fewer hemodynamic side effects than neuraxial blocks. Regional anesthesia can decrease the need for opioids and therefore result in decreased nausea, vomiting, and sedation. Regional anesthesia can also be used for surgical anesthesia as well as post-operative pain management. (Smith, 2008)

Prior to any block, the Anesthesiologist must first evaluate the patient. A review of the patient's medical history including an evaluation for preexisting neurologic injuries, medication history, capability to give informed consent, ability to cooperate for the procedure, availability of landmarks, ability to properly position the patient for the procedure, laboratory values (coagulation studies and platelet count), and finally the approval of the Surgeon to perform the block. A block has the potential to delay the diagnosis of a compartment syndrome and potentially worsen existing nerve damage, and therefore may not be safe in certain patients. (Smith, 2008)

Ultrasound guidance is recommended for the placement of any regional block, but especially in trauma patients, secondary to the maximal benefit of patient safety and comfort. The peripheral nerve stimulation technique can be painful and should be avoided. (Smith, 2008)

8.2.1 Upper limb blocks

Upper Limb Blocks	Indication	Concerns
Interscalene Brachial Plexus	Injuries of the shoulder and upper arm	• Associated with 100% incidence of diaphragm paresis which can last up to 6 hours • Difficult to place in patients with a cervical injury because of difficulty in positioning
Brachial Plexus Around the Clavicle	**Supraclavicular block**: injuries below the shoulder **Infraclavicular block**: injury below the shoulder; better for continuous catheter placement and in patients with cervical injury because the head may stay in a neutral position during placement	• Potential risk for pneumothorax
Axillary Brachial Plexus	Hand and forearm trauma Attractive for patients with coagulopathy secondary to the compressibility of the vessels in this location	• Must be able to abduct the arm • Failure to anesthetize the musculocutaneous nerve
Wrist	Radial, median, and ulnar nerves can be blocked at the wrist	

Table 38. Upper limb blocks (Miller, 2009; Smith, 2008)

8.2.2 Lower limb blocks

Lower Limb Blocks	Indication
Lumbar Plexus	• Patients with unilateral lower limb trauma that are not candidates for an epidural • Femur fracture • Hip fracture • Tibial plateau fracture
Femoral Nerve	• Femoral shaft fracture • ACL repair • Tibial plateau fracture
Fascia Iliaca	• Same indications as a femoral nerve block
Saphenous Nerve	• Medial aspect of the foot (ankle and forefoot fractures) • Tourniquet pain • Must be combined with the sciatic nerve block
Sciatic Nerve	• Analgesia to the posterior compartment of the thigh • Analgesia to most of the lower leg
Ankle	• Surgical procedures of the foot

Table 39. Lower limb blocks (Miller, 2009; Smith, 2008)

8.2.3 Intravenous (IV) regional anesthesia (Bier's block)

IV regional anesthesia is a simple, reliable, cost effective block that is good for short operative procedure on an extremity. Lidocaine is the recommended drug for this block, secondary to it being less cardiotoxic than bupivacaine. IV regional anesthesia requires exsanguination of the limb with a tight bandage, which may be very uncomfortable to an injured limb. Early deflation of the cuff used to keep the local anesthesia in the affected extremity can result in local anesthetic toxicity. (Smith, 2008)

8.2.4 Epidural anesthesia

Epidural anesthesia has been shown to provide superior dynamic analgesia for the treatment of post-operative hip fracture pain during rehabilitation. The patients are significantly less restricted by their pain. However, studies have shown that this decrease in pain does not significantly translate into enhanced rehabilitation. (Foss, 2005) Again, patients undergoing a hip fracture surgery have the highest risk of death from a pulmonary embolism. A spinal anesthetic is recommended for the actual surgery, but an epidural is rarely indicated for post-operative pain management secondary to the aggressive post-operative anticoagulation that will be initiated. (Miller, 2009)

8.2.5 Complications of regional anesthesia

Vascular Injury	• A risk/ benefit analysis is necessary in all patients: special concern if they are coagulopathic, have a low platelet count, are on blood thinners • Evolution of neurologic deficits from an expanding hematoma can take 4 hours to 3 days to manifest itself • Lack of treatment of a hematoma can lead to axon loss and sensory/ motor deficit • Consider pre-existing trauma or vascular injury before the placement of any block
Diaphragm Weakness	• The phrenic nerve lies close to the interscalene groove (easily blocked by the interscalene approach to the brachial plexus) • Unilateral diaphragm weakness is not usually significant in healthy patients, but it can be devastating in patients with chest trauma, poor pulmonary status, or a pneumothorax
Pneumothorax	• Serious complication of the supraclavicular brachial plexus block and intercostal nerve block • Rare after the interscalene and infraclavicular approach • Symptoms can be delayed and present as long as 6-12 hours after the procedure.
Intravascular Injection	• Most nerve plexuses are in the vicinity of a vascular structure • Intravascular injections can lead to convulsions • Careful vigilance, multiple aspirations, and slow fractionated injections are important • The addition of epinephrine to the local anesthetic helps to detect accidental intravascular injection
Horner's Syndrome	• The cervical sympathetic chain is in close proximity to the brachial plexus and can lead to Horner's syndrome • Symptoms: ptosis, miosis, anhydrosis, and unilateral conjunctival engorgement • Rate can be as high as 90% with interscalene and supraclavicular approaches
Infections	• No reported cases in single injections • Increased risk with catheters

Table 40. Complications of regional anesthesia (Smith, 2008)

9. Conclusion

Orthopedic trauma requires a coordinated approach between the Surgeon and the Anesthesiologist. Orthopedic cases can often be some of the most complex for the Anesthesiologist secondary to the associated co-morbidities of the patient and the potential for multiple simultaneous injuries.

Every patient requires a preoperative evaluation that is complete as possible in the time allowed. Airway management may be difficult secondary to the potential for associated cervical spine injuries, and the proper preparation and precautions should be taken. Every patient requires the standard ASA monitors for the procedure, whether the orthopedic procedure is performed in the operating room, emergency room, or angiography suite.

The anesthetic technique should be chosen after careful evaluation of the risks and benefits of regional versus general anesthesia. It is important to remember that often a combination of both will yield the best results.

The Anesthesiologist and the Orthopedic surgeon should be prepared for intra-operative complications including hypotension, blood loss, hypothermia, fat embolism, and compartment syndrome. Vigilance for these potential complications will lead to early diagnosis and treatment, and therefore a potentially improved outcome.

Finally, post-operative pain management also requires a multi-modal approach for the best results. Consider consulting the hospital's Acute Pain Management team for assistance. Untreated pain can lead to chronic pain syndromes and delayed rehabilitation in the orthopedic injury patient.

10. References

American Society of Anesthesiologists Committee on Standards and Practice Parameters. (2011). Practice Guidelines for Preoperative Fasting and the Use of Pharmacologic Agents to Reduce the Risk of Pulmonary Aspiration: Application to Healthy Patients Undergoing Elective Procedures. *Anesthesiology,* Vol. 114, No. 3, (March 2011), pp. 495-511.

Bassett M.D., Smith C.E. (2011). General Anesthesia for Trauma. In: Essentials of Trauma Anesthesia, Cambridge. In Press

Chung F. (2008). STOP Questionnaire. A Tool to Screen Patients for Obstructive Sleep Apnea. Anesthesiology 2008; 108:812–21

Fayad, A., Woo M. (2011). Echocardiography in Trauma. In: Essentials of Trauma Anesthesia, Cambridge. In Press

Fleisher, L.A., Beckman, J.A., Brown, K.A., et al. (2007). ACC/AHA 2007 Guidelines on the Perioperative Cardiovascular Evaluation and Care for Noncardiac Surgery: Executive Summary. *Circulation.*Vol. 116, (October 2007).

Foss, N.B., Kristensen, M.T., Kristensen, B.B., et al. (2005). Effect of Postoperative Epidural Analgesia on Rehabilitation and Pain after Hip Fracture Surgery: A Randomized, Double-blind, Placebo controlled Trial. *Anesthesiology.* Vol. 102, No. 6, (June 2005), pp. 1197-204.

Lovich-Sapola, J.A. (2010). *Anesthesia Oral Board Review: Knocking Out the Boards.* Cambridge University Press, ISBN 978-0-521-75619, Cambridge

Malinoski, D.J., Slater, M.S., Mullins, R.J. (2004). Crush Injury and Rhabdomyolysis. *Critical Care Clinics.* Vol. 20, (2004), pp. 171-92.

Miller, R.D., Eriksson, L.I., Fleisher, L.A., et al. (2009). *Miller: Miller's Anesthesia (7th ed.),* Churchill Livingstone, New York.

Nahm, N.J., Como, J.J., Wilber, J.H., et al. (2011). Early Appropriate Care: Definitive Stabilization of Femoral Fractures Within 24 Hours of Injury Is Safe in Most Patients With Multiple Injuries. *The Journal of Trauma.* [Epub ahead of print]

Olsen, S.A. & Glascow, R.R. (2005) Acute Compartment Syndrome in Lower Extremity Musculoskeletal Trauma. *Journal of the Acadamy of Orthopeadic Surgeons.* Vol. 1, No. 7, (November 2005), pp. 436-4.

Practice Guidelines for Perioperative Transesophageal Echocardiography. (2010). An Updated Report by the American Society of Anesthesiologists and the Society of Cardiovascular Anesthesiologists Task Force on Transesophageal Echocardiography. Anesthesiology 2010; 112:1084 –96

Robitaille, A., Williams, S., Tremblay, M.H., et al. (2008). Cervical Spine Motion During Tracheal Intubation with Manual In-Line Stabilization: Direct Laryngoscopy versus Glidesope Videolaryngoscopy. *Anesthesia and Analgesia.*Vol. 106. No. 3, (March 2008), pp. 935-41.

Smith, C.E. (2008). *Trauma Anesthesia.* Cambridge University Press, ISBN 978-0-521-87058-0, Cambridge.

Vallier, H.A., Cureton, B.A., Ekstein, C., et al. (2010). Early Definitive Stabilization of Unstable Pelvis and Acetabulum Fractures Reduces Morbidity. *The Journal of Trauma.* Vol. 69, No. 3, (September 2010), pp. 677-84.